Electroconvulsive Therapy in Children and Adolescents

Electroconvulsive Therapy in Children and Adolescents

Editors

Neera Ghaziuddin, MD, MRCPsych

Associate Professor of Psychiatry, University of Michigan

Garry Walter, MD, PhD

Professor of Child and Adolescent Psychiatry, University of Sydney

OXFORD
UNIVERSITY PRESS

OXFORD
UNIVERSITY PRESS

Oxford University Press is a department of the University of Oxford.
It furthers the University's objective of excellence in research, scholarship,
and education by publishing worldwide.

Oxford New York
Auckland Cape Town Dar es Salaam Hong Kong Karachi
Kuala Lumpur Madrid Melbourne Mexico City Nairobi
New Delhi Shanghai Taipei Toronto

With offices in
Argentina Austria Brazil Chile Czech Republic France Greece
Guatemala Hungary Italy Japan Poland Portugal Singapore
South Korea Switzerland Thailand Turkey Ukraine Vietnam

Oxford is a registered trademark of Oxford University Press
in the UK and certain other countries.

Published in the United States of America by
Oxford University Press
198 Madison Avenue, New York, NY 10016

Library of Congress Cataloging-in-Publication Data

Electroconvulsive therapy in children and adolescents / edited by Neera Ghaziuddin, Garry Walter.
p. ; cm.
Includes bibliographical references and index.
ISBN 978-0-19-993789-9 (alk. paper)
I. Ghaziuddin, Neera. II. Walter, Garry.
[DNLM: 1. Electroconvulsive Therapy. 2. Adolescent. 3. Child. 4. Mental Disorders—therapy. 5. Nervous System Diseases—therapy. WM 412]

RC485
616.89′122—dc23
2013017118

This material is not intended to be, and should not be considered, a substitute for medical or other professional advice. Treatment for the conditions described in this material is highly dependent on the individual circumstances. And, while this material is designed to offer accurate information with respect to the subject matter covered and to be current as of the time it was written, research and knowledge about medical and health issues is constantly evolving and dose schedules for medications are being revised continually, with new side effects recognized and accounted for regularly. Readers must therefore always check the product information and clinical procedures with the most up-to-date published product information and data sheets provided by the manufacturers and the most recent codes of conduct and safety regulation. The publisher and the authors make no representations or warranties to readers, express or implied, as to the accuracy or completeness of this material. Without limiting the foregoing, the publisher and the authors make no representations or warranties as to the accuracy or efficacy of the drug dosages mentioned in the material. The authors and the publisher do not accept, and expressly disclaim, any responsibility for any liability, loss or risk that may be claimed or incurred as a consequence of the use and/or application of any of the contents of this material.

9 8 7 6 5 4 3 2 1
Printed in the United States of America
on acid-free paper

Dedicated to young people, who should never be denied an opportunity to overcome problems and thrive.

CONTENTS

FOREWORD

The universe of psychiatric practice is broad and varied, including disciplines as different as forensic psychiatry, sleep-medicine psychiatry, consultation-liaison psychiatry, addictions psychiatry, geriatric psychiatry, child and adolescent psychiatry, and electroconvulsive therapy (ECT). This marvelous differentiation of subspecialties is both a blessing and a problem—a blessing because of the number of career choices available to the psychiatric trainee, a problem because of the limited cross-talk and cross-collaboration that occur among the sub-disciplines of psychiatry.

Such is the case with the application of ECT in children and adolescents. The vast majority of ECT providers come from a background of training in general psychiatry and/or geriatric psychiatry, with almost none trained in child and adolescent psychiatry. Similarly, very few child and adolescent psychiatrists provide ECT, and child and adolescent psychiatry training typically does not include a rotation on an ECT service. As a result, when a psychiatrically ill child or adolescent comes to the attention of either an ECT provider or a child and adolescent psychiatrist, neither practitioner is likely to have had specific training in responding to the needs of the young patient being considered for ECT. In this context, *Electroconvulsive Therapy in Children and Adolescents*, edited by Neera Ghaziuddin and Garry Walter, offers a most welcome, comprehensive compilation of all that we know about the use of ECT in minors, which will meet the needs of key practitioners from different backgrounds.

It is estimated that only 1% of all persons receiving ECT in the United States are younger than 18 years of age. Only a fraction of that proportion is less than 12 years of age. This means that a busy ECT service evaluating one or two new patients per week might evaluate one adolescent per year (probably less). This rate of accrual is too slow to allow the typical practitioner of adult ECT to gain any significant experience in child and adolescent ECT before mid-career, or later.

As a consequence, even the experienced ECT physician can feel lost when faced with the referral of a child or adolescent. Do the same diagnostic indications apply? For a given diagnosis, are the success rates the same as would be expected in an adult? What regulations apply regarding consent and assent? Is the technical approach for ECT the same or different as in an adult?

In the past, the ECT provider could consult the medical literature and would find a moderate amount of evidence dispersed over a broad territory of medical journals—but no systematic compilation of the evidence in the form of a textbook. Authoritative textbooks on ECT exist, such as the APA Task Force reports on ECT, but these textbooks have only summary information regarding children and adolescents. *Electroconvulsive Therapy in Children and Adolescents* is the first textbook to close this gap. The ECT provider who is not a child and adolescent psychiatrist will be reassured that there is more that is the same than is different in the application of ECT in children and adolescents as compared with adults. Still, there are some important distinctions, such as the critical role of ECT in catatonia and self-injurious behavior (SIB) in young people. SIB is a clear example of an indication that most psychiatrists with a general psychiatry background will not have encountered. SIB is one of those clinical entities that "needs to be seen to be believed," as the visual evidence of the injury makes the case for the severity of illness.

Electroconvulsive Therapy in Children and Adolescents is clear in drawing the lines between what is specifically and empirically known about ECT in youth, and what knowledge must be borrowed from studies in adults. The review of the child and adolescent psychiatry ECT literature is principally in the form of summarized case reports, case series, and retrospective chart reviews, peppered with the occasional prospective, systematic collection of data on a series of patients. There are no randomized clinical trials of ECT in children or adolescents. This in no way detracts from the material presented in *Electroconvulsive Therapy in Children and Adolescents*, nor should it produce therapeutic paralysis. To the contrary, the publication of *Electroconvulsive Therapy in Children and Adolescents* should assure ECT providers—and comfort parents of children being considered for ECT—that there is a collated body of knowledge that is consistent, hopeful, and consensus-driven. Whatever uncertainty remains in how to best provide ECT for mentally ill children and adolescents will continue to be worked out in the future. In the meantime, justice and beneficence demands that skilled ECT providers make this treatment available to relieve suffering in those children and adolescents for whom it is appropriate.

W. Vaughn McCall, MD, MS
Case Distinguished Professor and Chair
Department of Psychiatry and Health Behavior
The Medical College of Georgia, of Georgia Regents University
Editor, *The Journal of ECT*

PREFACE

The purpose of this book is to provide a scholarly overview of electroconvulsive therapy (ECT) in children and adolescents that draws on world leaders in the field. It is the first such book on the topic. It is written primarily for physicians and allied health professionals (psychologists, social workers, and nurses) who are interested in recommending or administering ECT, or simply learning more about the treatment, although we hope that young patients, parents, and caregivers may also find the information useful.

This book arose out of our clinical observations and sense of injustice. Respectively, we witnessed ECT to be a highly effective treatment in many young patients, while others in that age group who may have benefited from ECT were denied the opportunity to receive it, largely due to issues involving stigma and lack of professional knowledge. A typical case in the first category, prompting our efforts to publish the book, was as follows. A seriously depressed, 16-year-old patient was referred after failing a number of trials of psychotropic medication. While hospitalized for the ninth time, she was placed on "eye to eye" safety precautions intended for the most dangerously suicidal patients. With ECT, her depression improved, premorbid functioning was regained, and she was able to successfully engage in psychotherapy, which had previously not been possible when her symptoms were severe.

Included in this book are, to begin, chapters that examine the turbulent history of pediatric ECT, theories about the treatment's mechanism of action (including a feasible mechanism in young recipients), issues around stigma, and ethical and consent aspects. Given the myths abounding in relation to ECT—for example, that it is inherently cruel and causes permanent brain damage—which continue to pose a treatment barrier, we make no apology for focusing on matters pertaining to stigma and ethics. Also included are chapters that outline practical steps in the use of ECT, optimal administration of anesthesia, side effects (including how to minimize these), and ECT in those with comorbid neurological or other medical conditions; safety should be a paramount concern for all medical treatments, and hence our emphasis on this facet of ECT. The book concludes with chapters on various indications for the treatment in young patients, namely mood disorders, schizophrenia spectrum disorders, catatonia in autism, and self-injurious behavior. When "ECT" is mentioned to many mental health professionals, "depression" may immediately come to mind as the primary, and perhaps sole, clinical indication—these four concluding chapters highlight the dynamic state of the field, and the growing recognition that ECT is potentially beneficial for a range of conditions that may affect young people.

We have attempted to make the book not only scientifically and clinically rigorous, but also as user-friendly and "hands on" as possible, by including with each chapter a number of key points at the outset and a question and answer section at the end. Pervading all chapters is the recognition that there are gaps in our current knowledge base and that data for preadolescents are particularly limited. For the latter reason, the book focuses on adolescents rather than younger children.

The book would not have been possible without the energy and commitment of our esteemed chapter authors, emanating from North America, Europe, Australasia, and the Middle East, to whom we are indebted. We also salute their resolve and courage—championing the cause of ECT in young persons, notwithstanding the lifesaving nature of the treatment, does not win friends in every quarter. In addition, we acknowledge other professional colleagues for their staunch support over the years, and Dr. Nerissa Soh for administrative assistance. Finally, to our families—we are deeply grateful for your unwavering love, encouragement, and patience.

Neera Ghaziuddin
Ann Arbor, MI, USA
Garry Walter
Sydney, NSW, Australia

ABOUT THE EDITORS

Neera Ghaziuddin, MD, MRCPsych, is Associate Professor of Child and Adolescent Psychiatry at the University of Michigan Ann Arbor, appointed to the Faculty in 1992. She directs the Treatment Resistant Disorder clinic and trains future generations of child psychiatrists about severe, treatment resistant psychiatric disorders and about the use of electroconvulsive therapy in this age group. She has published extensively about ECT and adolescent mood disorders. She is the primary author of the American Academy of Child and Adolescent Psychiatry Practice Parameters for the use of ECT, published in 2004. In 2002 she received the ECT Investigator's Award from *The Journal of ECT* for the paper titled, "Electroconvulsive Therapy for Minors: Experience and Attitudes of Child Psychiatrists and Psychologists."

Garry Walter, MD, PhD, is Professor of Child and Adolescent Psychiatry at the University of Sydney and Clinical Director of Child and Adolescent Mental Health Services in Northern Sydney Local Health District, Australia. He is also Adjunct Professor at Dalhousie University, Canada. A child and adolescent psychiatrist, in 2002 he completed a doctorate on ECT in young people. He is the long-standing Editor of *Australasian Psychiatry*, International Editor-at-Large of the *Journal of the American Academy of Child and Adolescent Psychiatry,* and a member of several other editorial boards, including for over a decade *The Journal of ECT*. He has published over 300 papers and has received many prestigious research prizes, including for his studies on ECT, other psychiatric treatments, and stigma. In 2012 he was appointed a Member of the Order of Australia by the country's Governor-General for service to medicine in the fields of adolescent mental health, medical education, and publishing.

ABOUT THE EDITORS

CONTRIBUTORS

Bernard Biermann, MD, PhD
Medical Director, Child and Adolescent Inpatient Unit
University of Michigan C. S. Mott Children's Hospital
Department of Psychiatry,
University of Michigan Hospital and Health System
Ann Arbor, Michigan, USA

Yuval Bloch, MD
Director, Child and Adolescent Outpatient Clinic
Shalvata Mental Health Center
Senior Lecturer in Psychiatry
Sackler Faculty of Medicine, Tel Aviv University
Tel Aviv, Israel

William de Carvalho, MD
Director, ECT Department
Maison de Santé de Bellevue
Meudon, France

David Cohen, MD, PhD
Professor of Psychiatry
Université Pierre et Marie Curie
Head, Department of Child and Adolescent Psychiatry
Groupe Hospitalier Pitié-Salpêtrière
Paris, France

Angèle Consoli, MD, PhD
Director, Centre for Psychiatric Rare Diseases
Department of Child and Adolescent Psychiatry
Groupe Hospitalier Pitié-Salpêtrière
Paris, France

Dirk M. Dhossche, MD, PhD
Professor of Psychiatry
Medical Director of the Child Psychiatric Unit
University of Mississippi Medical Center
Jackson, Mississippi, USA

Max Fink, MD
Professor of Psychiatry and Neurology Emeritus
State University of New York at Stony Brook
Long Island, NY, USA

Neera Ghaziuddin, MD, MRCPsych
Associate Professor of Psychiatry
Director, Treatment Resistant Disorders Clinic,
Child and Adolescent Psychiatry Section
Department of Psychiatry
University of Michigan Hospital and Health System
Ann Arbor, Michigan, USA

Daniel E. Gih, MD
Clinical Assistant Professor of Psychiatry
Co-Medical Director, Michigan Comprehensive Eating Disorder Program
Department of Psychiatry,
University of Michigan Hospital and Health System
Ann Arbor, Michigan, USA

Polly Gipson, MA, PhD
Assistant Professor of Psychiatry,
Department of Psychiatry
University of Michigan Hospital and Health systems
Ann Arbor, Michigan, USA

Elise Hodges, MA, PhD
Clinical Assistant Professor
Associate Clinical Director, Neuropsychology Section
Department of Psychiatry
University of Michigan Hospital and Health Systems
Ann Arbor, Michigan, USA

Daniel F. Maixner, MD
Clinical Associate Professor
Director, ECT Program
Department of Psychiatry
University of Michigan Hospital and Health Systems
Ann Arbor, Michigan, USA

Andrew McDonald, B Med
Director of Clinical Services, Mental Health
Sydney Local Health District
Sydney, NSW, Australia

Joseph M. Rey, MD, PhD
Professor of Psychiatry
Notre Dame School of Medicine
Honorary Professor
Discipline of Psychiatry, Sydney Medical School, University of Sydney
Sydney, NSW, Australia

Michael Robertson, MD, PhD
Clinical Associate Professor
Centre for Values, Ethics and the Law in Medicine
University of Sydney
Sydney, NSW, Australia

Edward Shorter, PhD, FRSC
Jason A. Hannah Chair in the History of Medicine and Professor of Psychiatry
University of Toronto
Toronto, Ontario, Canada

Daniel Stein, MD
Director, Pediatric Psychosomatic Department
Edmond and Lily Safra Children's Hospital
The Chaim Sheba Medical Center, Tel Hashomer
affiliated with the Sackler Faculty of Medicine, Tel Aviv University
Tel Aviv, Israel

Emma Taylor, MB ChB
Consultant Anaesthetist
University Hospital Southampton NHS Foundation Trust
South Hampton, Hampshire, United Kingdom

Lee E. Wachtel, MD
Medical Director, Neurobehavioral Unit, Kennedy Krieger Institute
Associate Professor of Psychiatry
Johns Hopkins School of Medicine
Baltimore, Maryland, USA

Garry Walter, MD, PhD
Professor of Child and Adolescent Psychiatry
University of Sydney
Clinical Director, Child and Adolescent Mental Health Services
Northern Sydney Local Health District
Sydney, NSW, Australia

Electroconvulsive Therapy in Children and Adolescents

CHAPTER 1
The History of Pediatric ECT

EDWARD SHORTER

KEY POINTS

- More than seven decades of use and study suggest that ECT in children and adolescents is similar to ECT in adults in most respects, apart from the low frequency of use in young people; there are limited data in pre-adolescents.
- The safety and efficacy of ECT in young people were established early.
- After its introduction in the 1940s in the pediatric population, ECT was largely uncontroversial.
- The rejection of pediatric ECT that began in the 1960s occurred as a result of the cultural upheavals of the period and not as a result of negative new scientific findings.
- The use of psychoactive medications for some indications as an alternative to ECT often turned out to have disappointing results.
- A revival of pediatric ECT began in the 1990s as the dimensions of adolescent depression and other disorders responsive to ECT started to become apparent.
- Child psychiatry has, in the past, not been completely receptive to scientific data on the safety and efficacy of ECT.

OVERVIEW

Electroconvulsive therapy (ECT) in the adolescent and child population undergoes the same narrative arc over the last 50 years as in the adult population: initial acceptance after the introduction of ECT in 1938; rejection for social and cultural reasons in the turbulent protest movements of the 1960s and 1970s; then revival in the 1980s and afterward as scientific data make it apparent that the procedure is safe and effective in pediatric use (see Table 1.1). What is striking in the story addressed by this chapter is how little the rejection of

Table 1.1. KEY HISTORICAL DEVELOPMENTS IN PEDIATRIC ECT

Date	Development/Activity
1938	ECT introduced in Rome (2)
1940s–1950s	**Widespread acceptance, routine use in all age groups** **Psychoanalytic community divided (15)**
1941	First recorded pediatric use (epilepsy in 3yo) Hemphill & Walter, Bristol UK (1)
1943	First series in children and adolescents: n = 40, ages 5–19 ECT safe and effective, dramatic success in mania and melancholia Heuyer et al., Paris (4)
1947–1954	Large sample in pre-adolescents with follow-ups: n = 98, ages 4–12 ECT effective with "few side effects" in pediatric population with "childhood schizophrenia" Bender, New York (5–7, 10)
1951, 1954	Bender findings disputed: some patients "definitely worse" after ECT Diagnoses questioned: behavioral disorders, not "schizophrenia" Clardy, Orangeburg, NY (8–9)
1947–1957 (reported 1960)	Routine use of ECT and/or insulin coma therapy in diagnosis of "childhood schizophrenia" n = 23, ages 7–14; Hift et al., Vienna (13)
1960s–1980s	**Pediatric ECT becomes a rarity in response to the rise of psychopharmacology, ethical concerns and the spread of antipsychiatric attitudes from the counterculture into restrictive legislation and social abhorrence**
1963	Swedish clinicians reject ECT in a 7yo patient with severe "periodic catatonia" (21)
1973	NYU study finds that ECT has been supplanted by pharmacotherapy except for treatment of "catatonic states in adolescents" (26)
1975	*Wyatt v. Stickney* decision bans ECT on minors in Alabama, imposes tight restrictions on competent consenting adults (24) Film version of *One Flew Over the Cuckoo's Nest* spreads anti-ECT hostility into mainstream culture (2)
1980	British survey of 433 child psychiatrists finds that only 18% consider ECT even "occasionally" appropriate (33)
1978–1988	University of Rochester survey of over 1,000 ECT patients finds only 4 patients < 15 (31)
1983	26 US states forbid pediatric use of ECT, six others have established restrictive regulations (24)
1980s–1990s	**Pediatric ECT begins a comeback**
1978	First American Psychiatric Association (APA) task force grudgingly acknowledges acceptability of ECT in children and adolescents by "a small group of psychiatrists on rare and exceptional occasions" (39)

(continued)

Date	Development/Activity
Table 1.1 (CONTINUED)	
1990	Second APA task force accepts ECT in children < 12 for several indications, age no longer "an absolute counter-indication (40)
1990–1993	Retrospective case reviews confirm safety and effectiveness of ECT in minors (42–44)
1997	Comprehensive systematic review of 396 case reports finds little evidence of lasting cognitive effects; endorses ECT in minors; Rey and Walter, Sydney, Australia (46)
1998	Chapter on ECT in pediatric neuropsychiatry included in major American Psychiatric Press textbook (46)
2000s	**Expanding endorsements, lessening restrictions**
2000	Strong endorsement for ECT in adolescents, warning against unrealistic overprotectiveness: Cohen et al., Pitié-Salpêtrière child and adolescent service, Paris (48)
2001	APA task force report, 2nd edition: ethics restrictions lightened except in small children (41)
2004	American Academy of Child and Adolescent Psychiatry issues "Practice parameters" endorsing ECT for mood disorders in adolescents (51)
2010	ECT in young people and adults essentially the same, except for frequency of use; Walter et al., Australia (20)

ECT in the middle third of the twentieth century has to do with science, and how much it owes to cultural prejudices arising from the antipsychiatry movement and from the fictive reconstructions of Hollywood films.

BEGINNINGS

What is apparent in early accounts is their absolute matter-of-factness: the authors show no awareness that inducing seizures in children is any different from the procedure for adults; for these authors, the whole "question" of pediatric ECT is really a non-question. In one of the earliest accounts on record (1941), Robert Hemphill and W. Grey Walter at the Bristol City and County Mental Hospital stated in passing, as though neither statement was exceptional, that their eldest patient was "a lady of 74," their youngest a 3-year-old, "an epileptic in whom all else had failed to interrupt a series of minor attacks. . . . Neither of these patients came to any harm" (1). This complete indifference to age scarcely qualifies as "the introduction of pediatric ECT," yet historically Hemphill and Walter seem to have been the first to describe it, and only three years after the treatment had made its debut, in Rome, where Ugo Cerletti and Lucio Bini administered ECT to patient "Enrico X" (2).

In 1942, Georges Heuyer and associates at the Hôpital des Enfants-Malades (Hospital for Sick Children) in Paris began the systematic use of ECT in adolescents. On February 7, Heuyer, a prominent private practitioner in Paris who consulted at the Enfants-Malades, initiated the first of 11 stimuli on a 14-year-old patient who had a diagnosis of schizophrenia among oneiric, or dream-like, symptoms. The oneiria, at least, disappeared. Heuyer treated two further patients, one of whom, as a Jew in Paris under the Nazi occupation, had been traumatized by the arrest of his relatives and the taunting he had to endure at school; the boy's symptoms of melancholia, including an apparently catatonic mutism, were relieved by four ECT sessions. These three patients, treated amidst the most dramatic circumstances imaginable, represent the beginning of pediatric ECT (3).

The following year, 1943, Heuyer reported on what were now a total of 40 children treated with ECT, ranging in age from 5 to 19. The results in melancholic and manic illness were brilliant, in other disorders less so. Curious is Heuyer's account of success in patients with "tics": Jean Delay, shortly to become the professor of psychiatry in Paris, challenged the appropriateness of this indication in the subsequent discussion at the session of the Medico-Psychological Society at which Heuyer spoke. It is possible, however, that some of the "tics" were really stereotypies in catatonia (4).

LAURETTA BENDER

Credit for the introduction of pediatric ECT in the United States ECT belongs to Lauretta Bender, head of the Children's Ward of the Psychiatric Division of Bellevue Hospital in New York City and one of the founders of pediatric psychiatry, who in 1942 initiated convulsive therapy in patients ranging in age from 4 to 12. (It is worth noting that she also treated them with insulin coma therapy and LSD. [M. Fink, personal communication, Feb. 28, 2012].) Reporting on 98 "schizophrenic children," most of whom had received the full course of 20 electroconvulsive stimuli, once a day, she found, first, that ECT had few side effects in this child population. She noted a "lack of evidence of a lasting effect on the intellectual functioning and development of the child." Second, the procedure offered some benefit. Though there had been few full remissions, all hospital staff agreed that the children "were less disturbed, less excitable, less withdrawn, and less anxious.... They were more composed, happier, and were better able to accept teaching or psychotherapy." At follow-up after the war, 48 of these 98 were at home (almost all of them in school), 35 were in other psychiatric facilities, and 13 in institutions for children with mental retardation (5). In the discussion of this classic paper, given at the American Neurological Association in 1947, New York neurologist and psychiatrist Lothar Kalinowski, dean of American electrotherapists, noted that "children obviously are less confused" than adults receiving ECT (6). Thus, by this time it was clear that pediatric ECT could be administered safely and effectively with few concerns about harming the development of these young children. (Interestingly, pediatric ECT vanished from Bellevue after Bender left the service in 1956, soon to move to Columbia University.)

There was much agonizing about whether Bender's patients had undergone changes in mental function. While her studies were ongoing, psychologists Austin Des Lauriers and Florence Halpern on her service were evaluating the cognitive status of the children treated with ECT, and in 1947 (publishing findings first reported in 1946) said that they found "no change in reasoning and judgment." The children were less anxious, yet immediately following treatment the children also seemed "unafraid, but disinterested [sic] and flat" (7).

More hostile reports of the effects of ECT in the child population appeared. In 1951 Ed Rucker Clardy weighed in with a negative assessment of the kinds of patients, he said, whom Bender had been treating. Clardy, a physician, had previously worked in the area of mental retardation and the behaviorally disturbed youngsters of the training schools—and not in the world of child psychiatry per se—and was now in charge of the child guidance service at Rockland State Hospital in Orangeburg, New York. He said that a number of the children admitted to his service who had previously received ECT elsewhere—a number of them Bender's—had not done well at all (8). In 1954, he and a colleague condemned the treatment definitively: "In a number of cases, parents have told the writers that their children were definitely worse after EST [electro-shock therapy]." Clardy questioned the diagnosis of childhood schizophrenia and felt that many of the children had behavioral disorders (9). Since this was a selected population of children who had not responded well to ECT, it did not constitute a challenge to the efficacy of ECT as such. Yet it was widely cited.

The Clardy paper of 1951 evidently quite disturbed Bender (probably the 1954 paper as well), who in the early 1950s was leading a study sponsored by the National Institute of Mental Health (NIMH) on ECT in children. She apparently asked psychologists Saul Gurevitz and William Helme on the Bellevue children's service to undertake a follow-up study of the children aged 6–13 who had recently received ECT at Bellevue (she supported the study from her NIMH grant). The investigators' report was overwhelmingly positive. To be sure, just after treatment there seemed to be a decline in cognitive function. But subsequent testing at follow-up found that the children had recovered their "intellectual efficiency... in most cases being slightly higher than before shock" (10).

ECT IN EUROPE

In Europe as well as North America, there was a feeling that ECT in children was really quite routine and was not freighted with excessive concerns. Clinicians at a psychiatric clinic in in St-Sébastien, Spain, writing in 1950, described a psychotic 13-year-old girl with the symptoms of "acute catatonia," including severe motor agitation, negativistic thinking, and "the somatic symptoms that [Karl] Stauder reported in his [diagnosis of] 'lethal catatonia.'" She recovered over a period of several months following "shock treatments (insulin and electroshock)." A year later she was well, "despite a slight intellectual deficit" (11). The off-hand manner of the report suggests that by this time the treatment of psychosis in childhood with ECT must have been routine. (Stauder introduced the diagnosis of "lethal catatonia" in 1934 [12].)

In the 1950s, in the neuropsychiatric clinic in Vienna led by Professor Hans Hoff, children receiving the diagnosis "childhood schizophrenia" were automatically administered one of the shock therapies, either ECT or insulin coma therapy, the latter having been pioneered in Vienna. The diagnosis of childhood schizophrenia was not frequent; in the years 1947 to 1957 it was conferred only 23 times, the youngest patient being 7, the oldest 14. But of those 23 patients, 10 received insulin coma, 8 electroshock, and 5 a combination of the two. There was apparently no agonizing about bioethics—the term had not yet been invented—nor was parental reluctance reported (13). Shock therapy in Vienna seems to have been as self-understood as aspirin.

EARLY CONTROVERSY?

Pediatric ECT in the early days was not entirely uncontroversial. (Much like other treatments, such as lithium for mania, it was in widespread use, but was not universally accepted.) Within psychoanalysis, for example, opinion was divided. Psychoanalyst Margaret Mahler led the children's service of the New York State Psychiatric Institute. She apparently had little interest herself in ECT, but it was on her watch that, in the children's service, Bernard Pacella and Lothar Kalinowski, both noted electrotherapists, initiated in 1946 a study of ECT in children (14). It is impossible that such a study could have been conducted in a fortress of psychoanalytic thought if it had been highly controversial.

On December 8, 1947, the leadership of the psychoanalytically inspired Group for the Advancement of Psychiatry, known as GAP, informed the membership in a newsletter that GAP's committees on child psychiatry and on therapy had been asked to "study the use of electric shock therapy in children." Yet the committees had remained officially mute. Somehow among the membership, GAP said, "The opinion has been expressed that Electric Shock Therapy is harmful to children; this appears to be an area of disagreement that needs clarification" (15). This does not sound like a unified rejection front against ECT.

Alfred Gallinek, an émigré psychiatrist (fleeing the Holocaust) at Columbia-Presbyterian Medical Center in New York—which nested in a virtual hotbed of psychoanalysis—writing in the early 1950s, saw nothing troublesome in treating adolescents having "controversial indications" with ECT. One such indication was "pseudoneurotic schizophrenia," meaning severely neurotic but not psychotic, a diagnosis that his colleagues at the Psychiatric Institute of Columbia had just put in vogue. Yet it was apparent that, on the basis of the clinical picture, at least one of the adolescents Gallinek treated had catatonia; eight months of previous psychotherapy in his home town had proven fruitless, but this 14-year-old boy was completely restored after 15 sessions of ECT (16). Gallinek seems to have taken for granted that ECT was a straightforward treatment that required little hairsplitting about ethics.

Thus, within mainstream psychiatry and within society as a whole in the 1950s, pediatric ECT seems to have been accepted almost with complacence. John Campbell, who had a private psychiatric practice in Atlanta, reported in 1952 a series of 18 adolescent patients with "manic depressive psychosis," almost all of whom had responded well to ECT. In one case, the family refused seizure treatment on the grounds that the patient, a 14-year-old boy, was afraid of it. In another case, the patient, a 13-year-old girl, turned it down on the grounds that she had seen the movie *The Snake Pit*, a film starring Gloria De Havilland, in which ECT is depicted unsympathetically. Campbell did not report parents being apprehensive of memory loss or having their children's "brains burned" (17). Three years later, in 1955, as Campbell augmented his series, the youngest ECT patient was a girl of 11 (18).

ABSENCE OF COGNITIVE CHANGES?

None of the early reports mentions significant cognitive changes in pediatric ECT beyond a brief period of disorientation immediately following the stimulus. Georges Heuyer, author of the first accounts, said in 1943 of the 40 pediatric cases his team had treated in Paris, "Just as in adults, we have noted some disturbances of memory following ECT, but these disturbances have always been transitory and of short duration. After their disappearance, the children's intelligence shows no weakening, no abrogation of development" (4). In the 23 above mentioned patients in Vienna, "We were able to verify with repeated psychological testing that in all cases the amnestic syndrome was completely resolved" (13). Frantz Moise and Georgios Petrides said in 1996 of the 13 adolescent patients they had treated at the Stony Brook campus of the State University of New York, "None of the patients reported long-lasting memory difficulties or any experience that would indicate neurological impairment" (19). Looking back on half a century of experience with young people, Garry Walter and colleagues said in 2010, "There is no clear evidence that ECT has a negative impact on long-term cognitive functioning" (20). The notion that ECT causes long-term and devastating memory losses in children (and adults) is an urban myth (2).

THE WIND SHIFTS: THE DECLINE OF PEDIATRIC ECT IN THE 1960S AND AFTER

The relaxed and rather off-hand attitude to pediatric ECT that prevailed in many places before the 1960s gave way to a climate of grave ethical concerns and fears about brain damage. In 1963, Swedish clinicians were willing to use "insulin therapy" and anticonvulsants on a boy of 7 who suffered from severe "periodic catatonia." But ECT? "We have not given electro-convulsive therapy, as we do not generally use this method in children," they said (21).

Joseph Rey and Garry Walter puzzle over the decline of pediatric ECT in the 1960s and 1970s, attributing it to "apprehension about possible harmful effects as well as to the advent of psychotropic drugs" (22). Yet concern about adverse effects in the pediatric population were not new and go back to E. R. Clardy at the Children's Group in Rockland State Hospital (8). As for the supposed newness of psychotropic medications, one bears in mind that the barbiturates were introduced in 1903, the amphetamines for psychiatric indications in 1936 (23). Both drug classes had extensive pediatric use, and the cause for the great decline in pediatric ECT in the mid-twentieth century must be sought elsewhere.

Here is where accounts that depend solely on medical writing in tracing the arc of events become inadequate. One can understand this great decline only in the context of the determinedly antipsychiatric attitudes of the "flower children" and the entire revolt against the established order of the 1960s and 1970s. A team led by William Winslade, bioethicist at the Institute for the Medical Humanities at the University of Texas Medical Branch in Galveston, wrote in 1984, "One of the backwashes of that revolution was the patients' rights movement, and ECT became one symbol of the plight of patients allegedly at the mercy of the mental health establishment" (24). ECT came to stand for a devilish "medieval" holdover, mainly useful in disciplining patients and forcing them to toe the line of the establishment.

Simultaneously, the late 1950s and 1960s saw the introduction of new pharmacotherapeutic agents in child psychiatry, particularly such antipsychotics as chlorpromazine (also often referred to as "major tranquilizers"). Tricyclic antidepressants were less useful in disturbances in children (25). Yet the effectiveness of pharmacotherapy was often overestimated in these early days, and many children turned out to be "treatment resistant" to conventional psychopharmacology. Still, drug treatment carried the day over ECT; by 1973, Magda Campbell, a child psychiatrist at New York University Medical

Center, was able to write, "At present convulsive therapies have practically disappeared from practice, mainly due to the discovery of major tranquilizers. The use of electroshock treatment in catatonic states in adolescence constitutes about the sole remaining exception in child psychiatry" (26). (In general, pediatric psychiatry has been anything but reticent in the employment of pharmacotherapy. Yet some of the leaders in the field have been dubious about the use of pharmaceutical agents in this age group. One thinks of the quite negative assessment of Judith Rapoport, a senior investigator at the National Institute of Mental Health, in 1987: while not using the term "resistant," she nonetheless found most pharmacotherapy inapplicable in the pediatric population [27].)

LEGISLATION AND THE COURTS

The cutback on ECT began with a court decision, *Wyatt v. Stickney*, in 1975, in which a judge barred ECT in children and imposed elaborate ECT restrictions on state hospitals in Alabama governing ECT in adults. A group of legal scholars note, "The court permitted no one under the age of 18 to receive ECT, and competent consenting adults could not be given ECT without the Extraordinary Treatment Committee's approval" (28). Judicial indignation thus swept medical advice completely aside.

The 1970s saw a wave of laws and regulations in various state legislatures restricting pediatric applications of ECT, beginning with California in 1974 (not permissible in children age 12 and younger), Tennessee in 1976 (age 14), Colorado in 1977 (age 16), and Texas in 1993 (age 16). This was part and parcel of a larger legislative attack upon ECT in patients of any age. "By 1983," writes Winslade et al. (24), "26 states had passed such statutes," while six other states had established regulations governing ECT. The entire legislative stance oozed suspicion that doctors were determined to act against their patients' best interests by inflicting dangerous, drastic, and unproven remedies upon them.

For parents with afflicted children, navigating the way through this thicket of pointless and counterproductive regulation could be a nightmare. Journalist Peter Wyden describes family efforts to obtain convulsive treatment for their schizophrenic son amidst the bureaucratic impediments that the state of California had thrown up. Around 1987, Wyden and his wife penned the following letter to the judge who was supposed to grant the authorization but had somehow not yet done so: "You may be unaware of the intolerable hardship inadvertently imposed on my son Jeffrey Wyden, a ward of the Santa Clara Public Guardian's Office, by delaying in okaying electric shock treatments for him at El Camino Hospital. . . . Four Palo Alto psychiatrists recommended these treatments urgently. So do three teams of doctors at the

National Institute of Mental Health in Washington. Currently my son is unintentionally subjected to unnecessary torment because medications had to be withdrawn which would render electroshock treatments ineffective. Jeff's parents plead with you to stop delays at once. Society has created a terrible dilemma for this helpless person. Regulations designed to help are hurting him terribly" (29). This kind of scenario would be inconceivable were penicillin required. And ECT is the penicillin of psychiatry.

HOLLYWOOD

Such irrational legal initiatives, in which politicians believed themselves competent to make medical decisions, derived not from new findings in the medical literature but from cultural hostility to ECT stoked by such films as *One Flew Over the Cuckoo's Nest*, released in 1975. These externalist perspectives let us understand how the attitudes of an entire society, not just the medical evidence on safety, or lack thereof, shape the evolution of a treatment such as convulsive therapy. But in the context of the rabidly anti-ECT 1960s, performing the procedure on "defenseless" children was unthinkable!

This hostility of the counterculture to pediatric ECT, born of the 1960s, lingered on long after the tie-dye T-shirts and sandals with negative heels had been discarded. In 1985 a journalist noted in the Boston Globe, "While few deny that shock treatment has been misused, particularly with schizophrenics and disturbed children, many specialists now view it as the most effective available treatment for serious biological depression. . . ." (30). Thus, the looming rehabilitation of adult ECT did not embrace the procedure in children.

ECT IN CHILDREN BECOMES RARE

In a culture shaped by a Hollywood movie, ECT in children became extremely rare. (This offers an interesting insight into the role of culture vs. science in clinical decision-making.) In 1988, Laurence Guttmacher and Henry Cretella, psychiatrists at the University of Rochester, surveyed "all physicians at Strong Memorial Hospital who had used ECT in the last decade." How often in children? Of over 1,000 patients, only 4 had been younger than 15 (31). Eva Frommer, in charge of a children's psychiatric clinic at St. Thomas's Hospital in London, said in 1968 that among numerous outpatients, in five years of practice it had been necessary to use ECT only twice, once in a suicidal patient suffering from "schizoaffective psychosis," the other in a suicidal patient in a "severe phobic tension state" (32). A survey found that among 433 child psychiatrists in Britain in 1980, only 18% said that ECT was even "occasionally" appropriate. Others didn't use it at all, or only "rarely" (33).

There were, to be sure, isolated case reports from the 1970s and 1980s, the kinds of outcomes that should have set alert minds to work along the lines of, "Wait a minute. Maybe we could get those results too!" In 1986, reporting a series of 10 catatonia cases of all ages, a team of neurologists at Middlesbrough General Hospital in the United Kingdom mentioned a girl of 11 with "idiopathic familial catatonia" who recovered after 10 ECT sessions (34). In 1988, J. C. Powell, a consultant psychiatrist in charge of the adolescent unit of Crichton Royal Hospital, a psychiatric facility in Dumfries, Scotland, described a boy of 13 with "pre-pubertal depressive stupor" and a positive dexamethasone suppression test: "Following the first treatment, ECT was discontinued as the patient immediately began to eat and drink normally" (35).

Nonetheless, ECT remained anything but a conventional treatment for childhood depression and catatonia. In 1995, Max Fink and Gabrielle Carlson, psychiatrists at the State University of New York at Stony Brook, noted, commenting on a case of successful convulsive treatment in an 8-year-old girl, "The consideration of ECT in adolescents and children is a rarity" (36).

It was a measure of how deeply the well was poisoned that in 1995, when Beth Cizadlo and Allyson Wheaton, in the Department of Psychiatry of the University of Iowa College of Medicine, administered ECT to an 8-year-old girl with catatonia and depression, they believed the case to be the first in the English-language literature of treating a child with ECT for severe catatonia (37). (In fact, as we have seen, this was not true, but that they believed it to be so reflects how poorly established convulsive therapy was at the time in the pediatric population.)

PEDIATRIC ECT BEGINS A COMEBACK

Yet the weather vane was slowly turning. Reliable epidemiological data on the incidence of depressive illness in children and adolescents began to show the seriousness of the problem. According to statistics from the U.S. Center for Mental Health Services, in 2004 8.3% of adolescents aged 12–17 experienced a "major depressive episode" over the previous twelve months, and 4% of children ages 4–7 experienced "definite/severe difficulties" (38). A population in need of effective psychiatric treatment clearly existed.

From its first report on ECT in 1978 onward, the American Psychiatric Association (APA) warmed steadily to the idea of child and adolescent convulsive therapy. In 1978, the APA grudgingly conceded, "Even in children and adolescents, the use of ECT has been acceptable to a small group of psychiatrists on rare and exceptional occasions" (39).

By 1990, the APA had become considerably more permissive: ECT was now accepted for major depression, mania, catatonic schizophrenia, affective problems in schizophrenia, and possibly other psychoses as well. (This was written at a time when catatonia was still considered a subtype of chronic psychosis, or "schizophrenia.") The organization accepted ECT in children under 12 who were otherwise treatment-unresponsive or who could not be safely treated. "Age should not be considered an absolute counter-indication for the use of ECT," the task force of the APA determined (40). The customary strictures about elaborate collegial consultation and unresponsiveness to previous therapies were all present—as though one were about to administer really quite mild doses of cyanide to the small patients—yet the official voice of American psychiatry was clearly becoming more accepting.

By 2001, the APA had given up efforts to tightly circumscribe the indications. "In children and adolescents, ECT should be reserved for instances in which other viable treatments have not been effective or cannot be safely administered" (41). The number of outside consultants was now reduced to one for adolescents, remaining at two for small children. The ethics rituals, in other words, were becoming ever less cumbersome.

Clinical opinion began to swing around as well. In 1990, Mark Bertagnoli and Carrie Borchardt, pediatric psychiatrists at the University of Minnesota, reviewed the very sparse literature on the use of ECT in children and adolescents since the days of Heuyer and Bender—many with an N of 1. In 18 of the 21 studies, the patients were "improved" (42). So there seemed to be no doubt of efficacy.

Terry Schneekloth and collaborators reviewed in 1993 the 20 adolescent patients at the Mayo Clinic who had received ECT between 1983 and 1991, finding a significant benefit in patients with mood disorders and virtually no side effects (43) On the basis of similar data that he and Carlson had collected at Stony Brook, Fink penned in 1993 a forceful editorial in the journal *Convulsive Therapy*, spearing the field of child psychiatry for ignoring ECT at its meetings and in its textbooks. "There is no evidence," said Fink, "clinical, experimental, anatomic, or historical—to justify the attitude that ECT is unwarranted in the young" (44). *Convulsive Therapy*, alas, was not among the "must" readings in child psychiatry, but this was a first, powerful statement from a senior figure in the profession.

From the mid-1990s, a number of voices began endorsing convulsive therapy in adolescents and children. In a review of the 396 reported cases in the literature—overwhelmingly in adolescents rather than children—Joseph Rey and Garry Walter at the University of Sydney, writing in 1997, found little evidence of lasting cognitive effects: The commonest side effect was headache, the authors said (45). Thus a bugbear that had been brandished at the electrotherapists for 40 years vanished.

In 1998, Fink, at the Stony Brook Campus of the State University of New York, and C. Edward Coffey, in the Department of Psychiatry of the Henry Ford Health Systems in Detroit, contributed a chapter on ECT in pediatric neuropsychiatry to a major textbook published by the American Psychiatric

Press (46). This marked the moment in which pediatric ECT acquired, so to say, the keys to the city. In 1999, Fink and Madhavan Thuppal broke the barrier on ECT in mental retardation, concluding, "The benefits of ECT were similar to the benefits which occur in our patients without mental retardation." They likened it to previous treatments of adolescents with ECT: "At one time, poplar understanding argued that ECT was riskful and adolescents required compelling indications." Yet experience had shown that adolescents, too, could be treated by the same standard as adults (47).

In 2000, David Cohen, director of the child and adolescent psychiatry service at the Pitié-Salpêtrière hospital group in Paris, came out forcefully for ECT in adolescents and cautioned against medically non-indicated protectiveness. "The consequence of possible overprotection is that [the adolescent patient] may remain untreated because of unrealistic fears regarding ECT, even in cases of life-threatening conditions." Cohen and his associates concluded, "We consider that there is no ethical reason to ban ECT use in adolescents" (48). Such powerful voices were new.

Differences remained between children and adults in reasons for referral to ECT. In 2008, Yuval Bloch, leading a team of investigators at several Israeli child psychiatry centers, established that the major reason for child referrals to ECT was the severity of symptoms, particularly catatonia and suicidal behavior, while the major reasons for referral of adults was "lack of response to pharmacotherapy." This is actually good news, suggesting that clinicians are willing to recommend ECT for children because of the gravity of the illness while ECT in adults is considered a last-ditch recourse (49). (Other studies, however, suggest that child psychiatrists do in fact tend to regard ECT as a treatment of last resort, and most have had little training in the technique [50].)

Approvals mounted. In 2004, the American Academy of Child and Adolescent Psychiatry endorsed ECT for the treatment of mood disorders in adolescents "when more conservative treatments have been unsuccessful." The Academy task force noted that the response in such disorders as pediatric depression was on the order of 75–100%. (51). To put the recommendation in perspective, there is no drug with anything like the response rate of ECT, but most psychopharmacologic agents come with an array of side effects much greater than the (minimal) side effects of ECT. The task force remained mute on the subject of ECT in children, perhaps fearing to go a bridge too far and knowing that data in the pre-adolescent age group were limited. Yet the historical record of safety and efficacy in children as well as adolescents suggests that such cautiousness may result in withholding a powerful treatment from this population.

Garry Walter and colleagues asked in 2010, what were the real differences between ECT in young persons and adults? None, except for frequency of use, was the answer (20).

CONCLUSION

What conclusions may we draw from this brief survey?

One is that clinical decision-making in child psychiatry has been far less subject than one might imagine to the influence of scientific data. At the beginning of ECT's trajectory, data on the safety and efficacy of ECT in the pediatric population were actually quite considerable. Yet somehow this scientific evidence was simply brushed from the table in the hysteria about "putting electricity into the brains of helpless children" that arose from the counterculture in the 1960s. It was a hysteria that somehow washed over clinical psychiatry, sweeping away a large store of accumulated knowledge in the manner of the incoming tide. This is not supposed to happen in medicine, and yet it regularly occurs in psychiatry (52). The revulsion that greets the mention of "ECT" among many child psychiatrists today is ample evidence of this effect.

Is there unmet need here? Are there treatment-responsive pediatric populations that have not yet been offered ECT? The answer to this question is "yes." Consider the following letter that New York psychiatrist Eric London, a member of the scientific advisory board of the Autism Science Foundation, wrote to the *New York Times* in 2012, apropos the treatment of children with autism. (In the autism community, activists often pride themselves on avoiding pharmacotherapy.) "I recently saw a patient in a developmental center who wore a helmet because of constant head-banging. When I asked what medications had been tried, staff members proudly told me that they had successfully avoided medicating this patient. But this decision came at a terrible cost to him, as his constant head-banging caused detachment of both retinas and blindness" (53). There is early suggestive evidence that convulsive treatment is safe and effective in autistic children with symptoms of self-injury behavior, such as head-banging (54). Timely intervention might have avoided this tragic therapeutic outcome.

QUESTIONS AND ANSWERS

1. *Who reported the first series of young patients treated with ECT and what were the key findings?*

   In 1942 and 1943 in Paris, Georges Heuyer and colleagues reported the first series of young patients treated with ECT. Those patients with melancholia and manic illness showed a very favorable response to the treatment.

2. *What are the likely factors accounting for the decline in use of pediatric ECT in the 1960s?*

   A variety of factors may be implicated in the treatment's diminishing use in the 1960s, among them the "antipsychiatry" movement (arguably, the most important factor), concerns about the potential harmful effects of

ECT on the developing brain, and the emergence of other treatment methods, most notably pharmacotherapy. The release of the movie *One Flew Over the Cuckoo's Nest* in the following decade contributed to the treatment's marginalization.

3. *Why has pediatric ECT become a more acceptable treatment for many health professionals in the last 20 years?*

   There has been growing awareness, from reliable epidemiological studies, that depressive illness posed a serious health problem for which effective treatments were needed. In turn, this led to more permissive guidelines from eminent bodies such as the American Psychiatric Association and to further studies in pediatric ECT that appeared to demonstrate its effectiveness and safety.

ACKNOWLEDGMENTS

The author is grateful to Dirk Dhossche and Max Fink for their comments on an earlier version of this chapter.

DISCLOSURE

Prof. Edward Shorter has no conflicts to disclose. This research was funded in part by the Canadian Institutes of Health Research (CIHR), grant no. AMS-94689.

REFERENCES

1. Hemphill RE, Walter WG. The treatment of mental disorders by electrically induced convulsions. *Br J Psych*. 1941;87:256–75.
2. Shorter E, Healy D. *Shock Therapy: A History of Electroconvulsive Treatment in Mental Illness*. New Brunswick, NJ: Rutgers University Press; 2007.
3. Heuyer G, Bour, Feld. Electro-choc chez des adolescents. *Ann Méd Psychol.* 1942;100:75–89.
4. Heuyer G, Bour, Leroy. L'électro-choc chez les enfants. *Ann Méd-Psychol.* 1943.101:402–7.
5. Bender L. One hundred cases of childhood schizophrenia treated with electric shock. *Trans American Neurol Assoc*. 1947;72:165–9.
6. Kalinowski L. Discussion comment. *Trans American Neurol Assoc*. 1947;72:169.
7. Des Lauriers A, Halpern F. Psychological tests in childhood schizophrenia. *Am J Orthopsychiatry*. 1947;17: 57–67.
8. Clardy ER. A study of the development and course of schizophrenia in children. *Psychiatr Q*. 1951;25:81–90.
9. Clardy ER, Rumpf EM. 1954. The effect of electric shock treatment on children having schizophrenic manifestations. *Psychiatr Q*. 1954;28:616–23.

10. Gurevitz S, Helme WH. Effects of electroconvulsive therapy on personality and intellectual functioning of the schizophrenic child. *J Nerv Ment Dis.* 1954;120:213–26.
11. Bueno Ituarte R, Olaizola J. Les psychoses infantiles. In: Ey H, Marty P, eds. *Premier Congrès Mondial de Psychiatrie, Paris 1950*. Paris: Hermann; 1952. vol. 7, pp. 117–9.
12. Stauder KH. Die tödtliche Katatonie. *Arch Psychiatr Nervenkr.* 1934;102:614–34.
13. Hift E, Hift S, Spiel W. Ergebnisse der Shockbehandlung bei kindlichen Schizophrenien. *Schweiz Arch Neurol Neurochir Psychiatr.* 1960;86:256–72.
14. State of New York. *Eighteenth Annual Report of the Director of the Psychiatric Institute to the Department of Mental Hygiene for the Fiscal Year Ended March 31, 1947*. Utica: State Hospitals Press; 1947: pp. 8–9.
15. Group for the Advancement of Psychiatry. Circular Letter No. 63, 1947 Dec 8. Distributed among the membership in mimeographed form.
16. Gallinek A. Controversial indications for electric convulsive therapy. *Am J Psychiatry*. 1952;109:361–6.
17. Campbell JD. Manic depressive psychosis in children. *J Nerv Ment Dis.* 1952;116:424–39.
18. Campbell JD. Manic-depressive disease in children. *JAMA*. 1955;158:154–7.
19. Moise FN, Petrides G. Case study: electroconvulsive therapy in adolescents. *J Am Acad Child Adol Psychiatry*. 1996; 35:312–8.
20. Walter G, Robertson M, Rey JM, Soh N, Malhi G. ECT in young people and the pioneering spirit of Lauretta Bender. *Acta Neuropsychiatrica*. 2010; 22:253–4.
21. Annell A-L. Periodic catatonia in a boy of 7 years. *Acta Paedopsychiatr.* 1963;30:48–58.
22 Rey JM, Walter G. Half a century of ECT use in young people. *Am J Psychiatry.* 1997;154: 595–602.
23. Shorter E. *Before Prozac: The Troubled History of Mood Disorders in Psychiatry.* New York: Oxford University Press; 2009.
24. Winslade WJ, Liston ED, Ross JW. Medical, judicial, and statutory regulation of ECT in the United States. *Am J Psychiatry*. 1984;141: 1349–55.
25. Campbell M, Fish B, Shapiro T. Imipramine in preschool autistic and schizophrenic children. *J Autism Child Schiz*. 1971;1:267–82.
26. Campbell M. Biological interventions in psychoses of childhood. *J Autism Child Schiz*. 1973;4:347–73.
27. Rapoport JL. Pediatric psychopharmacology: the last decade. In: Meltzer H, ed. *Psychopharmacology: The Third Generation of Progress*. New York: Raven; 1987, pp. 1211–4.
28. Senter NW, Winslade WJ, Liston EH, Mills MJ. Electroconvulsive therapy: the evolution of legal regulation. *Am J Social Psychiatry*.1984;4:11–5.
29. Wyden P. *Conquering Schizophrenia: A Father, His Son, and a Medical Breakthrough*. New York: Knopf; 1982, p. 16.
30. Dietz J. Shock therapy's comeback: used against depression, it remains controversial. *Boston Globe*, January 14, 1987, p. 37.
31. Guttmacher LB, Cretella H. Electroconvulsive therapy in one child and three adolescents. *J Clin Psychiatry*. 1988;49:20–3.
32. Frommer EA. Depressive illness in childhood. In: *Recent Developments in Affective Disorders: A Symposium*. London: Royal Medico-Psychological Association; *British Journal of Psychiatry*, supp. no. 2, 1968, pp. 117–36.
33. Pippard J, Ellam L. *Electroconvulsive Treatment in Great Britain, 1980: A Report to the Royal College of Psychiatrists*. London: Gaskell; 1981, p. 13.

34. Barnes MP, Saunders M, Walls TJ. The syndrome of Karl Ludwig Kahlbaum. *J Neurol, Neurosurg Psychiatry*. 1986;49:991–6, tab 3.
35. Powell JC. Pre-pubertal depressive stupor: a case report. *Br J Psychiatry*. 1988;153:689–92.
36. Fink M, Carlson GA. Letter: ECT and prepubertal children. *J Am Acad Child Adol Psychiatry*. 1995;34:1256–7.
37. Cizadlo BC, Wheaton A. Case study: ECT treatment of a young girl with catatonia. *J Am Acad Child Adol Psychiatry*. 1995;34:332–5.
38. U.S., Substance Abuse and Mental Health Services Administration. Mental Health, United States, 2008, HHS Pub. No. (SMA) 10-4590. Rockville, MD: Center for Mental Health Services, SAMHSA; 2010, tab 1.1, p. 85; tab 1.2, p. 87.
39. American Psychiatric Association. *Report of the Task Force on Electroconvulsive Therapy*. Washington DC: APA; 1978, p. 162.
40. American Psychiatric Association. *The Practice of Electroconvulsive Therapy: Recommendations for Treatment, Training, and Privileging: A Task Force Report*. Washington DC: APA;1990, p. 15.
41. American Psychiatric Association. *The Practice of Electroconvulsive Therapy: Recommendations for Treatment, Training, and Privileging: A Task Force Report*. 2nd ed. Washington DC: APA; 2001, p. 58.
42. Bertagnoli MW, Borchardt CM. A review of ECT for children and adolescents. *J Am Acad Child Adol Psych*. 1990;29: 302–7.
43. Schneekloth TD, Rummans TA, Logan KM. Electroconvulsive therapy in adolescents. *Convulsive Therapy*. 1993;9:158–66.
44. Fink M. Editorial: Electroconvulsive therapy in children and adolescents. *Convulsive Therapy*. 1993;9:155–7.
45. Rey JM, Walter G. Half a century of ECT use in young people. *Am J Psychiatry*. 1997;154:595–602.
46. Fink M, Coffey CE. Electroconvulsive therapy in pediatric neuropsychiatry. In: Coffey CE, Brumback RA, eds. *Textbook of Pediatric Neuropsychiatry*. Washington DC: American Psychiatric Press; 1998, ch. 54, pp. 1389–408.
47. Thuppal M, Fink M. Electroconvulsive therapy and mental retardation. *J ECT*. 1999;15: 140–9.
48. Cohen D, Flament M, Taieb O. Electroconvulsive therapy in adolescence. *Eur Child Adoles Psychiatry*. 9;2000:1–6.
49. Bloch Y, Sobol D, Levkovitz Y. Reasons for referral for electroconvulsive therapy: a comparison between adolescents and adults. *Australas Psychiatry*. 2008;16:191–4.
50. Ghaziuddin N, Kaza M, Ghazi N. Electroconvulsive therapy for minors: experiences and attitudes of child psychiatrists and psychologists. *J ECT*. 2001;17:109–17.
51. American Academy of Child and Adolescent Psychiatry. Practice parameter for use of electroconvulsive therapy with adolescents. *J Am Acad Child Adol Psychiatry*. 2004;43: 1521–39.
52. Shorter E. *A History of Psychiatry, from the Era of the Asylum to the Age of Prozac*. New York: Wiley; 1997.
53. London E. Letter: Care of the disabled in state-run group homes. *New York Times*, Jan 2, 2012, p. A18.
54. Dhossche DM, Reti IM, Wachtel LE. Catatonia and autism: a historical review, with implications for electroconvulsive therapy. *J ECT*. 2009;25:19–22.

CHAPTER 2

The Mechanism of Action of ECT

MAX FINK

KEY POINTS

- The production of a generalized grand mal seizure is the key to effective treatment with ECT.
- Theories that seek to explain the mechanism of action of ECT have been in the following domains: psychological, electrophysiological, neurohumoral, neuroendocrine, receptor, GABA release, and neurogenesis.
- Arguably the best theory of the mechanism is the neuroendocrine theory, which focuses on the impact of seizures on the release of hypothalamic hormones.
- The efficacy of seizures is measurable by ictal and interictal EEG recordings and by releases of hypothalamic hormones into body fluids.
- Hormone changes associated with a single seizure are rapidly lost unless repeated.
- The neuroendocrine theory is a testable framework for understanding the mechanism of action of ECT in adults, as well as in children and adolescents.

OVERVIEW

Several decades of the use of electroconvulsive therapy (ECT) have enabled us to understand those elements of the treatment procedure that are associated with clinical efficacy. These decades also witnessed a variety of theories of its mechanism of action. We now know that the production of a generalized grand mal seizure is the key to effective treatment with ECT. The neuroendocrine theory is the most viable theory to explain the treatment's action, and that theory is particularly pertinent in childhood and adolescence, a period characterized by major endocrine changes.

In the 1930s, interest in biological mechanisms to treat psychiatric illnesses increased and ECT, insulin coma therapy, and lobotomy were introduced to the psychiatric hospitals. For two decades, ECT was the principal treatment of the severely psychiatric ill, accepted worldwide until the late 1950s, when an enthusiasm for psychoactive medications replaced it (1). Prescribing pills became the central theme of clinical psychiatry. In the 1970s, however, increasing rates of failure of medication treatment encouraged the recall of ECT to clinical use (2–4).

The efficacy of ECT is indisputable. Inducing repeated seizures relieves the syndromes of melancholic depression, malignant catatonia, and delirious mania. It does so rapidly, often within two to three weeks. But the effects may be transient, making necessary the continuation of treatments over many weeks and occasionally months. ECT reduces suicide risk and saves lives. Such dramatic changes stimulated many hypotheses as to how such a peculiar process could affect body physiology. Memory loss was the explanation proposed by psychologists; changes in the brain's electrophysiology as measured by electroencephalography (EEG) and by seizure thresholds were proposed by the neurology-minded; effects on the brain's neurotransmitters and neuroendocrines were the focus of psychopharmacologists; and "brain damage" was the rallying cry of anti-psychiatrists (4).

Almost all of our knowledge about ECT comes from studies in adults. Prejudice against the use of ECT in children and adolescents was sufficiently strong that, except for the experiments of Georges Heuyer and colleagues in Paris, and Lauretta Bender at Bellevue Psychiatric Hospital in New York City, ECT was not applied in children and rarely in adolescents, limiting the published experience to case reports (5). In the past decade, however, interest in ECT in children and adolescents, including those with mental retardation (6, 7) and autism, has increased (8, 9).

What we know about the mechanism of ECT is wholly derived from studies in adults. Despite positive and safe experiences with ECT in pediatric populations, the repeated misrepresentation of the treatment's risks frightened away potential prescribers and patients' families, ensuring widespread rejection. The alarm waves also inhibited studies seeking to understand the treatment mechanism (5, 10, 11).

Before assessing the merits of the hypotheses, we should discuss the known and well-documented facts of the treatment that must be accounted for.

WHAT WE KNOW ABOUT EFFECTIVE TREATMENTS

A cerebral seizure is essential. The repeated induction of grand mal seizures is the central event in the treatment's efficacy. The clearest benefit is seen when seizures are repeatedly induced, usually two to three times weekly.

Depressive and manic mood states, psychoses of diverse origins, motor disorders of catatonia, and the confusions of deliria are relieved, usually within 6 to 15 seizures (seizures were also an important event in insulin coma and lobotomy, now long discarded as outmoded) (12–14).

The significance of the grand mal seizure for ECT benefits is also demonstrated by the experience with the non-seizure brain stimulation methods that have been proposed as replacements for ECT. Prolonged sleep, subconvulsive stimulating electric currents, and prolonged coma induced by isoflurane anesthesia were enthusiastically hailed and then rejected as the results failed clinical efficacy. In the first decades of the twenty-first century, transcranial magnetic stimulation (TMS), vagus nerve stimulation (VNS), deep brain stimulation (DBS), and transcranial direct current stimulation (tDCS) are the present rages, each failing to demonstrate efficacy convincingly either in populations treated or in remission rates; the stimulation treatments remain unpersuasive as a substitute for ECT (15, 16).

One competitor remains. Inducing seizures by high-energy magnetic currents—magnetic seizure therapy (MST)—does seem to have the promise of inducing effective seizures. But magnetic seizure induction is singularly inefficient, like the injections with camphor that preceded inductions by electricity, seizures are poorly generalized and clinically inefficient. The methodology is also expensive so that seizures initiated by electricity are favored.

Different behaviors are relieved. Severely depressed mood is rapidly responsive to ECT, with remission rates from 50–90% within 3 to 4 weeks (17, 18). Remission rates are higher for the more severely ill, especially those with psychosis (19). The delusions of schizophrenia and psychotic mood states are relieved (20). The grandiosity and overactivity of delirious mania, rapid cycling mania, and mixed affective states are quickly reduced. The motor disorders of malignant catatonia, benign stupor, retarded catatonia, and the neuroleptic malignant syndrome are rapidly dissipated (21).

In each instance, the response is best measured in specific behaviors (e.g., depressed mood, insomnia, delusion, motor rigidity, mutism, suicidal thoughts) and not as resolution of a "disease" as codified by the American Psychiatric Association's *Diagnostic and Statistical Manual of Mental Disorders* (DSM) and the World Health Organization's *International Classification of Diseases* (ICD). Individual syndromes, not disorders or diseases, are altered by seizures.

Not all seizures are equally effective. The efficacy of seizures induced by electric currents varies with energy dosage, electrode placement, and the frequency and number of treatments. The quality and eventual efficacy of the seizures are measurable in the EEG recordings, both during the ictal events and in the interseizure periods (2). Clinical results are better when the EEG seizure occurs in both halves of the brain equally, and is of sufficient duration to show runs of high voltage slow waves mixed with spikes, followed by runs of high voltage slow waves and a sharp (precise) terminating end-point. Modern technology permits recording of the seizure while it occurs ("the monitored seizure"), allowing the therapist to decide whether the seizure is "effective" (and likely to be followed by beneficial effects) or "ineffective." An "ineffective seizure" can be immediately repeated, using better induction parameters, under the same anesthesia.

Not only is the elicited seizure reflected in the EEG recordings, but every seizure stimulates the release of hypothalamic-pituitary peptides into the blood and cerebrospinal fluid. The amount of hormones released varies with electrode placement, stimulation dose, and the number and frequency of treatments. Prolactin is rapidly released within the serum with a peak at 20 minutes. So characteristic is the prolactin release that it has been used to distinguish a grand mal seizure from that of a pseudoseizure (22).

Adrenocorticotropic hormone (ACTH), thyrotropin releasing hormone (TRH), and vasopressin are examples of well-studied hormones released by seizures (23). Indeed, it is the massive outpouring of these hormones that characterize the seizures in effective ECT. Lower levels of release mark the lesser effects with less efficient electrode placements and inadequate energy dosages. The lack of such release with the newly proffered brain stimulation methods cited earlier is a further signpost to their failed replacement for ECT.

EEG monitored treatment courses achieve higher remission rates than those in which such monitoring is not a feature. This is best seen in the reports by the Consortium for Research in ECT ("CORE") investigators in their treatment of major depression with bilateral ECT (24). Using EEG monitoring guidelines, their remission rates are 20% better than the rates reported in clinical trials based on unilateral ECT (25). Treatments based on bilateral electrode placement require shorter courses (26). In community settings where treatments are given with highly idiosyncratic and inefficient parameters, the treatment outcomes are less effective than those that assure effective treatments (27).

Seizures must be repeated for a benefit. The behavioral effects of seizures are incremental, requiring repetition until the pathological symptoms have cleared and new patterns of behavior have stabilized. ECT is not a surgical excision that removes the defect; it is more like the treatment of diabetes in which repeated administration of insulin and dietary control are needed to maintain healthy serum glucose levels. Discontinuing an ECT course at the first sign of relief or prescribing a fixed number of treatments at the onset of the course discourages effective treatment. Early termination ensures high relapse rates (28).

Contrast this model with the treatment practices using psychoactive medications, where neither the duration of treatment nor dosage are determined at the time of prescription. Treatment continues and is repeatedly changed as long as symptoms are detected, for weeks, months, and even years thereafter.

This tolerant attitude is not applied to ECT, where the minimum number of treatments is the proclaimed standard. Such limitation is particularly poignant in the treatment of pediatric patients,where each treatment is often attended by parental anxieties. Patients receiving short courses of ECT have high relapse rates compared to the experience in research studies where minimum numbers of treatments are preset (28).

Indeed, when depressed patients were treated with ECT and then maintained with medication or placebo, 80% relapsed within 6 months with placebo, 60% with nortriptyline alone, and 40% with the combination of nortriptyline and lithium (29). In a parallel study, continuation with a fixed schedule of ECT alone also reported a relapse of 40% (30). Similar high relapse rates are found in the treatment of depressed patients when antidepressant medication treatment is terminated prematurely (31).

Obtaining an effective seizure is the point of the treatments. Electricity is not the only effective way to induce seizures. Chemical inductions (e.g., flurothyl, pentylenetetrazol) are just as effective as those induced by electricity, indicating that electricity is not essential to our explanation. Neither anesthesia nor the electric current alone nor a single seizure is effective.

THOUGHTS ON MECHANISM

With these experiences in hand, we ask why and how do seizures relieve severe mental disorders? At the moment, we have no assured answer—we simply do not understand how ECT has the restorative capacity that it does. For that matter, no hypothesis for the mode of action of *any* psychiatric treatment—be it psychotropic medicines or the "talk" psychotherapies or brain stimulation—is satisfactory. For ECT, many hypotheses have been proposed (see Table 2.1).

Table 2.1. SOME THEORIES OF THE MECHANISM OF ACTION OF ECT

Theory	Suggested mechanism	Year	Proponent
Psychological	Memory loss	1950	Janis
Electrophysiological	Persistent brain function changes	1956	Fink, Kahn
Neurohumoral	Changes in brain neurotransmitters	1976	Modigh
		1978	Grahame-Smith et al.
Neuroendocrine	Release of hypothalamic peptides	1980	Fink & Ottosson
Receptor	Enhanced brain receptor activity	1982	Lehrer & Belmaker
GABA release	Change in seizure threshold	1983	Sackeim et al.
Neurogenesis	Increased gliosis and neurogenesis	1932	Meduna
		2000	Madsen, Bolwig, et al.
		2004	Ongür & Heckers

The first treatments, administered with high energy electric currents from the 1940s to the 1970s, were associated with immediate deliria and with periods of memory loss. At the time, psychiatric thought was dominated by the Freudian image of psychiatric illness as the response to recollections of infantile and childhood trauma. Psychological tests immediately after a course of treatments showed patients to have measurable deficits and, at the same time, they were relieved of depressed and manic moods, paranoid thoughts, and abnormal movements (32). The explanation that memory loss was the basis for the relief offered by seizures dominated clinical discussion. As treatment practices reduced the severity of the ictal deliria and the cognitive deficits, however, the hypothesis was no longer supportable (33).

In those years, EEG recordings during the course of ECT showed progressive slowing of frequencies of the rhythms, increased amplitudes, and bursts of seizure activity. But for many patients, these changes in EEG were not sustained, and evidence accumulated that more enduring changes were necessary for clinical benefit. The EEG changes were seen as necessary but not sufficient for a sustained ECT benefit. As well, many patients exhibited these changes and had not improved (34). In retrospect, the failure of the association is probably related to the heterogeneity of the patients treated. For those with melancholic depression, catatonia, or mania, the characteristic changes in EEG marked a successful treatment course; for those with hebephrenic psychoses, psychoneuroses, character pathology, and substance abuse, the EEG changes did occur but without clinical relief (2).

As psychopharmacology increasingly dominated clinical psychiatry, interest shifted to the brain's neurotransmitters of acetylcholine, epinephrine, norepinephrine, serotonin, dopamine, and gamma-aminobutyric acid (GABA). The efficacy of the drugs was attributed to changes in these substances. When the mechanism of ECT was considered, the same concepts of altered neurotransmitter concentrations were applied. In extensive studies in animals of the impact of seizures, the procedure identified as electroconvulsive shock (ECS) was undertaken, but these studies failed to find consistent changes, either in the levels of the transmitters (35, 36) or in the activity of the receptors (37). Occasional direct measures in patients failed to show abnormal functions before treatment, nor did the brain levels of the neurotransmitters change with seizures (38).

Another hypothesis was based on the occasional finding that the seizure threshold rose with repeated treatments, directing attention to the activity of GABA, the brain neurotransmitter believed to relate to seizure activity (39). When reliable studies showed that seizure thresholds did not consistently rise with treatment, the hypothesis failed (40).

The neurogenesis theory has its origin in the observations by Ladislas Meduna, the Hungarian originator of induced seizures for the relief of schizophrenia. A neuropathologist, he studied the concentration of brain glia in the mentally ill and found that concentrations of glia in postmortem brains were low in patients who died in schizophrenia and high in those who died in epilepsy. Clinical studies had reported that schizophrenia was uncommon in patients with severe and chronic epilepsy. He speculated that increasing gliosis might relieve schizophrenia (41). After determining that injections of camphor-in-oil induced grand mal seizures in animals, he went to Budapest's mental hospital at Lipótmezo and induced seizures in the more severely ill. Of the first 11 patients, nine were suffering from catatonia, the syndrome that is most responsive to induced seizures (42). Two were relieved sufficiently to leave the hospital, and in his trials in 110 patients over the next few years, more than half were relieved (43). The hypothesis of gliosis remained untested until the past decade, when new technology that permitted estimates of neurogenesis in animals demonstrated the increase in new brain cells after induced seizures (44, 45). The indirect confirmation of Meduna's hypothesis awaits verification in man.

The neuroendocrine theory was voiced in 1980 and over the decades has received considerable support (46–49). Among the more severely ill treated with ECT, the most immediate and beneficial effects of the procedure are seen on the body's vegetative functions of sleep and appetite. These functions direct attention to the hypothalamus, a brain region involved in the expression of emotions with profound control over the rest of the body through its actions on the pituitary gland. The hypothalamus and the pituitary gland produce hormones that circulate in the bloodstream and the cerebrospinal fluid, affecting other glands in the body (including the thyroid, parathyroid, adrenal, pancreas, ovaries, and testes) and other parts of the brain.

The importance of the hypothalamus in mental illness is consistent with the observation that hormonal functions in the mentally ill are wildly disordered (48). In the severely depressed, the entire axis linking the hypothalamus, pituitary gland, and adrenal and thyroid glands is dysfunctional, involving excesses of cortisol and other hormones. During ECT entailing bitemporal electrode placement—when electric currents pass from one temple to the other—the electric currents pass directly through the hypothalamus. (The lesser efficacy of unilateral electrode placement treatments—as suggested by many researchers in the field—may be largely due to their lowered stimulation of the hypothalamus and other centrencephalic tissues.) Hormones are released into the cerebrospinal fluid and into the bloodstream, with the amounts varying with the intensity of the gland's stimulation. How could such a release relieve mental disorders?

Consider the following scenario in a patient with abnormal cortisol functions. In an ensuing cascade of hormonal effects induced in the seizure, the hypothalamus releases its peptide and these stimulate the pituitary, which proceeds to alter the discharge of cortisol from the adrenal glands. The first effects of the stimulation are transitory, but by the fourth or fifth stimulus, the normal feedback actions of the hormones of the hypothalamic-pituitary-adrenal axis are again in place. Feeding and sleep become normal, and improvements in motor activity, mood, memory, and thought follow quickly.

In treating the mentally ill, the improved endocrine functions do not persist unless treatments are sustained. If the treatment duration is short, the glands quickly revert to their abnormal activities and the mental disorder is again evident. In such cases, continuation ECT is needed to sustain normal glandular functions and a normal mental state.

The position of neuroendocrine studies in psychiatry is a puzzle. Adrenal and thyroid functions are severely affected in the psychiatrically ill. These measures normalize when effective treatment achieves relief. When DSM-III dictated that manic depressive illness be split into syndromes of major depression and bipolar disorder, the hormone tests were discarded as markers of these conditions. This decision was premature. In data available to the DSM-III Task Force, these mood disorders were ill-defined and the samples were heterogeneous: there were some samples with hormone abnormalities and many without. This led to the failure to find specific and reliable tests as markers of these syndromes. The illness entities in DSM-III were determined by symptom checklists alone, without regard to physiology measures. As a result, the correlations between the hormone tests and clinical diagnoses were poor and hormone tests were rejected as diagnostically unrelated to the DSM criteria (48).

One should be optimistic that greater use of ECT in youth is likely to also increase interest in endocrine functions. It is timely to go back to the dexamethasone suppression test and thyroid function tests for a better understanding of the ECT mechanism (49).

CONCLUSION

While we cannot explain the connection between inducing seizures and relieving the syndromes of melancholia, catatonia, and mania, we know that our procedures are effective and safe. Our attention is focused on the neuroendocrine changes induced by seizures and the neuroendocrine dysfunctions of psychiatric illnesses. Childhood and adolescence are stormy periods of glandular changes, offering fascinating study opportunities. Now that increased attention is directed to ECT among youth, research of hormone changes should take center stage. Are the hormonal changes in adrenal and thyroid functions with seizures reported in adults also found in children and adolescents? The dramatic effects of seizures on hormone metabolism encourage such study.

ACKNOWLEDGMENTS

The chapter was abstracted from *Electroconvulsive Therapy: A Guide for Professionals and Their Patients* (New York: Oxford University Press, 2009). The author is grateful to Professor Edward Shorter of the University of Toronto for his collaboration and editing of an earlier draft.

QUESTIONS AND ANSWERS

1. *What are the characteristics of the ECT-induced seizure that are believed to be related to clinical effectiveness of the treatment?*

   Production of a generalized grand mal seizure is the key to the clinical effectiveness of ECT. Positive results are associated with the EEG seizure occurring in both halves of the brain equally, being of sufficient duration to show runs of high voltage slow waves mixed with spikes, followed by runs of high voltage slow waves, and having a sharp terminating end-point.

2. *What have been the main theories relating to the mechanism of action of ECT? (Please list.)*

   These theories have been in the following domains: psychological, electrophysiological, neurohumoral, neuroendocrine, receptor, GABA release, and neurogenesis.

3. *What is the rationale for the neuroendocrine theory for ECT's action?*

   Hormonal functions in mental illness are often disordered. For example, in severe depression, the axis linking the hypothalamus, pituitary gland, and adrenal and thyroid glands is dysfunctional, involving excesses of cortisol and other hormones. During ECT, particularly bilateral ECT, the electrical current passes though the hypothalamus, leading to the release of hormones into the cerebrospinal fluid and bloodstream. After several treatments, feedback action begins to restore normal hormonal function.

DISCLOSURE

Prof. Max Fink declares no conflicts of interest.

REFERENCES

1. Shorter E. *A History of Psychiatry*. New York: John Wiley & Sons; 1997.
2. Fink M. *Convulsive Therapy: Theory and Practice*. New York: Raven Press; 1979.
3. Fink M. *Electroconvulsive Therapy: A Guide for Professionals & Their Patients*. New York: Oxford University Press; 2009.
4. Shorter E., Healy D. *Shock Therapy: A History of Electroconvulsive Treatment in Mental Illness*. New Brunswick, NJ: Rutgers University Press; 2007.
5. Shorter E. The history of pediatric ECT. (Chapter 1 of this volume.)
6. Thuppal M, Fink M. Electroconvulsive therapy and mental retardation. *J ECT*. 1999;15:140–9.
7. Collins J, Halder N, Chaudhry N. Use of ECT in patients with an intellectual disability: review. *Psychiatrist*. 2012;36:55–60.
8. Dhossche DM, Reti IM, Wachtel LE. Catatonia and autism: a historical review, with implications for electroconvulsive therapy. *J ECT*. 2009;25:19–22.

9. Bailine SH, Petraviciute S. Catatonia in autistic twins: role of electroconvulsive therapy. *J ECT.* 2007; 23:21–22.
10. Fink M. Impact of the anti-psychiatry movement on the revival of ECT in the U.S. *Psychiatic Clinics N.A.* 1991;14:793–801.
11. Ottosson J-O, Fink M. *Ethics in Electroconvulsive Therapy*. New York: Brunner-Routledge; 2004.
12. Fink M. *A Beautiful Mind* and insulin coma: social constraints on psychiatric diagnosis and treatment. *Harvard Review of Psychiatry.* 2003;11:284–290.
13. Fink M, Shaw R, Gross G, Coleman FS. Comparative study of chlorpromazine and insulin coma in the therapy of psychosis. *JAMA.* 1958b;166:1846–50.
14. Valenstein ES (ed.): *The Psychosurgery Debate*. New York; San Francisco: WH Freeman; 1980.
15. Lisanby SH (ed.): *Brain Stimulation in Psychiatric Treatment*. Washington, DC: American Psychiatric; 2004.
16. Fink M. Transcranial magnetic stimulation is not a replacement for electroconvulsive therapy in depressive mood disorders. *J ECT.* 2011;27:3–4.
17. Fink M, Taylor MA. *Catatonia: A Clinician's Guide to Diagnosis and Treatment*. Cambridge, UK: Cambridge University Press; 2003.
18. Taylor MA, Fink M. *Melancholia: The Diagnosis, Pathophysiology and Treatment of Depressive Illness*. Cambridge, UK: Cambridge University Press; 2006.
19. Petrides G, Fink M, Husain MM, *et al.* ECT remission rates in psychotic versus non-psychotic depressed patients: A report from CORE. *J ECT.* 2001;17:244–253.
20. Fink M, Sackeim HA. ECT for schizophrenia? *Schizophrenia Bull.* 1996;22:27–39.
21. Fink M. Rediscovering catatonia: the biography of a treatable syndrome. *Acta psychiatr scand Supplementum.* 2013;441(127):1–50.
22. Trimble M. Serum prolactin in epilepsy and hysteria. *BMJ.* 1978;2:1682.
23. Fink M. Electroshock revisited. *Amer Scientist.* 2000;88(2):162–167.
24. Kellner CH, Knapp RG, Petrides G, et al. Continuation ECT versus pharmacotherapy for relapse prevention in major depression: a multi-site study from CORE. *Arch Gen Psychiatry.* 2006;63:1337–44.
25. Sackeim HA, Hasket RF, Mulsant BH, et al. Continuation pharmacotherapy in the prevention of relapse following electroconvulsive therapy: a randomized controlled trial. *JAMA.* 2001;285:1299–1307.
26. Fink M, Taylor MA. Electroconvulsive therapy: Evidence and challenges. *JAMA.* 2007;298:330–332.
27. Prudic J, Olfson M, Marcus SC, et al. The effectiveness of electroconvulsive therapy in community settings. *Biol Psychiatry.* 2004;55:301–12.
28. Wachtel LE, Hermida A, Dhossche DM. Maintenance electroconvulsive therapy in autistic catatonia: a case series review. *Prog Neuropsychopharmacol Biol Psychiatry.* 2010 May 30;34(4):581–7.
29. Sackeim HA, Hasket RF, Mulsant BH, et al. Continuation pharmacotherapy in the prevention of relapse following electroconvulsive therapy: a randomized controlled trial. *JAMA.* 2001;285:1299–1307.
30. Kellner CH, Knapp RG, Petrides G, et al. Continuation ECT versus pharmacotherapy for relapse prevention in major depression: a multi-site study from CORE. *Archives General Psychiatry.* 2006;63:1337–44.
31. Harvey BH, McEwen BS, Stein DJ. Neurobiology of antidepressant withdrawal: Implications for the longitudinal outcome of depression. *Biol Psychiatry.* 2003;54:1105–17.

32. Janis IL. Psychologic effects of electric convulsive treatments (post-treatment amnesias). *J Nerv Mental Dis.* 1950;111:359–382.
33. Abrams R. *Electroconvulsive Therapy*. 4th ed. New York: Oxford University Press; 2002
34. Fink M, Kahn RL. Relation of EEG delta activity to behavioral response in electroshock: Quantitative serial studies. *Arch Neurol Psychiatry (Chic.).* 1956; 78:516–525.
35. Modigh K. Long-term effects of electroconvulsive shock therapy on synthesis turnover and uptake of brain monoamines. *Psychopharmacology.* 1976;49:179–185.
36. Grahame-Smith DG, Green AR, Costain DW. Mechanism of the antidepressant action of electroconvulsive therapy. *Lancet.* 1978;1:254–256.
37. Lehrer B, Belmaker RH. Receptors and the mechanism of action of of ECT. *Biol Psychiatry.* 1982;17:497–511.
38. Fochtmann L. Animal studies of electroconvulsive therapy: foundations for future research. *Psychopharmacol Bull.* 1994;30:321–444.
39. Sackeim H, Decina P, Prohovnik I *et al.* Anticonvulsant and antidepressant properties of electroconvulsive therapy: a proposed mechanism. *Biol Psychiatry.* 1983;18:1301–10.
40. Fink M, Petrides G, Kellner CH, *et al.* Change in seizure threshold during ECT: a CORE study. *J ECT.* 2008;24:114–116.
41. Meduna L. Versuche über die biologische Beeinflussung des Ablaufes der Schizophrenie: Camphor und Cardiozolkrampfe. *Z ges Neurol Psychiatr.* 1935;152:235–62.
42. Gazdag, G, Bitter I, Ungvari GS, Baran B, Fink M. László Meduna's pilot studies with camphor induction of seizures: The first 11 patients. *J ECT.* 2009;25:3–11.
43. Meduna L. *Die Konvulsionstherapie der Schizophrenie*. Karl Marhold, Halle, 1937.
44. Madsen TM, Treschow A, Bengzon J, Bolwig TG, et al. Increased neurogenesis in a model of electroconvulsive therapy. *Biol Psychiatry.* 2000 Jun 15;47(12):1043–9.
45. Ongür D, Heckers S. A role for glia in the action of electroconvulsive therapy. *Harv Rev Psychiatry.* 2004 Sep-Oct;12(5):253–62.
46. Fink M, Ottosson J-O. A theory of convulsive therapy in endogenous depression: Significance of hypothalamic functions. *Psychiatry Res.* 1980;2:49–61.
47. Fink M. How does convulsive therapy work? *Neuropsychopharmacology.* 1990;3:73–82.
48. Shorter E, Fink M. *Endocrine Psychiatry: Solving the Riddle of Melancholia.* New York: Oxford University Press; 2010.
49. Fink M. Should the dexamethasone suppression test be resurrected? *Acta psychiatrica scandinavica.* 2005;112:245–9.

CHAPTER 3

ECT and Stigma

ANDREW McDONALD AND GARRY WALTER

KEY POINTS

- Goffman's pioneering work on psychiatric stigma, published in the 1960s, identified three targets for stigma: persons with physical deformities, persons with mental illness, or groups of minority status.
- The stigma encountered by those with mental illness can be exacerbated by certain treatments, such as ECT.
- Sources of information about stigma pertaining to ECT include the depiction of the treatment in movies and other media (portrayals that are generally noxious, and that include the depiction of ECT in young persons), biographical accounts, and a range of attitudinal studies that have examined the views of the public, health professionals, and patients (and their relatives).
- Studies of public opinion suggest that knowledge about ECT is generally inaccurate and attitudes toward it are highly negative.
- Among health professionals, a consistent research finding is that greater knowledge about ECT is associated with favorable attitudes and that psychiatrists, on the whole, have more positive views than other health professionals; differences in views between the various professional groups may be considerable.
- Overall, opinions of patients and family members about ECT are favorable.
- Effectively addressing the stigma surrounding the use of ECT in young persons remains challenging and will require both specific targeting of the treatment and a multifaceted approach.

OVERVIEW

This chapter defines stigma and its relationship to ECT, documents what those who receive ECT as well as their families, peers, and the wider community think of the treatment, explores the sources of this knowledge and these attitudes, and describes efforts to combat stigma. We will examine the proposition that more accurate knowledge about ECT is associated with more positive attitudes regarding its use, and will focus on one of the strongest challenges in tackling the stigma associated with ECT, namely, the wide disparity in the attitudes of mental health professionals.

In the early scenes of the 1980 movie *Ordinary People*, the central character, teenager Conrad Jarrett, returns home from hospital, having had treatment for depression following his suicide attempt. Attempting to reestablish the normal patterns of his life, Conrad resumes swimming training, where his coach takes him aside and asks whether he was "given shock out there." When Conrad indicates that he was, the coach tells him, "You know, Jarrett, I'm no doctor, but I would never have let them put electricity through my head" (1, p. 268).

This exchange may be fiction, but it encapsulates one of the reactions that a young person experiencing depression and receiving ECT may expect from friends and acquaintances. Already burdened with the weight of mental illness and the stigma that creates, it would appear that the *method* of treatment, however effective, may potentially magnify the stigma. What is "stigma," and how does it relate to ECT?

DEFINING STIGMA

The term "stigma" is ubiquitous in the contemporary professional and lay discourse regarding mental illness, has sprouted a burgeoning literature over nearly half a century (2), and is the focus of numerous public and professional campaigns (3, 4). And yet the term is often left to speak for itself, loosely defined if at all, and therefore taking on many different meanings in different contexts. When we talk of stigma, we might all know what we mean, but are we all talking about the same entity?

In ancient Greece, *stigmata* were marks on the skin of discredited individuals—slaves, traitors or criminals—that signified their devalued status. While stigmata assumed more positive connotations for some in the Christian era, with lesions on the palms and feet associating the sufferer with the wounds of Jesus and therefore bestowing positive status, the modern re-coining of the word implies a negative evaluation. In the 1960s, the Canadian sociologist Erving Goffman wrote a seminal work on stigma, describing it as a mark that defined an individual, or group, as discredited (5). He identified three targets for stigma: physical deformities, mental illness, and an association with groups of minority status based on race, religion, or other beliefs or characteristics. The developments of Goffman's work within the social and medical sciences has identified stigma very much as a social process involving a power gradient between a dominant group that bestows stigma on less powerful individuals or groups. Hinshaw (6) describes stigma as a "global devaluation of certain individuals on the basis of some characteristic they possess, related to membership of a devalued, disgraced or disfavored group . . . an internal mark of deep degradation to the individual who carries it and a licence to the social majority to perpetuate or escalate judgmental attitudes and responses" (pp. 23–24). Without delving into clashing arguments regarding the development of stigma, there is some consensus about its constituent parts, which includes cognitive processes (stereotypes), emotional processes (prejudice), and behavioral processes (discrimination). In this formulation, stereotypes are generalized beliefs about social groups, not necessarily pejorative but a means of providing some order to a complex world. When these beliefs take on negative emotions, or ignore evidence of their falsehood, they become prejudices, which Hinshaw defines as "unreasoning, unjustifiable, overgeneralized, negatively tinged attitudes toward others on the basis of group membership" (p. 22). When individuals or groups act, or fail to act, on the basis of their prejudices, they practice discrimination—unfair treatment or harmful actions based on an individual's group membership.

The above describes the stigmatizing of devalued individuals and encompasses a number of overlapping conceptualizations including "public," "experienced," or "enacted" stigma, entailing discrimination in many domains, such as restricted access to employment, accommodation, and health care. The corollary of "public" stigma is "personal" stigma, in which individuals may apply some of the same misconceptions about mental illness to themselves (sometimes referred to as "self-stereotypes"), experience negative emotions such as sadness or guilt ("self-prejudice"), and behave by, for example, not applying for jobs they assume will be barred to them ("self-discrimination"). An individual may also anticipate stigma in others ("perceived," "felt," or "anticipated" stigma), leading to self-isolation and slowness to seek help.

Thus, stigma is something that happens to individuals or groups of individuals. Can stigma happen to a physical treatment, such as ECT? Certainly, there are many examples in the literature where ECT is referred to as itself being the subject of stigma (7, 8). In many cases, stigma is used synonymously with a wide range of terms such as "opprobrium" and "vilification" on the one hand, and negative evaluations that characterize it as a barbaric, discredited, or archaic treatment on the other hand. While all such representations appear extensively in the literature, stigma in this chapter will refer specifically to a process experienced by groups and individuals. In this context, ECT adds to the stigma experienced by those who receive it, in the case of young people by their parents who provide consent for it, and by the health professionals who deliver it. An often quoted but potent illustration of this point is the fate that befell vice presidential candidate Thomas Eagleton in the 1972 US presidential elections. Once the fact of his past history of mental illness—in particular, his treatment with ECT—became known, he was marked as damaged and was publicly stigmatized, despite having served as lieutenant governor of Missouri and as a senator both during and after his period of psychiatric treatment. Eagleton was considered too great a risk to be "one heartbeat away" from the presidency, and he was dropped from the Democratic ticket (9, p. 6).

KNOWLEDGE OF AND ATTITUDES TOWARD ECT

How does one measure stigma? In the absence of a "stigma-manometer," the majority of the literature uses the proxy measures of stigmatizing knowledge and attitudes. This requires that one accepts the formulation of stigma as comprising cognitive, emotional, and behavioral components and, further, the often implicit assumption that problems of knowledge (such as stereotypes) or problems of negative emotions (prejudice) result in stigmatizing behavior.

To examine the evidence of stigma related to ECT in young people, let us return to the example of Conrad Jarrett from the film *Ordinary People* (10), and imagine his back story to the point of his reunion with his swimming coach, following Conrad's pathway from illness through his ECT treatment and toward recovery. Along the way, we consider the stigmatizing obstacles that block his path: the beliefs and attitudes of his peers toward the mentally ill; what the mental health professionals whom the Jarretts approach for help think of ECT; how Conrad and his parents might react to the recommendation for ECT given attitudes of the general public toward the treatment; what those who, like Conrad, have been treated with ECT think of it; and what his parents are likely to have thought of their son's course of ECT.

A review of community attitudes to mental illness in general is beyond the scope of this chapter. We will present a representative review of the evidence regarding stigma in mental illness more generally, and provide a comprehensive review of evidence linking ECT with stigma. We will explore the hypothesis, often implicit and not invariably confirmed, that the provision of accurate information regarding ECT and personal exposure to those who have received the treatment are associated with more positive and less stigmatizing beliefs regarding mental illness and reduced discriminatory behavior toward sufferers.

YOUNG PEOPLE'S VIEWS ABOUT MENTAL ILLNESS

Even before Conrad became depressed, research suggests that he would have emerged from early childhood with negative attitudes about mental illness (11), and as an adolescent boy would have been more prone to regard his incipient feelings of depression as signs of personal weakness, and may have attempted to conceal his symptoms or refuse his parents' entreaties to accept help. There has been a proliferation of research into the attitudes of young people toward mental illness, much of it based on public surveys in which subjects are asked their response to a series of clinical scenarios. This research has sought to detect problems with knowledge (such as stereotypes) or problems with attitudes (such as prejudices) that may lead to stigmatizing responses or behavior. One of the main limitations of this research has been acknowledged by several investigators, in their conclusion that "most work on stigma has been beside the point," namely, that it is based on surveys which assume that statements regarding knowledge, attitudes, and behavioral intentions are linked with actual behavior, rather than studying behavior directly, and therefore the research provides no clear implications or guidance regarding how to intervene (3).

In a survey of 303 high school students in California, published in 2005, Corrigan et al. (12) explored student attitudes toward adolescents with mental illness and alcohol abuse; it was found that students believed the mentally ill carried personal responsibility for their illness, and those with alcohol abuse even more. In addition, it was found that the students associated mental illness with dangerousness, pity, and fear, and that anger toward the mentally ill increased with the attribution of personal responsibility, while pity decreased. Corrigan's finding that stigma in adolescents is multifaceted was confirmed in a survey of 415 Chicago school students, with boys holding more stigmatizing ideas (13).

A subsequent Australian telephone survey by Jorm and Wright (14) of young people and their parents supported Corrigan's conclusion that the construct of stigma is multidimensional, and that it applies in different degrees and in different ways, depending on the type of mental illness—for example, psychosis, depression, and alcohol misuse were seen as more dangerous and unpredictable, and elicited greater social distance, while social phobia was more likely to be seen as a weakness. Direct contact with mental illness reduced some, but not all, aspects of stigma, confirming Corrigan's observation that contact may either reinforce or negate negative stereotypes, depending on the nature of the contact—for instance, a young person encountering an aggressive mentally ill person will have the stereotype that the mentally ill are by nature violent reinforced.

The results of a partial repeat of Jorm's survey (15) with a telephone sample of 3,021 Australian young people aged 15–25 years, but adding items about attitudes to post-traumatic stress disorder (PTSD), were consistent with the earlier study; it was found that perceptions of dangerousness and unpredictability and a desire for greater social distance were generally higher for psychosis/schizophrenia, while social phobia was considered a sign of personal weakness. Respondents rated perceived stigma much higher than personal stigma—possibly through a social desirability bias, where respondents were more willing to attribute negative evaluations to others than to themselves, or perhaps because individuals overestimated the level of discrimination in others. A further Australian survey of 1,375 students aged 12–17 years also identified higher levels of perceived versus personal stigma, as well as reinforcing earlier findings that male sex, younger age, and lack of personal and family experience were associated with increased personal stigma (16).

PUBLIC ATTITUDES TO ECT

Once Conrad and his parents have approached professionals for help and it has become clear that he is suicidally depressed, is not responding to other forms of treatment, and his doctor recommends ECT, how are Conrad and his parents likely to react? Reviewing the literature on public attitudes regarding ECT may give us some idea. Given that public and professional views of ECT have received widespread coverage over many years in the lay media, it is intriguing that this has been the subject of so little empirical investigation. Table 3.1 summarizes the rather meager number of publications in peer reviewed journals. All employ unique methodologies and questionnaires. With two exceptions (17, 18), sample numbers are generally small, and sampling bias is a problem in all but one study (18). Half compare lay to professional attitudes. Unsurprisingly, findings are quite inconsistent and difficult to generalize, other than to note that attitudes to the treatment are overwhelmingly negative in all but one (19). A number ask about exposure to different sources of information about ECT, for example personal experience and media/film, but other than noting the association, none examines causation.

Kalayam and Steinhart (19) compared the views of 224 people from three lay groups to those of patients who had received ECT and the views of a range of mental health professionals (the latter described in more detail below). The study provides little detail of the public opinions, other than to note that the public agreed that ECT was appropriate in specific conditions, was associated with clinical improvement, and was not likely to cause memory loss, although public views were, together with those of psychologists, closest to being undecided. The public were more fearful of the treatment than patients, but significantly less fearful than psychologists. The authors wondered what the fuss regarding negative public attitudes was all about. Kerr et al. (20), in their survey of general hospital visitors to patients not treated with ECT, found much less positive views, with these visitors significantly more likely to have negative general attitudes to the treatment than visitors to patients treated with ECT, who in turn had more negative attitudes than patients—62.5% dreaded or feared the treatment compared to ECT visitors (38.7%) and patients

Table 3.1. STUDIES OF PUBLIC ATTITUDES TO ECT

Study	Year	Country	Sample (RR)	Sample Characteristics	Comparison Groups
Kalayam and Steinhart (19)	1981	US	224 (56.3%)	3 Convenience samples • Randomly telephoned • Visitors to surgical ward • Hospital employees	• Patients • Mental health professionals
Kerr et al. (20)	1982	Australia	62	Convenience sample Hospital visitors to patients not receiving ECT	• ECT patients • Visitors to ECT patients
O'Shea and McGennis (21)	1983	Eire	100 (100%)	Convenience sample Dublin industrial facility employees	—
Jorm et al. (22)	1997	Australia	2031 (85%)	Random sample Adults 18–74 in private dwellings	—
Lauber et al. (18)	2005	Switzerland	1737 (63%)	Random sample Swiss residents aged 16–76	—
Teh et al. (17)	2007	Australia	381 (63%)	Convenience sample Students <19 yrs (31%) Adults 19–64 yrs (35%) Adults >64 yrs (34%)	—
McFarquhar and Thompson (23)	2008	UK	70 (86.4%)	Convenience sample Non-health employees	• Medical students • MRCPsych students

RR = response rate

(18.4%). Both visitor groups were more likely to have misconceptions regarding the treatment—for example, the beliefs that patients were zombies after ECT (44.6% general visitors, 58.1% ECT-patient visitors, 26.7% patients) and that ECT is given to patients who "don't behave" (42.9%, 24.2%, 22%, respectively), although visitors to ECT patients held fewer erroneous beliefs. O'Shea and McGennis (21) surveyed 100 workers in a Dublin factory and found that 24% would refuse the treatment for themselves outright, 47% would advise against a relative consenting to ECT in the face of a medical recommendation (the same percentage giving the opposite advice), and 60% would refuse to give consent for a sick and incapable relative. Only 6% were aware that the treatment involved a general anesthetic and muscle relaxants. None had received ECT themselves, but 13% had relatives who had received the treatment, and of these respondents, 69% considered that their relative had benefited. Sixty-one percent had seen the 1975 film *One Flew Over the Cuckoo's Nest* (24) and, of these, 65% said they had been "put off" ECT by the film.

Jorm et al. (22) reported on the first random sample of public views regarding ECT, in a telephone survey of a representative national sample of private householders in urban and rural Australia. Subjects were given a vignette of a person experiencing either schizophrenia or depression, were asked of their knowledge regarding the conditions, and what treatments would be harmful and helpful. Thirty-nine percent correctly identified the depression vignette, and 27% the schizophrenia vignette, although around three-quarters correctly identified some form of mental distress. Respondents tended to favor alternative rather than traditional treatments—for example, vitamins and special diets were rated more helpful than antidepressants and antipsychotics. ECT was rated as most harmful in both scenarios, more so in depression (72%) than schizophrenia (66%).

The first survey to focus specifically on ECT was the Swiss telephone survey by Lauber et al. (18), and therefore its report of the overwhelmingly negative public views of ECT might cause some alarm. A sample of 1,737 adults aged 17–37 were presented with two clinical scenarios depicting persons with schizophrenia or depression, and were given 18 possible treatment options; the survey also inquired about general attitudes to mental illness and treatment. Of the 18 treatment options offered, ECT was the least accepted—it is worth noting that alternative treatments included "taking fresh air and relaxing," "taking vitamins," and "seeing a naturopath"; 56.9% of the sample considered ECT as harmful, and only 1.2% considered it a helpful treatment. Increasing age was significantly correlated with reduced perception of harm. Notably, contact with a mentally ill person was significantly correlated with increased perception of harm, contradicting earlier findings (20, 21).

Teh et al. (17) conducted a survey in three distinct age groups—high school students, adults attending health and social centers, and older adults in community groups and centers and retirement villages. These researchers assessed knowledge of ECT technique and indications, the sources of knowledge, and attitudes to the treatment. Between one-quarter and one-half did not know the correct answers to the knowledge questions. Of the 85% who had heard of ECT, respondents cited television (45.6%), movies (42%), books (24.5%), and newspapers (24.5%) as sources of information. Less than 10% cited family experience, and less than 3% personal experience. Subjects were given a series of clinical scenarios involving different diagnoses and ages, as well as being asked if they would accept the treatment themselves. Fifty to seventy-five percent were opposed across all scenarios, and a greater number opposed involuntary treatment. No significant relationship was found between knowledge and attitudes.

The study by Teh et al. (17) is the only one to address public views of ECT in young people, and indeed the weight placed on this topic, despite it being only a small part of the survey, suggests a particular desire on the part of the authors to influence the debate. It was noted that a greater number were strongly opposed to treatment for a 7-year-old in a scenario containing three alternative ages—the authors submit that their results, combined with uncertainty about the effects on ECT on the developing brain, indicate the need to reconsider the use of ECT in children and adolescents. In a finding that runs contrary to the authors' caution, adolescent respondents were more likely to support treatment for themselves, but this is dismissed as the result of teenage perceptions of invincibility—hence they "may not consider the risks involved with ECT appropriately"—or as teenage experimentation.

On a more modest scale, McFarquhar and Thompson (23) compared the knowledge and attitudes of 70 non-medical employees to those of medical students and psychiatric trainees. As might be expected, in most cases the public sample tended to be less knowledgeable and show less support, with psychiatric trainees at the opposite end of both spectrums and medical students somewhere in the middle. The general public sample were significantly less likely to seek ECT for severe depression than both students and trainees, and a significantly greater proportion indicated concern about brain damage, pain, and not knowing what can happen, as well as being more likely to be concerned about what other people would think. This may suggest that perceived stigma was more common in the general public, but encouragingly over 80% of the public did not consider it so. The public sample was significantly least likely to advise a family member to have the treatment. Seventy percent of the total sample reported having seen ECT portrayed in films. None of the participants made positive comments about the portrayals, and the public sample were much less likely to consider the portrayal "outdated/inaccurate."

While taking account of the limited quality and varied methodologies of studies of public opinion, knowledge generally appears to be inaccurate and attitudes highly negative. In the two random surveys comparing ECT to other treatments, ECT was judged the most harmful and the least helpful. Only one survey found more neutral or favorable responses, and its methodological shortcomings limit its generalizability. If we accept the proposition that the negative attitudes are often based on misconceptions or misinformation, and that such prejudicial opinions can lead to stigmatization and consequent negative outcomes, how might this adversely affect young persons for whom ECT is recommended? Let us return once again to Conrad and his parents, and assume that as members of the public their views may overlap with research findings—how are they likely to respond to the recommendation for ECT?

At this point, it is worth considering the concept of family stigma associated with mental illness, which contains stereotypes of shame, blame, and contamination. In a review of the limited research on the subject, Larson and Corrigan

(25) noted that 25–50% of family members believe that they should hide their relationship with a family member with mental illness to avoid bringing shame to the family, 20–33% reported that a family member with mental illness caused strain or distance in relationships with extended family or friends, and 20–30% reported low self-esteem because they have a relative with mental illness. The consequences of such perceived stigma are illustrated in a US study involving 156 spouses or parents of patients with psychosis having their first psychiatric admission (26). While it was encouraging that 85% of family members reported experiencing no avoidance by family or friends, almost 40% acknowledged telling no one or limiting communication with family or friends. Contrary to the authors' expectations, concealment was less frequent in patients with more severe illness and those living with their relatives. A later US study of adult attitudes to treatment of mental illness in children goes some way to explaining family efforts to conceal. In-person surveys of 1,062 adults were conducted as part of the General Social Survey, and four questions were related to perceived stigma. Forty-five percent agreed or strongly agreed that getting mental health treatment would make the child an outsider at school, 41% felt that a child would suffer as an adult when others learned he or she had received mental health treatment, 57% did not trust that confidentiality would be respected, and 36% considered that getting mental health treatment would make the parent feel like a failure. While the authors acknowledged that the study did not indicate that respondents were more likely to discriminate against children with mental illness, it posited that perceptions of stigma alone may be enough to delay parents or caregivers in recognizing mental health problems and seeking treatment for their children (27).

MENTAL HEALTH PROFESSIONALS AND ECT

Having received a treatment recommendation for ECT, what views are the Jarretts likely to receive from the professionals involved in Conrad's care? This section will examine first the views of mental health professionals in general toward ECT, then child and adolescent professionals, further exploring the proposed relationship between knowledge and attitudes.

Research on mental health professionals over the last 30 years has been more consistent in methodology than that of research on the general public, and it may be taken as a sign of concern that views within different professional groups remain remarkably consistent and fixed (see Table 3.2). All studies are cross-sectional and all but one compare different professions. As noted above, Kalayam et al. (19) compared the views of a number of professional groups to those of patients and members of the public. Although their paper provides few details, it notes that all professionals agreed that ECT is appropriate, safe, and effective, but psychologists, along with the public, were closest

Table 3.2. MENTAL HEALTH PROFESSIONALS' ATTITUDES TO ECT

Study	Year	Country	Sample (RR)	Sample Characteristics	Key findings
Kalayam et al. (19)	1981	US	300	76 psychiatric residents 85 psychiatric nurses 67 psychologists 72 social workers	All professionals endorsed positive views Psychologists closest to undecided and most fearful
Janicak et al. (28)	1985	US	195	60 physicians 39 nurses 39 psychologists 40 social workers	⇑ positive attitudes correlated with ⇑ knowledge and experience
Gass (29)	1998	UK	167 (48%)	Mental health nurses	⇑ knowledge associated with more positive views
Lutchman et al. (30)	2001	UK	198 (74%)	114 (74% RR) psychiatrists 37 (69%) psychologists 52(75%) nurses 25(85%) social workers	Psychiatrist most and psychologist least accurate knowledge and positive views
Byrne et al. (31)	2006	Ireland	593 (100%)	383 med students and doctors 210 nurses	Direct association better knowledge and positive attitudes in doctors, not nurses

RR = response rate

to being undecided. Psychiatrists most strongly agreed with the statements. Patients anticipated less fear from the treatment than psychiatrists, while psychologists and social workers expressed the most, with psychologists significantly more fearful than the public. Psychologists most strongly disagreed that ECT is like minor surgery. Janicak et al. (28) found that knowledge was significantly associated with clinical experience for professionals as a whole, and while not significant in any of the individual professions, there was a trend toward significance in doctors, nurses, and social workers, but not in psychologists. Acceptance was assessed by inquiring whether the professionals would themselves undergo ECT if depressed—among respondents as a whole, those who would allow themselves to undergo ECT if very or extremely depressed had significantly higher mean knowledge scores than those who would not.

The study by Gass (29) is the only one not to compare different professional groups, concentrating on a sample of mental health nurses in Wales, and using the research instruments designed by Janicak et al. (28). It was found that positive attitudes were significantly correlated with place of work and exposure to patients receiving the treatment (29). Knowledge was associated with length of experience and place of work. Replicating the findings of Janicak et al. (28), knowledge scores were positively correlated with more positive attitudes. Lutchman et al. (30) posted surveys to psychiatrists, nurses, social workers, and psychologists in North London, achieving satisfactory response rates across all groups, and using a new questionnaire, ominously titled QuAKE ("Questionnaire on the attitudes and knowledge of ECT") which proved to have good psychometric properties. Although the results were not seismic, neither were they particularly reassuring. In the attitude questions, the authors note that a consistent pattern emerges in which the disciplines are ranked in order of agreement with "positive" and disagreement with "negative" statements, as follows: psychiatrists, nurses, social workers, and psychologists. Differences between professions were highly significant (p values <0.0001) for all but one statement. Psychologists showed significant differences from the other three groups on several attitudes: fewer than 15% believed that ECT would more likely benefit than harm a patient or be unlikely to cause brain damage, and 51% considered that ECT was a cruel treatment, with the same percentage stating there was no real evidence that it works. Overall, 12% of all professionals thought that ECT should be banned, with psychologists (27%) contributing most to this figure, and psychiatrists (2%) the least. In knowledge questions, the same ranking applied—nurses being closest to psychiatrists in most correct answers, and social workers scoring more correct responses than psychologists in all but one item.

Byrne et al. (31) confirmed the association between better knowledge and more positive views in a sample of Irish medics, but not in the comparison group of nurses and nursing students. Nurses had lower levels of knowledge and more negative attitudes to ECT—they were eight times more likely to see ECT as a last resort and nine times more likely to underestimate its efficacy. While the authors considered that endorsement of "last resort" was the incorrect answer, it is worth noting that this accords with the UK National Institute for Clinical Excellence (NICE) (32) recommendations as discussed below.

Research on child and adolescent professionals provides a different picture, with all professionals demonstrating lower levels of knowledge about the treatment and more equivocal attitudes regarding its use in younger persons (see Table 3.3). Only one of the papers (35) compares views between different professional groups. Parmar (33) sent questionnaires to all child and adolescent psychiatrists in 5 UK regions in northern England and Scotland. She first tested the acceptance of the concept of depression in this population, finding that 85% of the sample considered the concept useful in adolescents, and 60% useful in children. She gave three diagnoses across three different age groups, under 12 years, 12–17 years, and over 17 years, and sought views on which treatments would be unhelpful. For example, in psychotic depression, the only scenario reaching statistical significance, respondents felt that ECT would be unhelpful in 42%, 19%, and 5% of the respective age groups. This

Table 3.3. CHILD AND ADOLESCENT MENTAL HEALTH PROFESSIONALS' ATTITUDES TO ECT

Study	Year	Country	Sample (RR)	Sample Characteristics
Parmar (33)	1993	UK	99 (79%)	Child and adolescent psychiatrists in 5 northern UK regions
Walter et al. (34)	1997	Australia and NZ	206 (83%)	All members child and adolescent faculty RANZCP
Ghaziuddin et al. (35)	2001	US	635 (39%)	417 (38% RR) psychiatrists 177 (35%) psychologists
Walter and Rey (36)	2003	Australia and NZ	129 (54%)	As with Walter et al. 1997

RR = response rate

did not reflect a bias against physical treatments in general, as in the same scenario only 0–1% did not support the use of medication. Of the 79% who had never used ECT in younger persons, the main reasons given were lack of evidence in this age group (22%) and the belief that other treatments would be effective (18%).

In the mid-1990s, Walter et al. (34) mailed a survey to all members of the child and adolescent faculty of the Royal Australian and New Zealand College of Psychiatrists, achieving an impressive response rate (83%). Forty percent rated their knowledge of ECT in younger persons as nil or negligible, with only 7% considering their knowledge more advanced or sophisticated. Only 21% had experience of ECT in patients under 19 years. Having had patients treated with ECT was the strongest predictor of possessing some knowledge. The fact that around 90% perceived ECT as an effective treatment in adult depressive disorders excludes the possibility of a more pervasive anti-biological bias. Thirty-nine percent considered ECT unsafe in children, compared to 17% for adolescents and 3% for adults. Seventy-one percent disapproved of the use of ECT in children, compared with 32% in adolescents and 3% in adults. Nearly three-quarters considered that ECT should only be given as a last resort. Walter and Rey (36) repeated the same survey with the same group four years later, achieving a lower response rate (54%), placing some doubt on the interpretation of changes in views since the first survey. There was a significant increase in the report of prescribing medication. A similarly low percentage had experience of ECT in younger persons (28% vs. 21% four years previously). Psychiatrists were significantly less likely to rate their knowledge as "nil or negligible" and more likely to have "some" or "more advanced" knowledge. Despite this, there was no significant change in the proportion comfortable to provide a second opinion. Twenty-eight percent considered ECT unsafe in children (39% in earlier survey), 10% (17%) in adolescents, and still 3% in adults. A significantly greater number (76% vs. 63%) were likely to support the use of ECT in adolescents. The authors suggest that their findings indicate that psychiatrists' views are amenable to change.

Ghaziuddin et al. (35) surveyed a random selection of American child and adolescent psychiatrists and psychologists—a significantly lower percentage of psychologists worked exclusively in child and adolescent practice (8% vs. 31%). The response rate of 39% meant that it was not possible to exclude sampling bias. Over half the respondents stated that they had "minimal knowledge" of ECT in younger persons, while only 16% knew a patient who had received the treatment. Those with some or advanced knowledge were significantly more likely to approve of its use in children and adolescents. Psychologists were significantly more likely than psychiatrists to state that they had little knowledge of ECT, and were less likely to support its use and safety. A majority of respondents considered ECT as a treatment of last resort, with no significant difference between the professions.

So what conclusions can we draw from these surveys? It might provide some comfort that a consistent finding is the relationship between increasing knowledge and positive views toward ECT, but what is of concern is that there seems to have been little if any shift in the levels of knowledge and attitudes between various professions over the last 30 years. A consistent finding of surveys of adult clinicians was a steep gradient in knowledge and support, with psychiatrists at the top and psychologists at the bottom, and Ghaziuddin's survey of child and adolescent clinicians supports this. While the lack of clinical exposure of other mental health professionals to ECT in their training might explain some of this difference, it is unlikely to be a sufficient explanation. One might conclude that views regarding ECT that psychiatrists might consider stigmatizing (such as "ECT is a cruel treatment" and "in this day and age ECT should be banned" (30, p. 144)) are endorsed almost as articles of faith by their professional colleagues. This impression is reinforced in the biographical accounts of two psychologists who themselves received ECT for depression (1). The Canadian psychologist Norman Endler wrote in *Holiday of Darkness* (37) of his treatment for two depressive episodes of bipolar disorder with ECT. After worsening and paralyzing melancholia and failed pharmacological attempts at treatment, his psychiatrist recommends ECT. Endler explains his initial aversion to the treatment as a combination of a traumatic observation of unmodified ECT as a student, and a professional bias against what he considered a poorly targeted and ill-understood treatment. Just prior to his first treatment, a psychologist colleague tries to talk Endler out of accepting the treatment: "He wanted to know why I was willing to 'get half my brains burned out'" (p. 73). Despite experiencing side effects, Endler accepts a second course and strongly endorses the treatment as safe, humane, and effective. In *Undercurrents, A Life Beneath the Surface*, another clinical psychologist, Martha Manning (38), describes her treatment with ECT and her struggles with personal and public stigma as a result. Like Endler, she battles to overcome her professional bias against accepting the treatment, and after a successful course of ECT, she experiences stigmatizing responses from friends to whom she reveals the treatment, such as, "How could you let them do that to you?" (p. 165). Her clinical response to ECT leads her to support its use, "... lately I've been thinking, 'Damn it, I didn't rob a bank. I didn't kill anybody. I have nothing to be ashamed of'" (p. 165). "In choosing the hospital and ECT, I chose to fight for my life" (p. 186).

Professionals who find themselves side by side in the battle against the stigma of mental illness would appear to hold widely divergent views regarding one of the most stigmatizing of psychiatric topics. With the clinical reality that all members of the modern multidisciplinary team are likely to influence patient and parent choices regarding treatment, this remains a major and important challenge in addressing the stigma surrounding ECT.

ADULT PATIENT ATTITUDES TO ECT

Having received a course of ECT treatment, how are Conrad and his parents likely to view the treatment? Before looking at the small number of studies of adolescent recipients of ECT, it is worth exploring the much more substantial literature regarding adult patient attitudes. In 2003, Rose et al. (39) published a systematic review of patient attitudes to ECT that covered most, but not all, published studies on the subject to that point. This survey is noteworthy for a number of reasons and therefore worth dwelling on. First, it was funded by the UK Department of Health to inform NICE guidelines on ECT (32) that were then under development. While reviewing peer-reviewed articles on the subject, it also incorporated seven independently published or unpublished surveys completed by or with the assistance of patients, and then applied an idiosyncratic weighting to methodological variables, such as interval between treatment and interview, number of questions, venue of interview, and nature of interviewer. The review explicitly excluded articles concerning children and adolescents for reasons that are not explained. The ultimate effect of these editorial decisions is to undercut the academic research up to that point in time, introducing a degree of relativism and concluding that "the levels of perceived benefit differed between patient led and clinician led studies because different methods were used and because in many cases these methods did not allow an adequate description of the complexity of the subjective experience" (39, p. 4). The review sought to identify positive responses to treatment based on the response to the statements "ECT is helpful" or "I would have ECT again," and found a wide discrepancy between peer-reviewed articles and patient-contributed (non-peer-reviewed) studies: "helpful" 70–85% in the former and 30–40% in the latter, and "would have again" 60–98% in the former and 18–41% in the latter. The study also noted that one-third of patients reported memory loss, and it criticized the methodology of clinical research for focusing on anterograde amnesia, when patient concerns tended to focus on gaps in biographical memory. This review had a significant influence on the NICE committee (which did not include any psychiatrists) and, as a result, the guidelines published in 2003 recommended restrictions on the use of ECT to depressive illness when other treatments had failed (40).

A number of studies are not included in Rose et al.'s review for reasons that are not entirely clear. For example, Malcolm (41) questioned 100/102 consecutive patients prior to and after their course of ECT in northern England, exploring attitudes and finding that 60% expressed fear of ECT prior to and 55% post-treatment. Sestoft et al. (42) mailed surveys to all patients from six psychiatric departments in Denmark who had been admitted over a two-year period with a diagnosis of depression; 359 (54.9% response rate) returned completed questionnaires, of whom 113 had been treated with ECT and 246 without ECT. There were no statistical differences in levels of satisfaction, with 75.2% of ECT and 68.3% of non-ECT patients believing the treatment effective, and 52.2% of ECT and 50% of non-ECT indicating they would recommend the same treatment to someone in the same situation as them. When asked their preferred treatment option in a future episode, 29.2% of ECT patients indicated ECT compared to only 3.7% of the non-ECT sample. The authors suggest that ECT is a commonly used treatment in Denmark, where it has not attracted the same degree of controversy as elsewhere.

Since Rose's review, there have been a small number of new studies, brief details of which appear in Table 3.4, which describes the key findings.

ADOLESCENT PATIENT ATTITUDES TO ECT

In contrast to the relative abundance of adult patient surveys, there have been only four surveys of the experience and attitudes of adolescent ECT recipients and/or their parents (see Table 3.5). All have small sample sizes and were conducted some time after ECT was given.

Walter et al. (47) found generally positive views among 36 individuals who were on average 17 years old at the time of ECT treatment. Sixty-nine percent believed ECT to be a treatment for depression and none thought it a punishment. Fifty percent thought ECT had been helpful and 27% detected no change, while 12% thought it made things worse. Sixty-nine percent would have the treatment again. Forty-two percent felt they had received adequate information and 88% considered it a legitimate treatment, but 23% considered it cruel. Fifty-eight percent remembered being a little or very fearful prior to treatment and 50% during treatment. When asked what was worst, 73% felt it was the illness and 8% the ECT. The parents of the same sample (48) also expressed positive views. Twenty-one out of 28 believed they had

Table 3.4. RECENT STUDIES OF PATIENT ATTITUDES TO ECT

Study	Year	Country	Sample Size (RR)	Study details	Key Findings
Brodaty et al. (43)	2003	Australia	81	Consecutive ECT inpatients Dementia/psychosis excluded Mean age 67.2 years Interviewed pre- and post-ECT HRSD and GAF pre and post	Pre- 39.7% & 68.8% post believed ECT would/had improve/d condition Patients poor judges of outcome Greater improvement associated with more positive views
Arshad et al. (44)	2007	Pakistan	190	Convenience sample of in/ out-patients	140 (74%) aware of ECT, 25 (13%) had received ECT 37% ECT inhumane/ form of torture 86% ECT effective 62% believed serious side effects Authors noted continued use of unmodified ECT in Pakistan
Bustin et al. (45)	2008	Canada, UK, Argentina	75 (91%)	Methodological problems—small number, no sampling info, varied info gathering 30 England, 30 Argentina, 15 Canada Outpatients who had NOT received ECT	Small numbers limit interpretation of results overall and between groups 41% thought ECT unsafe 80% thought ECT for control or punishment >2/3 incorrect ECT knowledge Knowledge highest Canada and lowest Argentina
Chakrabarti et al. (46)	India	2010	—	Review of evidence from 16 studies in 6 developing countries + Japan Wide variation in samples & methodology	Relatives better informed, more positive views, more satisfied 35–76% fear of ECT High rates of perceived coercion Wide range of satisfaction

RR = response rate

Table 3.5. ATTITUDES AND ADOLESCENT ECT

Study	Year	Country	Sample Size	Methodology
Walter et al. (47)	1999a	Australia	26/45 (58% RR)	Telephone survey Subsample of all adolescents receiving ECT 1990–1998 in NSW, Australia Interview on average 3 years post-ECT
Taieb et al. (49)	2001	France	10 patients 18 parents	Semi-structured interview Interview average 4.5 years post-ECT
Walter et al. (48)	1999b	Australia	28/45 parents (62%)	Parents of above Walter et al. sample Telephone survey
Kalman et al. (50)	2008	Israel	13/32 patients (41%)	Face to face semi-structured interview—extension of Walter et al 1999a questionnaire All adolescents (<19 years) receiving ECT in university institution 1990–2003 Interview average 4.9 years post-ECT (vs. 8.5 years in patients not interviewed)

RR = response rate

received adequate information prior to the treatment, 17 out of 28 considered ECT had been helpful, while 9 felt it had been unhelpful and one believed it had made the situation worse. Only 2 out of 28 believed that ECT was used to control behavior and none considered it a punishment. Twenty-four would support ECT again on the advice of a doctor, while 22 would have the treatment themselves. Taieb et al. (49) interviewed in person an even smaller sample of 10 adolescents and 18 of their parents on average 4.5 years but as long as 9 years after ECT. Both groups found the treatment frightening, although this is not quantified. Sixty percent of adolescents and 83% of parents would accept the treatment again. Only one individual from each group considered they had full information. When asked whether they could have refused treatment, 89% of parents said yes, while 80% of adolescents were unsure. In Kalman's survey of 13 patients, 69% considered ECT an effective and legitimate treatment. This study chose to focus on consent procedures, and suggested a relationship between perceived efficiency of the treatment and the understanding of the adolescents that they could have refused treatment, but the small sample size, low response rate, and significant differences in diagnosis, age, and period since treatment of those interviewed versus those not interviewed limit the generalizability of its findings (50).

So what, in summary, do we learn from a review of attitudes to ECT? First, public attitudes are overwhelmingly negative, professional views are mixed, and patient views are most positive when measured by clinicians and less positive when measured by peers, but even then are substantially more positive than the attitudes of the general public. The limited information regarding attitudes of adolescent patients and their parents suggests generally positive attitudes in both groups, although the small sample sizes make it difficult to reach firm conclusions.

At every stage of Conrad Jarrett's pathway from adolescent depression through hospitalization and back into the community, he is likely to have faced stigma and discrimination. As an adolescent male, he is more likely to have judged the onset of his depressive symptoms as a sign of personal failure or weakness, and anticipating prejudicial responses from family and friends, he may have concealed his problems and delayed seeking help. If his peers perceived a change in his behavior, they may have ostracized or avoided him. After Conrad's attempted suicide, his parents might have feared shame and blame that their son was ill and may have kept the fact of his illness from family and friends. When Conrad's doctor suggested ECT, he and his parents' first response may have been horror, and if they sought advice from other professionals involved in his care, they may have received information of widely divergent accuracy and seemingly irreconcilable opinions, which may have delayed his receiving the treatment and may have prolonged his illness. Once he returned home, his disclosure that he had received ECT attracted public stigma.

TACKLING THE STIGMA SURROUNDING ECT

This final section will explore options for tackling the stigmatizing attitudes toward ECT that prevail within younger persons, the general public, and mental health professionals. The last 30 years have seen an exponential growth in efforts to tackle stigma surrounding mental illness, with advocacy groups, national and international professional associations, and governments launching numerous campaigns utilizing a variety of strategies (51, 52). These strategies broadly fall under three headings: protest, education, and contact (53). Protest as a tactic has been influenced by the experience of civil rights movements and efforts to address stigma against minority groups, but within mental health runs the risk of reinforcing rather than redressing stigmatizing attitudes. Educational campaigns that aim to "focus on replacing emotionally charged myths surrounding mental illness with facts that counter the myths" (p. 115) have been shown to have positive outcomes, but have yet to demonstrate sustained attitude change over time. In line with the observation, not admittedly universally endorsed in the surveys reviewed above, that people who have had contact with people with mental illness tend to hold less prejudicial attitudes, anti-stigma strategies that have incorporated elements of contact have demonstrated attitude change that is sustained over time and is associated with change in behavior (53).

Campaigns targeting younger persons have mainly focused on education and contact, both in the media and through school-based interventions. Mass media campaigns include the "Change Your Mind" campaign in the United States in 2000 that broadcast public service announcements on MTV channels with the aim of increasing adolescents' use of mental health services. These announcements attracted large audiences and a volume of traffic to its website (54). School-based education programs have produced short-term positive effects but have failed to demonstrate sustained effects. For example, a secondary school intervention in the United Kingdom drew upon education and contact components. While attitude scores were more positive at both one week and six months after the sessions, improvements in mental health literacy weakened at six-month follow-up. Higher baseline scores and a history of personal contact were associated independently with positive change (55). Programs directed toward at-risk younger persons may achieve superior outcomes and satisfaction, but at the expense of increased perceived stigma (56). As far as can be determined, ECT is not addressed directly in any such intervention—this might be explained by the infrequency of use in this population or the potential for perceived stigma of targeted campaigns in the face of prevailing community attitudes. However, returning to one of the central challenges in addressing stigma surrounding ECT, given the leadership of such campaigns from a broad range of health and social science disciplines, there is no guarantee that those responsible for such campaigns would see ECT as a subject fit for de-stigmatization.

Efforts so far to address stigma within the general public appear more reactive than proactive in nature. While prominent advocates for the treatment have used mass media to defend the treatment (9), this has often been in response to sensationalized and intuitively appealing media portrayals of the treatment. This highlights a central dilemma in attempting to address stigmatizing attitudes to ECT in the general public, that the venue for such efforts, the print and visual media, are themselves purveyors of many of the negative messages regarding the treatment. As noted above, the media and films remain major sources of information for many people regarding ECT (17, 57). A number of studies of media portrayals have confirmed the general impression that overall media coverage of ECT is negative. Euba et al. (58) examined all references to ECT in the British press between 2000 and 2007, and found that 11% of these were positive, 31.9% negative, and the remainder neutral. "Cruelty" and "tool of repression" were recurring themes. Hivon et al. (59) examined portrayals of a number of controversial treatments in Canadian newspapers and magazines between 2000 and 2006. These researchers particularly examined the sources that journalists used in preparing their reports, and how by striving to "provide readers with a balanced story, one in which extreme and often opposite points of view are given equal weight, without providing any hint as to how representative of the general community these viewpoints really are," readers can end up misinformed. In the example of ECT, they found that scientific experts were cited in 31% of reports, and lay experts in 26%. Of the lay expert opinions, only 11% were positive. They comment that groups which are politicized, such as anti-ECT groups, are, by virtue of being more visible to journalists, more likely to be called upon to provide "balance" and therefore ultimately do the opposite. A review of ECT accounts in American popular magazines between 1940 and 2005 demonstrates that ECT actually enjoyed a positive if sensationalized portrayal in the first 30 of those years, but that this shifted substantially during the 1970s, particularly following the disendorsement of Thomas Eagleton in the 1972 US presidential election, after which ECT was labeled as an archaic, barbaric tool of oppression: "Public discussions of the treatment became a battleground in which opponents and advocates expressed their beliefs about aggressive psychiatric treatment and about psychiatry's traditional power over patients" (9). The effect of the release in 1975 of the film *One Flew Over the Cuckoo's Nest* was clearly to provide those on one side of this battle with a powerful and endlessly reloading weapon (60); the 2012 whimsical movie *Moonrise Kingdom* served to add to the anti-ECT ammunition, and indeed drew attention to the treatment in the young (61). While the efforts of vocal advocates such as Max Fink and Harold Sackeim, among others, have provided a greater degree of balance in media coverage, with the emphasis on the refinements of ECT practice divorcing it from what is acknowledged as ill-targeted and excessive past practice, it has been left to such prominent voices to confront the weight of opposing information in the media without the resources and infrastructure afforded to the anti-stigma campaigns described above. ECT therefore remains marginalized at best, and demonized at worst, within the press and popular media.

However, a relatively recent development is the emergence of public figures acknowledging their treatment with ECT and using their celebrity status and their visibility within mass media to advocate for ECT. While works written by ECT recipients such as Norman Endler, Martha Manning, and Laura Kivler have promoted positive messages, their readership and therefore the reach of their message have remained relatively limited. The advocacy of figures such as Kitty Dukakis and Carrie Fisher has reached considerably further. Dukakis (62) has appeared in the media repeatedly and has co-authored an account of her successful treatment with ECT (*Shock: The Healing Power of Electroconvulsive Therapy*). While reporting persistent lacunae in her memory, she strongly endorses the treatment as lifesaving and humane. More recently, Carrie Fisher has applied her wit and verbal flair to her account of successful maintenance ECT for depression, *Shockaholic* (63). Having acquired her opinions of ECT from her voracious movie-viewing, she shares many of the fears and misconceptions about the treatment, yet ultimately endorses ECT: "Your whole life you hear about this terrifying treatment that turns you into a vegetable, only to finally find out that it had all the charming qualities of no big deal. Sort of like getting your nails done, if you nails were in your cerebral cortex." (p. 20) It remains to be seen, but it may be that the powerful endorsement of celebrities will shift public opinion in ways that earnest advocacy has failed to accomplish over the last 30 years.

Finally, it is worth briefly considering what can be done to rebalance the steep gradient in knowledge and attitudes within the health professions. The only evidence with any relevance involves the training regarding ECT of medical students, which demonstrates that students enter their psychiatric term with many of the same misconceptions of the general public regarding ECT, as well as indicating many of the same influences such as movies and TV (57, 64–66), and that didactic teaching and/or witnessing of ECT can have a substantial effect on knowledge and attitudes (65, 67, 68). Although it is by no means the case that medicine has its house in order with regard to the stigma of mental illness (69, 70)—the term "iatrogenic stigma" has even been coined to denote the potentially stigmatizing effects of some elements of psychiatric practice (71)—evidence as described above would suggest that medicine is the profession least in need of attention with regard to ECT. This evidence suggests the importance of advocating for more balanced ECT information within social work, nursing, and psychology training, admittedly a suggestion that is unlikely to meet with a warm embrace. Contrasting psychiatry and psychology, attitudinal evidence suggests that the two disciplines continue to invoke parallel narratives of a safe, advanced, and effective remedy on the one hand, and a crude and brutalizing anachronism on the other. This raises the prospect that some of the most ardent campaigners against the stigma of mental illness themselves hold views toward ECT that could be interpreted as stigmatizing. When it comes to discussion of ECT in young people, opposing positions become even more stubbornly reinforced.

One of the successes of the campaigns addressing stigma has been the joining of forces in common purpose of professional organizations with individuals and families who have lived experience of mental illness and the detrimental effects of the stigma it attracts. The same sadly cannot be said of efforts thus far to address stigmatizing attitudes around ECT in general and ECT in young people, yet hope should never be abandoned. Measures that will not go astray include renewed efforts to educate the full range of stakeholders about the treatment; working with the various media to promote more authentic portrayals and reports of ECT (in the process, seeking every opportunity to be proactive rather than reactive); ongoing advocacy by prominent ECT recipients (one day, perhaps even a person of renown who benefited from ECT in their youth); relentless research of the mechanisms underpinning the illnesses requiring ECT for a young person and of the mode of action, effectiveness, and side effects of the treatment; and further refinements in ECT technique and administration to make it as slick and scientific as possible. Such efforts cannot harm.

CONCLUSION

A young person receiving ECT is liable to experience stigma on the basis of his or her age, illness, and treatment. Negative attitudes toward ECT contribute to this stigma, which may result in a range of negative consequences such as concealment of illness, delays in accessing professional care, and social exclusion. Misconceptions regarding ECT are associated with negative attitudes toward it, and when people who hold these misconceptions are provided with accurate information or come into contact with individuals who have received the treatment, they view the treatment in a more positive light. Despite the established link between knowledge and attitudes, and the generally positive regard of those who are treated with ECT, views in the general community and among mental health professionals have changed little over the last 30 years. This suggests that efforts to this point to demonstrate the safety and effectiveness of ECT, and remove some of the "baggage" attached to it during the antipsychiatry movement, have had little effect. Campaigns that have targeted mental illness in younger persons have mostly bypassed the subject of ECT, which may reflect the relative rarity of its use, the even greater ambivalence to its use among health professionals, and greater negativity within the general public. It is timely to "regroup" and adopt a multifaceted approach in an effort to change this bleak picture.

QUESTIONS AND ANSWERS

1. *What is the origin of the word "stigma" and when was it first applied in relation to the field of psychiatry?*

   Derived from the Greek *stigmata*, the term was applied in the 1960s by Irving Goffman to denote a mark that defined an individual or group, including those with mental illness, as discredited. There is growing recognition that the stigma encountered by persons with mental illness may be exacerbated by certain forms of treatment, such as ECT.

2. *Which two of the following sources of information about stigma pertaining to ECT have found largely negative attitudes or depictions? Movie depictions, community surveys, psychiatrist surveys, patient surveys, and recent biographical accounts.*

   Movie depictions and community surveys.

3. *What strategies may be employed in an effort to improve the stigma associated with ECT in young people?*

   (a) Educating the full range of stakeholders about the treatment; (b) working with the various media to promote more authentic portrayals and reports of ECT; (c) ongoing advocacy by prominent ECT recipients; (d) further research of the mechanisms underpinning the illnesses requiring ECT for a young person and of the mode of action, effectiveness, and side effects of the treatment; and (e) further refinements in ECT technique and administration.

DISCLOSURES

Dr. Andrew McDonald has no conflicts of interest to declare.

Prof. Garry Walter has received research support from Lundbeck and AstraZeneca for a study titled "Psychiatric Evaluation in Primary Care."

REFERENCES

1. McDonald A, Walter G. The portrayal of ECT in American movies. *J ECT.* 2001 Dec;17:264–74.
2. Payne NA, Prudic J. Electroconvulsive Therapy: Part II. A biopsychosocial perspective. *J Psychiatr Pract.* 2009;15:369–90.
3. Mehta N, Thornicraft G. Stigmatisation of people with mental illness and of psychiatric institutions. *Ethics in Psychiatry.* 2010;45:11–32.
4. Abbey S, Charbonneua M, Tranulis C, Moss P, Baici W, Dabby L, et al. Position paper: stigma and discrimination. *Can J Psychiat.* 2011;56.
5. Goffman E. *Stigma: Notes on the Management of Spoiled Identity.* New York: Simon & Schuster; 1963.
6. Hinshaw SP. *The Mark of Shame: Stigma of Mental Illness and an Agenda for Change.* New York: Oxford University Press; 2007.
7. Fink M. Prejudice against ECT: competition with psychological philosophies as a contribution to its stigma. *Convulsive Therapy* 1997;13:253–65.
8. Wilkinson D, Daoud J. The stigma and the enigma of ECT. *Int J Geriatr Psych.* 1998;13:833–35.
9. Hirshbein L, Sarvananda S. History, power, and electricity: American popular magazine accounts of electroconvulsive therapy, 1940-2005. *J Hist Behav Sci.* 2008;44:1–18.
10. Redford R. *Ordinary People*; 1981. Paramount Pictures.
11. Wahl O, Wood A, Zaveri P, Drapalski A, Mann B. Mental illness depiction in children's films. *J Commun Psychol.* 2003;31:553–60.
12. Corrigan PW, Demming LB, Goldman HH, Slopen N, Medasani K, Phelan S. How adolescents perceive the stigma of mental illness and alcohol abuse. *Psychiat Serv.* 2005;56:544–50.
13. Watson AC, Miller FE, Lyons JS. Adolescent attitudes towards serious mental illness. *J Nerv Ment Dis.* 2005;193:769–72.

14. Jorm AF, Wright A. Influences on young people's stigmatising attitudes towards peers with mental disorders: national survey of young Australian and their parents. *Brit JPsychiat.* 2008;192:144–9.
15. Reavley NJ, Jorm AF. Young people's stigmatizing attitudes towards people with mental disorders: findings from an Australian national survey. *Aust NZ J Psychiat.* 2011;45:1033–9.
16. Calear A, Griffiths KM, Christensent H. Personal and perceived depression stigma in Australian adolescents: magnitutde and predictors. *J Affect Disorders.* 2011;129:104–8.
17. Teh SPC, Helmes E, Drake DG. A Western Australian survey on public attitudes toward and knowledge of electroconvulsive therapy. *Int J Soc Psychiatr.* 2007;53:247–73.
18. Lauber C, Carlos N, Wulf R. Lay beliefs about treatments for people with mental illness and their implications for antistigma strategies. *Can J Psychiat.* 2005;50:745–52.
19. Kalayam B, Steinhart MJ. A survey of attitudes on the use of electroconvulsive therapy. *Hosp Commun Psychait.* 1981;32:185–8.
20. Kerr RA, McGrath JJ, O'Kearney RT, Price J. ECT: Misconceptions and attitudes. *Aust NZ J Psychiat.* 1982;46:43–9.
21. O'Shea B, McGennis A. ECT: Lay attitudes and experiences—a pilot study. *Irish Med J.* 1983;76:40–3.
22. Jorm AF, Korten AE, Jacomb PA, Christensen H, Rodgers B, Pollitt P. "Mental health literacy": a survey of the public's ability to recognise mental disorders and their beliefs about the effectiveness of treatment. *Med J Australia.* 1997;166:182.
23. McFarquhar T, Thompson J. Knowledge and attitudes regarding electroconvulsive therapy among medical students and the general public. *J ECT.* 2008;24:244–53.
24. Forman B. *One Flew Over the Cuckoo's Nest*; 1975.
25. Larson JE, Corrigan P. The stigma of families with mental illness. *Acad Psychiatr.* 2008;32:87–91.
26. Phelan JC, Bromet EJ, Link BG. Psychiatric illness and family stigma. *Schizophrenia Bull.* 1998;24:115–26.
27. Pescosolido BA, Perry BL, Martin JK, McLeod JD, Jensen PS. Stigmatizing attitudes and beliefs about treatment and psychiatric medications for children with mental illness. *Psychiat Serv.* 2007;58:613–8.
28. Janicak PG, Jason M, Trimakas KA, Gibbons R. ECT: An assessment of mental health professionals' knowledge and attitudes. *J Clin Psychiat.* 1985;46:262–6.
29. Gass JP. The knowledge and attitudes of mental health nurses to electroconvulsive therapy. *J Adv Nurs.* 1998;27:83–90.
30. Lutchman RD, Stevens T, Bashir A, Orrell M. Mental health professionals' attitudes towards and knowledge of electroconvulsive therapy. *J Ment Health.* 2001;10:141–50.
31. Byrne P, Cassidy B, Higgins P. Knowledge and attitudes toward electroconvulsive therapy among health care professionals and students. *J ECT.* 2006;22:133–8.
32. National Institute for Health and Clinical Excellence. TA59: Guidance on the use of electroconvulsive therapy. http://publications nice org uk/guidance-on-the-use-of-electroconvulsive-therapy-ta59 2003 (cited 2012 Sep 27)].
33. Parmar R. Attitudes of child psychiatrists to electroconvulsive therapy. *Psychiat Bull.* 1993;17:12–3.

34. Walter G, Rey JM, Starling J. Experience, knowledge and attitudes of child psychiatrists about ECT in the young. *Aust NZ J Psychiat.* 1997;31:676–81.
35. Ghaziuddin N, Kaza M, Ghazi N, King C, Walter G, Rey JM. Electroconvulsive therapy for minors: experiences and attitudes of child psychiatrists and psychologists. *J ECT.* 2001;17:109–17.
36. Walter G, Rey JM. How fixed are child psychiatrists' views about ECT in the young. *J ECT.* 2003;19:88–92.
37. Endler NS. *Holiday of Darkness: A Psychologist's Personal Journey out of His Depression* (rev. ed.). Toronto, ON, Canada: Wall & Thompson; 1990.
38. Manning M. *Undercurrents: A Life Beneath the Surface.* San Francisco: Harper; 1994.
39. Rose D, Fleischmann P, Leese M, Bindman J. Patients' perspectives on electroconvulsive therapy: systematic review. *Brit Med J.* 2003;326:1363.
40. Scott AIF. College guidelines on electroconvulsive therapy: an update for prescribers. *Adv Psychiatr Treat.* 2005;11:150–6.
41. Malcolm K. Patients' perceptions and knowledge of electroconvulsive therapy. *Psychiat Bull.* 1989;13:161–5.
42. Sestoft D, Pederson L, Bendsen BB, Hancke B, Larsen SAL, Mikkelsen S, et al. The effect of electroconvulsive therapy on patients' attitude to treatment of depression. *Nord J Psychiat.* 1998;52:31–7.
43. Brodaty H, Berle D, Hickie I, Mason C. Perceptions of outcome from electroconvulsive therapy by depressed patients and psychiatrists. *Aust NZ J Psychiat.* 2003;37:196–9.
44. Arshad M, Arham A, Arif M, Bano M, Bashir A, Bokutz M, et al. Awareness and perceptions of electroconvulsive therapy among psychiatric patients: a corss-sectional survey from teaching hospitals in Karachi, Pakistan. *BMC Psychiatry.* 2007;7:27.
45. Bustin J, Rapoport MJ, Krishna M, Matusevich D, Finkelsztein C, Strejilevich S, et al. Are patients' attitudes towards and knowledge of electroconvulsive therapy transcultural? A multi-national pilot study. *Int J Geriatr Psychiat.* 2008;23:497–503.
46. Chakrabarti S, Grover S, Rajagopal R. Perceptions and awareness of electroconvulsive therapy among patients and their families: a review of the research from developing countries. *J ECT.* 2010;26:317–22.
47. Walter G, Koster K, Rey J. Electroconvulsive therapy in adolescents: Experience, knowledge, and attitudes of recipients. *J Amer Acad Child & Adoles Psychiatry.* 1999;38:594–9.
48. Walter G, Koster K, Rey J. Views about treatment among parents of adolescents who received electroconvulsive therapy. *Psychiat Serv.* 1999;50:701–2.
49. Taieb O, Flament MF, Corcos M, Jeammet P, Basquin M, Mazet P, et al. Electroconvulsive therapy in adolescents with mood disorder: patients' and parents' attitudes. *Psychiat Res.* 2001;104:183–90.
50. Kalman N, Luria I, Ratzoni G, Lefkovitz Y, Braw Y, Linder M, et al. Electroconvulsive therapy in adolescents: patient attitudes, satisfaction and informed consent procedures. *Int J Child & Adoles Health.* 2008;1:199–205.
51. Walter G, Rose A. Psychiatric stigma and the role of the psychiatrist. *Australas Psychiatry.* 1997;5:72–4.
52. Rosen A, Walter G, Casey D, Hocking B. Combating psychiatric stigma: an overview of contemporary initiative. *Australas Psychiatry.* 2000;8:19–26.

53. Corrigan PW. Target-specific stigma change: a strategy for impacting mental illness stigma. *Psychiatr Rehabil J.* 2004;28:113–21.
54. SAMHSA (Substance Abuse and Mental Health Services Association). Change your mind about mental health. http://www promoteacceptance samhsa gov/ campaigns/Program_Details aspx?ID=15. 2000.
55. Pinfold V, Toulmin H, Thornicroft G, Husley P, Farmer P, Graham T. Reducing psychiatric stigma and discrimination: evaluation of educational interventions in UK secondary schools. *Brit J Psychiat.* 2003;182:342–6.
56. Rapee RM, Wignall A, Sheffield J, Kowalenko N, Davis A, McLoone J, et al. Adolescents' reactions to universal and indicated prevention programs for depression: perceived stigma and consumer satisfaction. *Prev Sci* 2006;7:167–77.
57. Walter G, McDonald A, Rey JM, Rosen A, Walter G, McDonald A, et al. Medical student knowledge and attitudes regarding ECT prior to and after viewing ECT scenes from movies. *J ECT.* 2002 Mar;18:43–6.
58. Euba R, Crugel M. The depiction of electroconvulsive therapy in the British press. *J ECT.* 2009;25:265–9.
59. Hivon M, Lehoux P, Denis JL, Rock M. Marginal voices in the media coverage of controversial health interventions: how do they contribute to the public understanding of science? *Public Underst Sci* 2010;19:34–51.
60. McDonald A, Walter G. Hollywood and ECT. *Int Rev Psychiatry.* 2009;21:200–6.
61. Anderson W. *Moonrise Kingdom*; 2012. Scott Rudin Productions.
62. Dukakis K, Tye L. *Shock: The Healing Power of Electroconvulsive Therapy.* New York: Penguin Books; 2006.
63. Fisher C. *Shockaholic.* New York: Simon and Schuster; 2011.
64. Andrade C, Kumar NSR. Medical students' attitudes toward electroconvulsive therapy: An Indian perspective. *J ECT* 1996;12:86–90.
65. Szuba MP, Guze BH, Liston EH, Baxter LR, Roy-Byrne P. Psychiatry resident and medical student perspectives on ECT: influence of exposure and education. *Convulsive Therapy* 1992;8:110–7.
66. Clothier J, Freeman T, Snow L. Medical student attitudes and knowledge about ECT. *J ECT* 2001;17:99–101.
67. Benbow SM. Medical students and electroconvulsive therapy: Their knowledge and attitudes. *Convulsive Therapy* 1990;6:32–7.
68. Kinnair D, Cawson S, Perera R. Electroconvulsive therapy: medical students' attitudes and knowledge. *Psychiatrist* 2010;34:54–7.
69. Summerfield D. Does psychiatry stigmatize? *J Royal Soc Med.* 2001;94:148–9.
70. Walter G. The attitudes of health professionals towards carers and individuals with mental illness. *Australas Psychiatry.* 1998;6:70–2.
71. Sartorius N. Iatrogenic stigma of mental illness. *Brit Med J.* 2002 Jun 22;324:1470–1.

CHAPTER 4

Ethical and Consent Aspects

MICHAEL ROBERTSON, JOSEPH M. REY, AND GARRY WALTER

KEY POINTS

- Values-based child and adolescent psychiatry requires the provision of ECT that is clinically indicated, of high quality, accessible, responsive to the needs of the patient and his or her family, and well integrated with other treatments and service components.
- Against a background of widespread antipathy toward the use of ECT in children and adolescents, child psychiatrists, particularly those in high-income Western countries, may face significant challenges in their moral deliberations over the use of ECT in this age group.
- Like any treatment decision in medicine, the use of ECT in a young person is subject to a risk-benefit analysis.
- Applying the method of "principles-based ethics," consent to ECT by children and adolescents often entails prima facie tension between the principle of respect for patient autonomy and the principles of beneficence ("doing good") and non-maleficence ("not harming").
- Relevant to children and adolescents are the notions that the capacity to make autonomous decisions about health evolves with the child's development, that parents and guardians are generally involved in the consent process, and that "assent" rather "informed consent" applies in the case of minors.
- Clinicians may enhance a young patient's and family's understanding of ECT prior to the treatment in several ways: face-to-face discussion; recommending video/DVD descriptions of ECT; showing the young person and family the ECT suite, ECT apparatus, and recovery area; having the young patient and family speak to previous teenage recipients and families about the treatment; and providing practical information in writing.
- Policy, procedures, and legislation about the use of ECT in young persons vary from country to country (and between jurisdictions in the same country) and are continuously changing; clinicians need to familiarize themselves with the laws and practices that apply to them.

OVERVIEW

In this chapter, we consider first the value system of child psychiatry as a basis for moral deliberation over the use of electroconvulsive therapy (ECT) in children and adolescents. We then describe, in turn, the context of the impassioned public debate over biological treatments in child psychiatry, risk-benefit considerations of ECT in children and adolescents, complexities in relation to consent for the treatment, processes of consent in different countries and different jurisdictions, core elements of the consent process irrespective of regional differences, and the ethical dilemmas surrounding *not* providing ECT to this patient group. Because ECT is an extremely rare procedure in children younger than 12 years, most of the information presented here refers to adolescents, that is, people aged 12–18 years.

INTRODUCTION

The notion of a child or teenager being administered ECT will be challenging—conceptually and ethically—for most laypersons. The Internet is replete with accounts of the "barbarity" of ECT from some of its "survivors" (1). The language used in such discourse is as emotive as it is hyperbolic, as one website indicates:

> Is there any limit to the depravity of the psychiatrists who use or promote the use of electroshock on children? If there is such a place as hell, surely its hottest places are reserved for those psychiatrists. (2)

Occupying much less space in readily accessible media are positive statements about ECT in young persons, such as the one below (by GW, the third author) in an Australian newspaper:

> It [ECT use in young people] is rare but . . . it can be lifesaving. (3)

Even within the psychiatric profession, there is dissension about the use of ECT in children and adolescents. For example, again in Australia, a prominent senior psychiatrist declared in the lay press, in response to reports of the increase use of ECT in children under age 12:

> I am shocked and amazed that children that young are being treated this way. (4)

The issue of stigma attending this area is examined in Chapter 3. Apart from the more extreme views about ECT, attitudes that ECT is restricted to a dramatic, end-stage treatment of last resort still prevail in both medical and community circles (5). Such opinions add to the challenges that child psychiatrists face when contemplating the ethical and consent aspects of ECT in young people. Consideration of the values of child and adolescent psychiatry will provide a useful starting point for psychiatrists' deliberations about this treatment and will help to crystallize their thinking.

THE "VALUES" OF CHILD AND ADOLESCENT PSYCHIATRY AND THEIR RELEVANCE FOR THE PROVISION OF ECT

"Ethics" essentially exists and acts according to a particular axiological (value) system. At the time of writing, there was no substantive statement from a global body, such as the World Psychiatric Association (WPA) or International Association for Child and Adolescent Psychiatry and Allied Professions (IACAPAP), regarding a values-based practice and "craft" of child and adolescent psychiatry. In lieu of such a document, one can look to the American Academy of Child and Adolescent Psychiatry (AACAP), which has formulated a system of values in relation to the characteristics of mental health services providing care for children and adolescents. According to the AACAP, these services should be (6):

- "child focused" and "family driven";
- culturally sensitive and integrated;
- timely, effective and evidence based; and
- integrated with other systems of care (e.g., the foster care system).

From this axiological standpoint, several fundamental elements have been articulated, including service coordination, early intervention and screening, planned and coordinated transitions between different parts of a service, advocacy and protection in keeping with human rights concerns, access to comprehensive services, individualized clinical care, community-based approaches to care, family involvement in all phases of clinical care, and integration of care across all services dealing with the needs of children. Within these identified elements are numerous annotations regarding more specific concerns, such as consent and representing the wishes of the child patient in treatment decisions.

In broad terms, the values of the child and adolescent psychiatric profession turn upon the provision of competent clinical services that are both sensitive to the needs of the child and family and occur against a background of those traditional ethical principles regulating medical practice: the expectation of helping (beneficence), doing no harm (non-maleficence), due attention to patient autonomy (allowing for differences in the younger age group—addressed later), and justice (7, 8). Applied to the administration of ECT, a values-based child and adolescent psychiatry requires the provision of ECT treatment and services that are clinically indicated (i.e., used for conditions for which they are effective), of high quality, accessible, responsive to the needs of the patient and his or her family, and well integrated with the other components of the child and adolescent mental health sector. The discussion that follows will approach the ethical dilemmas raised from this perspective.

THE CONTEXT OF PUBLIC DEBATE OVER BIOLOGICAL TREATMENTS IN CHILD PSYCHIATRY: AN UNFAVORABLE CLIMATE FOR ECT IN MANY JURISDICTIONS

In recent times, the seemingly "anti–child psychiatry" public discourse has focused upon the issue of psychotropic drug use in children and adolescents. The use of psychotropic drugs, particularly stimulants and antidepressants, in child and adolescent psychiatry patients has trebled from 1987 to 1996 (9). This has been especially worrisome in relation to children of preschool age (10). Matters are not helped by the fact that much of the prescribing has been off-label (11).

This area has been fertile ground for critics of psychiatry (see, e.g., 12), several of whom have called into question many of the widely accepted diagnostic categories, particularly attention deficit hyperactivity disorder (ADHD), or have queried the apparent high frequency of some diagnoses, for example early onset bipolar disorder. Opponents of the discipline have also emphasized the apparent Faustian pact between child psychiatrists and pharmaceutical companies, who have allegedly conspired to influence the evidence base supporting the use of psychotropics in children with certain disorders (13–15). Such rancor in the community often culminates in large-scale, albeit frequently unsuccessful, class litigation, exemplified by the infamous action launched in the United States against the American Psychiatric Association and a pharmaceutical company Novartis, which markets Ritalin (16).

In such an environment, any public or professional discourse over ECT in children and adolescents is likely to be emotive, rhetorical, and unbalanced. Weighing into the field of ECT in young patients, Breggin argued:

> The ECT lobby is much larger and stronger than the lobotomy lobby, and much better organized, with its own journal and shock advocates positioned in high places in medicine and psychiatry. To impede this medical steamroller called shock treatment will require public outrage, organized resistance from survivor groups and psychiatric reformers, lawsuits, and state legislation. (17)

It needs to be emphasized, however, that such antipathy is not universal. It is largely culture-bound and is voiced mostly in high-income Anglo-Saxon countries (18). Standards and practices in low-income countries are quite different. For example, in India more than half of those treated with ECT in teaching hospitals have unmodified ECT (ECT without anesthesia and muscle relaxants)—prohibited practice in developed nations, due to the complications of that method—and about 1.4% of all ECT recipients are younger than 18 years (19).

Against this background, child psychiatrists, particularly those in high-income Western countries, may face significant challenges in their moral deliberations over the use of ECT in children and adolescents. These changes and deliberations may overlap with those associated with other biological treatments, although use of medication, once frowned upon, is currently more acceptable and is much less tinged by negative connotations.

USE OF ECT IN ADOLESCENTS AND RISK-BENEFIT ANALYSIS

The general consensus is that ECT may be underutilized for adolescents (20). ECT is an effective and safe treatment (21) for serious psychiatric disorders, and recent years have seen the development of detailed practice guidelines for its use in young people by professional bodies in the mental health field (e.g., 22). Due to the rarity of administration, the evidence base for the effectiveness and safety of ECT in pre-adolescents is much less than that for teenagers (23). As in adults (24), the commonest indication for ECT in young people is severe mood disorder, although ECT may also be used for other conditions, for example, psychotic disturbance, catatonia, and selected types of self-injurious behaviors (SIB). In some countries, use is common in schizophrenia (19). Invariably, young patients who receive ECT are very unwell immediately before their first ECT treatment, and their autonomy and capacity to consent may thus be significantly impaired. This raises concerns about the distress caused by practices such as restraint, which may have been required as part of the overall management strategy prior to ECT, the difficulties of explaining the ECT procedure to adolescents, and the pressure to "act," given the urgency of a clinical situation such as catatonia or non-response to other treatments. In these circumstances, child psychiatrists tend to focus upon the relief of distress and the mitigation of immediate risk, having balanced these with the need for proper adherence to axioms such as appropriate consent and scrutiny of practice, careful monitoring of the state of the patient and his or her family, and, where possible, allowing the patient and his or her family as much agency as possible in the use of the treatment.

It follows that, as in any treatment decision in medicine, the administration of ECT to a young person is subject to a risk-benefit analysis. Though ECT is in general argued to be a safe and effective treatment, a primary concern is the harm that ECT may potentially cause to the developing brain, and this issue needs to be addressed in any examination of the ethical dilemmas. Some researchers (e.g., 25) have reported memory impairments observed in young patients who have undergone ECT. Breggin contends that there is evidence that ECT in children and adolescents leads to a loss of autobiographical memory, impaired new learning and reduced psychomotor speed, resulting in a decline in "overall mental function" (17). However, such claims are not supported by the scientific literature, which does not provide evidence of brain injury or impairment attributable to ECT in young people (23, 26), nor of long-term adverse cognitive effects in this age group (27–29). In adults, some persistent neuropsychological deficits after an ECT course have been demonstrated, and have been found to vary with technical aspects of the treatment (30).

CONSENT TO THE TREATMENT

The issue of consent to ECT occupies a large amount of literature in the adult ECT field. In one study, a third of surveyed adults believed that they did not give adequate consent to ECT (31). It has been argued that "true" informed consent to ECT is impossible, given the power differential that characterizes the dynamic of psychiatry, particularly with the prospect of involuntary treatment in some of these patients (32). The severity of illness that is usually associated with the use of ECT in all patient age groups heightens prevailing concerns about consent to treatment and in itself, as previously mentioned, further diminishes patient autonomy.

Autonomy is influenced by time and task. In relation to the former, the capacity for an 8-year-old child to consent to treatment is clearly different from that of an adolescent of 15 years. This is potentially even more fraught in situations where, for example, a child is growing up with a developmental or intellectual disability. Regardless, in the eyes of the law and according to the tenets of best practice, a patient who is legally a "minor" cannot consent to treatment; only a parent or guardian can consent. (We have referred here to "minors" instead of "children and adolescents" because in many countries people older than 16 years are able to consent to treatment themselves—the specific issue of consent and its legality need to be considered in this context.)

With most children, the child's capacity to make autonomous decisions about their health evolves with their cognitive and emotional development. Evolving or "future" autonomy (33) is significant to clinical decision-making (34). Indeed, some countries recognize "mature minors" (usually 14- to 16-year-olds) for the purposes of consent to treatment, although rarely is this extended to consent for ECT.

Much of the discourse over consent to treatment by children and adolescents draws upon the method of "principles-based ethics" (8, 35), in particular, the prima facie tension between the patient's autonomy and the principles of beneficence ("doing good") and non-maleficence ("not harming"). This is especially problematic in psychiatry, where there may be sustained or acute impairment of patient autonomy, and it becomes even more challenging in the setting of *developing* autonomy (36). Unlike a decision to participate in family psychotherapy, attend a school for children with special needs, or even commence psychotropic medication, many decisions around the use of ECT in young people tend to be made—for better or worse—in extreme circumstances. In such clinical situations, this further reduces the weighting given to the child's emerging autonomy.

It should be highlighted that autonomy is not a categorical entity, and thus unsurprisingly some of the general treatment literature in child and adolescent psychiatry has considered the viability of the construct of "informed consent" in childhood, in particular how decisions made by parents or guardians on behalf of the child or adolescent should reflect the wishes of the young person (37, 38). Relevant here is the notion of "assent" (agreement): a parent or legal guardian has the legal authority to "consent" for a minor, but it is normally desirable to (also) obtain the minor's "assent," even though that is not legally necessary. Wherever possible, in all branches of medicine, the preferences or concerns of a child or adolescent should be considered and integrated into clinical decision making. In many decisions around the use of ECT, however, the acuity and risk posed by extreme suicidality or psychosis, or the additional impairment arising from catatonic excitement, diminish the impact of the wishes of the child.

The above clinical scenarios and background considerations promote the role of the parent or guardian as proxy for autonomous choice for the child. Given analogous concerns about impaired autonomy in late life and childhood, the evidence that family participation in consent for ECT in elderly patients is "extremely valuable" (39) suggests that this approach may apply at least equally in the use of ECT in children and adolescents. In this setting, the role of the psychiatrist is one of juggling the complex relationship between a child's confidentiality, his or her capacity for consent, assent, and the role of advocate for the child's interests in light of the views of the parent or family (40). Of course, the therapeutic relationship in child psychiatry is unique in that it frequently casts the therapist in the role of de facto parent or authority figure (41), functioning as an additional proxy for autonomy.

PROCESSES OF CONSENT IN DIFFERENT COUNTRIES AND JURISDICTIONS

Policy, procedures, and legislation about the use of ECT in young persons vary considerably from country to country—indeed even between jurisdictions (e.g., states or regions) in the same country—and are continuously changing. Overall, use and consent procedures are becoming increasingly more restrictive. For example, the Mental Health Act of India 1987 is currently being revised; the draft of the new Act prohibits ECT in minors, although it remains to be seen whether this will be kept in the final form of the Act (42).

Nevertheless, it represents a quite dramatic change from previous Indian legislation and practice. Thus, clinicians need to familiarize themselves with the laws and practices in their own country.

Use of ECT is strictly regulated in most Anglo-Saxon countries (e.g., US, Canada, UK, and Australia), yet quite liberal in others (e.g., Scandinavian and most low-income countries). The use of both anesthesia and muscle relaxants is now accepted and recommended practice. However, in a few countries, such as Japan, India, Romania, Spain, and Nigeria, unmodified ECT is still in use (19). It is worth noting that the World Health Organization has called for a worldwide ban on unmodified ECT. It also warrants mentioning that in Slovenia and Luxembourg, ECT is not available to treat people of *any* age—patients must travel to neighboring countries to receive the treatment (43).

In the US, there is great variability between states in the laws that govern the use of ECT in minors. For instance, in the state of Michigan, ECT may be administered if there is consensus among three child and adolescent psychiatrists. In the neighboring state of Illinois, ECT for a minor may only be authorized by a court order, which often specifies the number of permitted treatments and the time period in which these must be administered. Such a practice is likely to delay treatment and may undermine an individualized treatment plan. The reader is referred to a case (44) in which, after protracted litigation, treatment with ECT was permitted for a young female with psychosis and catatonia. However, the Probate Court ordered that only 12 treatments were permitted and that these were to be administered over 90 days. Clearly, allowing the legal system to determine the number of treatments and/or duration of treatment is unlikely to be in the best interests of a seriously ill adolescent. Similar age-related restrictions are found in the Mental Health Code for California, Tennessee, Colorado, and Texas. This judicial scrutiny of ECT has created both clinical and ethical dilemmas in an emerging climate and expectation of the right to receive effective treatment (45).

Because ECT is very uncommon in the young—representing only about 1% of all ECT courses administered—many child psychiatrists and other mental health professionals are not familiar with the procedure, its administration, or the laws regulating its use. For example, in a survey of 625 child and adolescent psychiatrists and psychologists in the United States, 93% of respondents stated that they possessed little knowledge about the use of ECT in children and adolescents (46), while 40% of participants in a similar study in Australia and New Zealand rated their knowledge about ECT as minimal (47). The lack of knowledge and experience about ECT among child and adolescent psychiatrists and the requirement, in some jurisdictions, for two or three child psychiatrists to agree on the treatment have created a uniquely restrictive environment for ECT that is unmatched for almost any other medical treatment.

Keeping in mind the shifting regulatory environment, consent procedures for ECT across countries can be summarized as follows.

Children younger than 12 years:

- ECT in prepubertal children is extremely rare. While the majority of countries do not ban the treatment's use in children, a few legislatures specifically forbid the use of ECT in this age group. For example, in the state of Texas, ECT is banned for people younger than 16 years; there are similar age-related restriction in Colorado, California, and Tennessee.

Youth aged 12–16 years (or below the age of consent for medical treatment in the specific country, e.g., 18 years):

- The majority of countries require only parental consent for the administration of ECT, as for any other medical or surgical procedure.
- Some countries, however, specifically state that parents or relatives cannot consent for ECT on behalf of adolescents. If adolescents are unable to give consent themselves (either because of their illness or because they are not "mature minors"), consent is given by a magistrate or by a psychiatrist, usually after obtaining the opinion of a second psychiatrist. For example, in the Australian state of Western Australia, parents or guardians cannot give consent for a minor to receive ECT. Minors must give consent themselves, irrespective of their age, if the treating psychiatrist believes they are mature enough to make their own health care decisions. Otherwise, these young patients are treated as if they were involuntary patients: treatment requires the approval of a second psychiatrist. Failure to adhere to this process may result in up to 2 years of imprisonment for practitioners.
- When parents are the people authorized to give consent, it is good practice in many countries to also seek the young person's "assent."
- While in the majority of countries, consent for ECT is understood as consent for a *course* of 6 to 12 administrations, that is not true everywhere. Some countries—such as Italy, Ireland, and Latvia in Europe—require separate written consent before each ECT administration. Most countries allow for consent to be withdrawn at any stage, except in the case of involuntary patients.
- In most legislatures, consent covers not only the ECT itself but also the associated procedures such as anesthesia. However, some countries require a separate consent for anesthesia (e.g., Spain, Austria, Slovakia, Greece, Switzerland, and Germany) (43).

Involuntary patients:

- For patients receiving treatment against their wishes, it is required to follow the specific procedures for involuntary treatment in the specific country. For example, in some Australian states this means the approval of an independent "mental health tribunal."

CORE ELEMENTS OF THE CONSENT PROCESS

Notwithstanding the regional differences in consent policy, procedures, and legislation noted above, there are four key pieces of information to be imparted, through discussion, in the clinical process of consent, irrespective of location. Thus, wherever possible, (1) the rationale for ECT, (2) treatment procedure, (3) alternatives to ECT, and (4) the natural course of illness without treatment should be explained to the patient and patient's family (48). These areas should also be broached with parents alone if, for example, the young patient's mental state precludes his or her comprehension of the information, as well as in cases where assent, rather than consent, is sought from the ECT recipient. (Obtaining "assent" entails clinicians helping children gain a developmentally appropriate understanding of the nature of their illness by explaining what they can expect [good and bad] with the treatment, evaluating young patients' understanding of the situation, including whether they feel inappropriately pressured, and seeking an expression of the patients' willingness to accept the treatment [49].) In *all* cases involving children and adolescents, age-appropriate language should be used. In isolated cases—these would be extremely rare—an older adolescent estranged from family may be competent to make all treatment decisions and elect to not have the family involved. Finally, it is worth highlighting that both consent and assent are not a single event or moment in time, but rather a *process*; for example, adolescents unable to consent at the commencement of the ECT course may be able to do so after one or more treatments (50).

To complement face-to-face discussion and enhance a young patient's and family's understanding of ECT prior to the treatment, a number of educational tools should be made available (48). These include video/DVD descriptions of ECT; showing the young person and family the ECT suite, ECT apparatus, and recovery area; having the young patient and family speak to previous teenage recipients and families about the treatment (51); and providing practical information in writing. An example of the last is provided in Appendix 4.1 (48). An example of a written consent form is shown in Appendix 4.2.

ETHICAL IMPLICATIONS OF RESISTING ECT IN MINORS

In the light of the scientific literature, it is an unavoidable conclusion that ECT in children and adolescents is a safe, effective, and lifesaving treatment. Moreover, the treatment is usually seen as a beneficial aspect of the management of severe mental health problems in these patients—most young ECT recipients would have ECT again, if clinically indicated, as well as recommend it to others, and their parents have similar positive views (52, 53). Delays in receiving ECT may lead to significant deterioration in the psychiatric illness for which the treatment is administered. The disruption to the child's emotional, educational, and interpersonal development that may be brought about by delays in treatment is a further, compelling counterargument to the assertion that ECT for children and adolescents with certain disorders is in some way barbaric or immoral (54). Thus, alongside the principles of respect for autonomy (and its above-described nuances in a young person), beneficence, and non-maleficence, due attention to the principle of "justice" (8) provides a relevant rejoinder to those who wish ban ECT in young persons. Both "distributive justice" (fair distribution of a resource, in this case ECT treatment) and "rights-based justice" (respect for people's rights, here the right to ECT) are germane (55).

One of the corollaries of a comparative lack of expertise in the use of ECT in children and adolescents is the comparative paucity of scientific literature in the field. As it stands, much of the evidence base for ECT in the young is in the form of case studies or retrospective reviews (56), although there has been a systematic review of published studies that support the use of ECT in patients in this age group (57). While these are valid methodologies, and despite the fact that the ethical notion of "casuistry" (58) would suggest that experience with even a small number of cases can still usefully inform ethical deliberations, the quality of research data in the field of child and adolescent ECT encounters the dilemma of a "deficiency of evidence" being confounded by "evidence of deficiency." In order for the practice to evolve, child psychiatrists need to abide their values and their axioms in terms of advocating and conducting such research in the most rigorous way possible. Given the prevailing climate in which psychiatry, in particular child psychiatry, exists, this is a most challenging prospect.

CASE VIGNETTE: ANDY

Andy was a 13-year-old boy who was in the care of a foster family. Andy suffered from moderately severe autism and since puberty had been prone to aggressive outbursts toward his foster parents. Over a period of six weeks, Andy became withdrawn and increasingly unresponsive. His foster parents eventually brought him to the Emergency Department in a state of catatonic stupor.

Andy was admitted to the pediatric ward and given I.V. fluids. After consultation with a child psychiatrist, Andy had several injections of lorazepam with only limited benefit in reducing his catatonic symptoms. Given the gravity of the clinical situation, Andy's clinicians sought approval for ECT from the relevant authorities. As there were no specific facilities for pediatric mental health, Andy's ECT was to be given in the ECT suite of the adult psychiatric ward. After two ECT treatments, Andy's catatonic symptoms improved, but then deteriorated progressively over a period of five days. When Andy was brought to the ECT suite for the third ECT session, he became agitated, fearful, and resistive. Andy was physically restrained, was given anesthetic, and subsequently received ECT.

Following this incident, staff at the ECT suite expressed concern about further treatments with ECT, particularly in light of the distress Andy exhibited during the session. Taking into account the failure to control Andy's catatonic symptoms by other means, it seemed that ECT remained the only treatment option.

The child psychiatrist arranged a meeting with the staff of the pediatric ward, the ECT suite, the anesthetist, and Andy's foster parents. At the meeting, the child psychiatrist explained the nature of catatonia and the evidence for the efficacy of ECT in its treatment. The staff agreed that Andy's distress at being taken to the ECT suite could be best alleviated by him having a sedative antipsychotic medication prior to the treatment. Using this approach, Andy had a further course of 5 treatments of ECT, following which his catatonia resolved.

This vignette raises a number of issues related to the ethics and value system of a child psychiatrist, alongside other health professionals. In the first instance, there was a need for decisive and life-saving treatment. This required coordination of the efforts of a number of parties and the management of negative responses by some components of the health system. Andy's distress at having ECT needed to be balanced against the requirement for him to have the treatment; the process of defusing the negative responses around this aspect of the situation represented a form of advocacy by the child psychiatrist. In broader terms, the clinical setting of a general pediatric ward relying on an adult ECT suite represented a need for advocacy to provide more appropriate clinical services sensitive to the needs of the child and his caregivers.

CONCLUSION

In the past decade, interest in the use of ECT in children and adolescents has continued to grow. Alongside calls for a blanket ban on the treatment in young people (59) are published guidelines articulating the situations in which the treatment may be very helpful, and indeed potentially lifesaving, in this age group and how it is to be used (22). Sometimes lost in the heat of the battle and stridency of viewpoints is the plight of a young patient who may stand to benefit from a treatment that has been shown to be effective in similar patients of similar age in the past, with few if any side effects. Consideration of "values-based" psychiatric practice, along with due attention to the principles of respect for autonomy (and its nuances in children and adolescents), beneficence, non-maleficence, and justice, suggests that ECT has a potentially important role in suitable young patients. It behooves practitioners in the child and adolescent mental health field to ponder the myriad ethical issues attending ECT use in children and adolescents, and to become familiar with the various aspects pertaining to consent to the treatment in their jurisdiction.

QUESTIONS AND ANSWERS

1. *Name four core ethical principles that should inform a clinician's decision-making in relation to the use of ECT in children and adolescents.*

   Respect for autonomy, beneficence, non-maleficence, and justice.

2. *How does autonomy differ in young people compared to adults regarding consent and decisions about a person's health?*

   A child's capacity to make autonomous decisions about his or her health is not static but evolves with cognitive and emotional development. Although a parent or legal guardian may have the legal authority to consent for a minor, it is normally desirable, though not legally necessary, to (also) obtain the minor's "assent" (agreement).

3. *List four pieces of information that should be conveyed to young patients and/or family in seeking consent for ECT.*

   (1) The rationale for ECT; (2) treatment procedure; (3) alternatives to ECT; and (4) the natural course of illness without treatment.

4. *List some of the ways in which a clinician may enhance a young patient's and family's understanding of ECT prior to the treatment.*

   This may be achieved in several ways: face-to-face discussion; recommending video/DVD descriptions of ECT; showing the young person and family the ECT suite, ECT apparatus, and recovery area; having the young patient and family speak to previous teenage recipients and families about the treatment; and providing practical information in writing.

DISCLOSURES

A/Prof. Michael Robertson has no conflicts to disclose.

Prof. Joseph M. Rey has no conflicts to disclose.

Prof. Garry Walter has received research support from Lundbeck and AstraZeneca for a study titled "Psychiatric Evaluation in Primary Care."

REFERENCES

1. Joshi N. Internet electroconvulsive therapy. *Psychiat Bull.* 2009;33:155.
2. Frank L. Electroshocking children. http://psychiatrybuster.blogspot.com/2007/06/electroshocking-children-by-leonard-roy.html. 2007.
3. Masters C. Shock treatment back. *Daily Telegraph* Nov 18, 2006.
4. Hale E. Child shock therapy. *Sunday Herald Sun* Jan 25, 2009.
5. Morrison L. Shocked beyond belief. *Australas Psychiatry.* 2009;17:164–7.

6. American Academy of Child and Adolescent Psychiatry. AACAP/CWLA Foster Care Mental Health Values Subcommittee. http://www.aacap.org/cs/root/policy_statements/aacap/cwla_foster_care_mental_health_values_subcommittee. 2002 [cited Jan 8, 2012]; http://www.aacap.org/cs/root/policy_statements/aacap/cwla_foster_care_mental_health_values_subcommittee.
7. Robertson M, Walter G. Overview of psychiatric ethics I: professional ethics and psychiatry. *Australas Psychiatry.* 2007;15:201–6.
8. Robertson M, Ryan C, Walter G. Overview of psychiatric ethics III: principles-based ethics. *Australas Psychiatry.* 2007;15:281–6.
9. Olfson M, Marcus S, Weissman M, Jensen P. National trends in the use of psychotropic medications by children. *J Am Acad Child & Adoles Psychiat.* 2002;41:514–21.
10. Zito J, Safer D, dosReis S, Gardner J, Boles M, Lynch F. Trends in the prescribing of psychotropic medications to preschoolers. *JAMA.* 2000;283:1025–30.
11. Lakhan S, Hagger-Johnson G. The impact of prescribed psychotropics on youth. *Clinical Prac Epidem Ment Health.* 2007;3:21.
12. Breggin P. *Toxic Psychiatry.* New York: St Martin's Press; 1994.
13. Kolata G. Boom in Ritalin sales raises ethical issues. *New York Times* May 15, 1996.
14. Sparks J, Duncan B. The ethics and science of medicating children. *Ethical Human Psychol Psych.* 2004;6:25–39.
15. Citizens Commission on Human Rights International. The corrupt alliance of the psychiatric-pharmaceutical industry. http://www.cchrint.org/cchr-issues/the-corrupt-alliance-of-the-psychiatric-pharmaceutical-industry. 2009. (cited 2012 Sep 26).
16. Hausman K. Last of ritalin-based lawsuits against APA comes to a close. *Psychiatric News.* 2002 Apr 5;37:1.
17. Breggin P. ECT damages the brain: Disturbing news for patients and shock doctors alike. *Ethical Human Psychol Psych.* 2007;9:83–6.
18. Agarwal AK, Andrade C. Indian psychiatrists' attitudes towards electroconvulsive therapy. *Indian J Psychiatry.* 1997;39:54–60.
19. Chanpattana W, Kunigiri G, Kramer BA, Gangadhar BN. Survey of the practice of electroconvulsive therapy in teaching hospitals in India. *J ECT.* 2005 Jun;21(2):100–4.
20. Shoirah H, Hamoda H. Electroconvulsive therapy in children and adolescents. *Expert Rev Neurother.* 2011;11:127–37.
21. Stein D, Weizman A, Bloch Y. Electroconvulsive therapy and transcranial magnetic stimulation: can they be considered valid modalities in the treatment of pediatric mood disorders? *Child Adoles Psychiat Clinics N Am.* 2006;15:1035–56.
22. Ghaziuddin N, Kutcher S, Knapp P. Practice Parameter for Use of Electroconvulsive Therapy With Adolescents. *J Am Acad Child Adoles Psychiat.* 2004;43:1521–39.
23. Walter G, Rey JM, Ghaziuddin N, Loo C. Electroconvulsive therapy, transcranial magnetic stimulation, and vagus nerve stimulation. In: Martin A, Scahill L, Kratochvil CJ, eds. *Pediatric Psychopharmacology: Principles and Practice.* 2nd ed. New York: Oxford University Press; 2011, pp. 363–73.
24. Bloch Y, Sobol D, Levkovitz Y, Kron S, Ratzoni G. Reasons for referral for electroconvulsive therapy: a comparison between adolescents and adults. *Australas Psychiatry.* 2008;16:191–4.
25. Reisner A. The electroconvulsive therapy controversy: evidence and ethics. *Neuropsychol Rev.* 2003;13:199–219.

26. McClintock S, Husain M. Electroconvulsive therapy does not damage the brain. *J Am Psychiat Nurses Assoc* 2011;17:212–3.
27. Cohen D, Taieb O, Benoit N, Chevret S, Corcos M, Fossati P, et al. Absence of cognitive impairment at long term follow-up in adolescents treated with ECT for severe mood disorders. *Am J Psychiat.* 2000;157:460–2.
28. Ghaziuddin N, Laughrin D, Giordani B, Ghaziuddin N, Laughrin D, Giordani B. Cognitive side effects of electroconvulsive therapy in adolescents. *J Child Adoles Psychop.* 2000;10:269–76.
29. Jap S, Ghaziuddin N. Catatonia among adolescents with Down syndrome: a review and 2 case reports. *J ECT.* 2011;27:334–7.
30. Sackeim H, Prudic J, Fuller R, Keilp J, Lavori P, Olfson M. The cognitive effects of electroconvulsive therapy in community settings. *Neuropsychopharmacol.* 2007;32:244–54.
31. Rose D, Wykes T, Bindman J, Fleischmann P. Information, consent and perceived coercion: Patients' perspectives on electroconvulsive therapy. *Brit J Psychiat.* 2005;186:54–9.
32. Breeding J. Electroshock and informed consent. *J Humanist Psychol.* 2000; 40:65–79.
33. Green J, Stewart A. Ethical issues in child and adolescent psychiatry. *J Med Ethics.* 1987;13:5–11.
34. Reiter-Thiel S, Eich H, Reiter L. The ethical status of the child in family and child psychotherapy. *Praxis der Kinderpsychologie und Kinderpsychiatrie* 1993;42:14–20.
35. Beauchamp T, Childress J. *Principles of Biomedical Ethics.* 5th ed. New York: Oxford University Press; 2001.
36. Reiter-Thiel S. Autonomy and beneficence: Ethical issues in electroconvulsive therapy. *Convulsive Therapy* 1992;8:237–44.
37. Pearce J. Consent to treatment during childhood. *Brit J Psychiat.* 1994;165:713–6.
38. Dickenson D, Jones D. The philosophy and developmental psychology of children's informed consent. *Psychiat Psychol Philo.* 1995;2:287–303.
39. Levine S, Blank K, Schwartz H, Rait D. Informed consent in the electroconvulsive treatment of geriatric patients. *Bull Am Acad Psych Law.* 1991;19:395–403.
40. Black D, Subotsky F. Medical ethics and child psychiatry. *J Med Ethics.* 1982;8:5–8.
41. Koocher G. Ethical issues in psychotherapy with adolescents. *J Clin Psychol.* 2003;59:1247–56.
42. Balhara YPS, Mathur S. ECT Prohibition for children and adolescents in mental health care act of India: a step in the right direction? *J ECT.* 2012;28:1–2.
43. Gazdag G, Takács R, Ungvari G, Sienaert P. The practice of consenting to electroconvulsive therapy in the European Union. *J ECT.* 2012;28:4–6.
44. Circuit Court of Champaign County. No. 4-98-0826. *In the Matter of A. M. P., a Minor, Cora Plank and Eli Plank, Petitioners-Appelles, v A. M. P., a Minor, Respondent-Appellant.* http://www.state.il.us/court/opinions/appellatecourt/1999/4thdistrict/march/html/4980826.htm. March 26, 1999 (cited 2012 Dec 24).
45. Leong G, Eth S. Legal and ethical issues in electroconvulsive therapy. *Psychiat Clin N Am.* 1991;14:1007–20.
46. Ghaziuddin N, Kaza M, Ghazi N, King C, Walter G, Rey JM. Electroconvulsive therapy for minors: experiences and attitudes of child psychiatrists and psychologists. *J ECT.* 2001;17:109–17.

47. Walter G, Rey JM, Starling J. Australian and New Zealand child psychiatrists' knowledge and attitudes about ECT in young people. *Aust NZ J Psychiat.* 1997;31:676–81.
48. Walter G, Rey J, Mitchell P. Practitioner review: Electroconvulsive therapy in adolescents. *J Child Psychol Psych.* 1999;40:325–34.
49. Committee on Bioethics of the American Academy of Pediatrics. Informed consent, parental permission, and assent in pediatric practice. *Pediatrics.* 1995:95:314–317.
50. Walter G, Ghaziuddin N. Using other biological treatments: electroconvulsive therapy, transcranial magnetic stimulation, vagus nerve stimulation and light therapy. In: Rey JM, Birmaher B, eds. *Treating Child and Adolescent Depression.* Baltimore, MD: Lippincott Williams & Wilkins; 2009, pp. 87–97.
51. Kutcher S, Robertson HA. Electroconvulsive therapy in treatment resistant bipolar youth. *J Child Adol Psychop.* 1995;5:167–75.
52. Walter G, Koster K, Rey J. Electroconvulsive therapy in adolescents: experience, knowledge, and attitudes of recipients. *J Am Acad Child Adol Psychiat.* 1999;38:594–9.
53. Walter G, Koster K, Rey J. Views about treatment among parents of adolescents who received electroconvulsive therapy. *Psychiat Serv.* 1999;50:701–2.
54. Ottoson J, Fink M. *Ethics in Electroconvulsive Therapy.* New York: Brunner-Routledge; 2004.
55. Gillon R. Medical ethics: four principles plus attention to scope. *Brit Med J.* 1994; 309: 184–188.
56. Walter G, Rey J. Has the practice and outcome of ECT in adolescents changed? Findings from a whole-population study. *J ECT.* 2003;19:84–7.
57. Rey J, Walter G. Half a century of ECT use in young people. *Am J Psychiat.* 1997;154:595–602.
58. Robertson M, Ryan C, Walter G. Overview of psychiatric ethics IV: the method of casuistry. *Australas Psychiatry.* 2007;15:287–91.
59. Funk M, Drew N, Saraceno B. *WHO Resource Book on Mental Health, Human Rights and Legislation.* Geneva: World Health Organization; 2005, page 64.

Appendix 4.1: EXAMPLE OF WRITTEN INFORMATION ABOUT ECT THAT MAY BE GIVEN TO YOUNG PATIENTS AND FAMILIES (ORIGINALLY IN [48], REPUBLISHED AND ADAPTED WITH PERMISSION)

ELECTROCONVULSIVE THERAPY (ECT) IN YOUNG PEOPLE

What is electroconvulsive therapy?
Electroconvulsive therapy (ECT) is a treatment for certain mental disorders that was discovered almost 60 years ago. It is given by a team of specialist doctors and nurses. One of the doctors, an anesthetist, puts the patient to sleep for a short while with an anesthetic. While the patient is asleep, an electric current is applied to the head by another doctor. A brief seizure, which can hardly be noticed because the muscles are relaxed, follows. The patient is then taken to a recovery room and is looked after there by trained nurses. The whole procedure takes about 10 minutes. ECT is usually given two or three times weekly. Most patients need 6 to 12 treatments, but a few patients require more.

How does ECT work?
An imbalance of chemicals is thought to cause most mental disorders for which ECT is given. ECT corrects this imbalance, though how it actually does this is not known. A lot of research is currently being done to discover this.

Is ECT an approved treatment?
All major medical and psychiatric organizations, including the American Psychiatric Association, Royal College of Psychiatrists (UK), and Royal Australian and New Zealand College of Psychiatrists, approve the use of ECT and have guidelines for how it should be given.

Why do young people have ECT?
The main reason is severe depression. Young people with this condition may feel unhappy, be unable to enjoy anything, sleep poorly, and feel suicidal. ECT is also sometimes used to treat mania, schizophrenia, and other conditions.

How often is ECT given to young people?
ECT is used more often in adults but the treatment is occasionally used for young people. About 1% of people who have ECT are teenagers. When used, it is generally after medication and other treatments have not helped or have caused serious side effects.

How effective is ECT?

More than half of the young people who have ECT improve a great deal or recover fully from their symptoms. This is very pleasing given how unwell the person is just before ECT and the fact that other treatments did not work. ECT does not stop the person from becoming unwell again. It is thus important that most people start taking medication again after ECT and be followed-up by their doctor.

How safe is the treatment?

ECT is very safe. The risks are the same as those for an operation needing a brief anesthetic. When thinking about safety, it is also worth keeping in mind the bad effects of other treatments as well as the risks of not treating the condition at all. Suicide, for example, is not rare in people who are severely depressed.

What are the main side effects of ECT?

The side effects of ECT are mild and don't last long. Some people complain of headache after waking from the anesthetic but this is brief and goes away with analgesics. A few people complain of muscle aches for a short while. Some people complain of memory problems. This stops once the treatment has finished.

Does ECT damage the brain?

There is no evidence to suggest this. Studies of brain structure and function show that ECT does not injure the brain.

Who gives consent for ECT?

The doctor recommending ECT will discuss this treatment with the patient and the patient's family and provide time for them to ask questions about the treatment. If the patient and family choose to go ahead with ECT, the patient will then sign a consent. When patients can't understand what they are told about ECT (usually because of their illness), a panel made up of a doctor, a lawyer, and a patient representative will consider whether ECT should go ahead.

Why has ECT had such a bad image?

After ECT was discovered, it was used for all mental disorders. Drug treatments were not around at the time and there were few other treatments. Also, muscle relaxants were not given, resulting in more side effects from the seizure. Movies such as *The Snake Pit* and *One Flew Over the Cuckoo's Nest* gave negative accounts of ECT, and this helped to create a bad image. As practiced these days, ECT is a safe, even lifesaving treatment, used for particular illnesses and according to strict guidelines.

Appendix 4.2 EXAMPLE OF AN ECT CONSENT FORM

Dr ________________________________ has told me that I have the following condition:

____

The doctor has therefore recommended electroconvulsive therapy as an appropriate treatment.

The doctor has explained to me that:

a. The treatment generally consists of the following: I will be taken to a treatment room in the morning before breakfast. I will be attended by an anesthetist and a physician. A needle will be placed in my vein through which an anesthetic will be injected and I will become drowsy and fall asleep. Then I will receive a muscle relaxant. I will be given oxygen through a mask and it may be necessary for the anesthetist to assist my breathing.

   The electroconvulsive therapy will take place while I am anesthetized. Brief electric currents will be passed through electrodes placed on my scalp. The electric currents will stimulate my brain. Treatments are given every other day and I may require a number of treatments. The average number of treatments required is 9, although some patients require fewer and others require more. The treatment is designed to reverse my present condition.

b. The following risks are involved with this treatment:

   There are two separate types of risk. First, there are some risks related to the anesthesia. These risks consist of the following: respiratory arrest, cardiac arrest, and even death. Second, there are some risks related to the treatment itself: memory for recent events may be disturbed and dates, names of friends, public events, telephone numbers and addresses may be difficult to recall. In most patients, memory returns to normal within 4 weeks after the last treatment, but in some cases memory problems remain for months and even years. Additionally, in very rare cases, there is the risk of seizures, bone fractures, and even death. This risk is negligible (less than one in 10,000 cases) but has been documented.

c. My condition could also be treated in the following ways, but they are not recommended at this time:

   ____

d. There is no guarantee that this treatment will improve my condition.

   I understand that this consent form covers the maximum of twelve (12) treatments to be administered in a series over a four-week period. However, since the average number of treatments administered is nine (9), I may not require all twelve treatments.

I understand that I may discontinue treatment at any time although my physician would like me to continue until an adequate course is completed.

I understand the treatment and have discussed it with Dr. _________ who has answered all of my questions.

I therefore permit the physician (and such other persons as are needed to assist) to administer the treatment to me. I further permit the anesthetist (and such other persons as are needed to assist) to administer anesthetic to me in connection with the procedure.

_______________	_______________	_________
PATIENT	WITNESS	DATE

The patient is unable to consent because:

And I, as his/her legally authorized representative, therefore consent for the patient:

_______________	_______________	_________
LEGALLY AUTHORIZED REPRESENTATIVE	WITNESS	DATE

____

RELATIONSHIP TO PATIENT

THIS SIGNED CONSENT IS VALID UNTIL

____

DATE

CHAPTER 5

A Practical Guide to Using ECT in Minors

NEERA GHAZIUDDIN, POLLY GIPSON, AND ELISE HODGES

KEY POINTS

- ECT may be administered to a minor using the guidelines of the American Academy of Child and Adolescent Psychiatry, or other similarly recognized guidelines.
- Adolescents should be hospitalized for initiating a course of ECT.
- Second opinion for ECT should be given by an independent psychiatrist, who has adequate experience with using ECT in minors.
- Consent of the legal guardian and assent of the patient (whenever possible) should be obtained.
- A pre-ECT evaluation should include a psychiatric history, target symptoms, laboratory tests, brain imaging, neuropsychological evaluation (to be repeated on completion of ECT) and assessment by an anesthesiologist.
- Consultation with other medical specialties should be decided on a case-by-case basis.
- A treatment course generally includes an index course (2 to 3 times per week), which may be followed by an individually determined continuation course.
- The number of treatments during the index or the continuation course should be based on clinical response and not based by a determined number.
- Close follow-up is necessary during ECT and on completion of the course.
- Patients and their families benefit from psychosocial support during the treatment.
- Pharmacotherapy should be started toward the end of the ECT course. Psychotherapy may be beneficial for some patients on completion of ECT.

OVERVIEW

The goals of this chapter are to describe practical aspects necessary for the safe and effective administration of electroconvulsive therapy (ECT); selection of patients who may benefit from ECT; pre-ECT workup, description of the device and the treatment procedure; and optimum monitoring during and following an ECT course. We begin this chapter with suggested training requirements for child and adolescent psychiatrists and allied professionals who treat this population, including psychologists, social workers, nurses, and other medical specialists such as pediatricians and neurologists. Adequate training and hands-on experience among professionals appear to be important factors, so that youth who need this treatment may receive it in the safest and most effective manner. Readers should bear in mind that there are no controlled ECT trials in patients below the age of 18 years. [It should be noted that terms such as "children," "youth," and "minors" are used interchangeably and refer to patients younger than 18 years. "Adolescents" refers to individuals who range in age from 12 to 18 years, whereas pre-pubertal children are those below age 12. Due to paucity of data in pre-pubertal children, the majority of the information presented in this chapter is based on experience with adolescents.]

TRAINING

Child Psychiatry Fellows, Pediatric Specialists, and Medical Students

Adequate training is essential for the appropriate use of ECT in children and adolescents. With proper training, ECT may be demystified by child and adolescent psychiatrists who will be able to offer the treatment to severely ill youth who are not responding to other interventions. Many advanced level psychiatric trainees (known as Child Fellows in the United States) may enter a training program after having received cursory training about ECT during their adult psychiatry residency. Medical students, too, often have inadequate exposure to ECT, and may enter a psychiatry residency program with minimal knowledge and/or negative views.

Negative views about this treatment are widely held, both within and outside psychiatry, which have powerful historical underpinnings (see Chapter 1, "The History of Pediatric ECT"). Other likely reasons are the absence of systematic prospective studies in this age group and the lack of controlled ECT trials in children and adolescents below 18 years of age; negative stereotypes perpetuated in the popular media (see Chapter 3, "ECT and Stigma"); inadequate opportunities to observe, firsthand, a treatment that is quick, painless, and humane; and the lack of longitudnal experience in following up patients who receive this treatment. Lack of experience among child and adolescent psychiatrists who train future generations is also a significant factor. For instance, a study completed in the United States found that the majority of child and adolescent psychiatrists and psychologists lacked experience with ECT, including when the procedure may be indicated. Additionally, across both disciplines, professionals expressed negative views about ECT treatment (1). It was noted, however, that negative views were directly proportional to a lack of adequate experience (1). Similarly, in a survey conducted in Australia by Walter and colleagues (1997), it was found that the majority of child and adolescent psychiatrists lacked experience in using ECT and held negative attitudes about ECT (2). However, in a subsequent survey published in 2003, there were encouraging results among a subgroup of the original participants, namely that child and adolescent psychiatrists had self-rated improvement in knowledge of ECT (3).

Data, albeit limited, indicate that exposure to ECT, including observing the procedure, must start early during psychiatric training. However, these recommendations have not been adequately incorporated in many training curriculums. For instance, recommendations by the American Psychiatric Association (APA) to include training in ECT have been followed by less than one-third of adult residency programs that had participated in a survey (4). The APA recommendations include that adult residents should receive four hours of didactic training, participate in at least 10 treatments and provide care to three patients receiving ECT.

It is also important that other pediatric specialists who treat children and adolescents, especially with comorbid psychiatric and chronic medical disorders, are knowledgeable about ECT. The rationale is that these providers may then appropriately refer an adolescent for ECT, and will be able to give accurate information if the adolescent/family wish to discuss this treatment option. Therefore, in addition to familiarity with conventional psychiatric treatments, it is important that pediatric specialists have sufficient knowledge and training regarding ECT. Unfortunately, a lack of adequate familiarity about ECT has been noted among internists who treat adults (5) and is likely to be even more common among pediatric specialists.

In the experience of the authors, patients with depression comorbid with other Axis I psychiatric diagnoses, those with chronic physical problems (such as chronic pain), or cases with catatonia, who could benefit from ECT are either overlooked or misdiagnosed resulting in prolonged treatments that may be ineffective or possibly harmful in some cases.

Essential components of a successful child and adolescent fellowship training experience should include hands-on experience in use of ECT (i.e., when to refer for ECT, patient selection, administering ECT, managing a patient during ECT, and providing follow-up on completion of ECT) along with guided study of the literature.

Psychologist, Neuropsychologists, and Other Allied Mental Health Professionals

The lack of training in ECT and negative attitudes appear to extend to nursing students and nursing staff, psychologists, and possibly to other allied mental health professionals. This is particularly problematic because allied mental health providers, as members of any multidisciplinary treatment team, are likely to be closely involved in helping youth and their families consent to treatment, tolerate the procedure, set realistic expectations of efficacy and side effects, and play an important role in treatment compliance. These key treatment components may be inadvertently undermined when there is inadequate knowledge and training. For instance, a study conducted in British Columbia found that only a minority (8.5%) of nursing students and nursing-aid students reported having adequate knowledge of ECT (6). Consequently, it is necessary that steps be taken to rectify the information gap for clinicians across disciplines and provide adequate training and experience. Based on currently available data, the necessary ingredients for residents to become skillful in delivering ECT are guided study, observing the procedure and direct involvement with the care of the patient (7); these training components likely apply to trainees from other disciplines.

Several surveys indicate that psychologists in particular report little to no knowledge or experience with ECT as a treatment option for patients who had failed to respond to conventional treatments (1, 2, 8). Furthermore, anecdotal observation does not indicate a substantial shift in knowledge or practice to close this gap among child psychologists in training. Psychologists can potentially play a key role due to their more frequent contact with the patient. Typically, any experience garnered by psychologists about ECT will occur during placement within a psychiatry department, if such experience is available. With adequate training, psychologists could identify patients who may benefit from an ECT referral, provide supportive psychotherapy to youth and their families during the treatment and during the follow-up period, and play a key role in detecting any early signs of relapse.

Neuropsychology training programs, similar to psychology programs, are likely to provide limited information about ECT at the pre-doctoral internship level, unless trainees are introduced during training within a hospital setting. Psychopathology courses in a doctoral program may include a discussion of ECT, but the extent of the discussion is likely to be restricted in scope and may be limited to the treatment of specific disorders such as major depression or bipolar disorder (9). Specialized training experiences such as the pre-doctoral internship or postdoctoral fellowship, particularly in a hospital setting, are more likely to provide didactics and experience in evaluation and treatment of patients referred for ECT. As such, trainees should be knowledgeable about the neuropsychological deficits anticipated to be observed at both pre- and post ECT time points.

Suggested areas of training and continuing education opportunities will vary by discipline, but may include (a) familiarity with practice guidelines about patient selection and referral resources for adolescents who need an ECT evaluation; (b) discipline-specific requirement that several ECT procedures are observed, so that questions from potential patients and their families can be answered in a consistent way by the entire treatment team; (c) attendance and participation in didactics, grand rounds, or conference presentations; (d) knowledge of therapeutic interventions for youth and families during and after ECT (support for the patient and their family during treatment, appropriate psychotherapy on completion of the treatment course, liaise with school to assist with reintegration, etc.); (d) knowledge of side effects of ECT; and (e) guided study.

PATIENT SELECTION

ECT is indicated for children or adolescents who meet diagnostic criteria for severe psychiatric disorders (e.g., mood disorders, psychosis, catatonia, or severe self-injurious behaviors) and/or have failed to respond adequately to conventional treatments. Although both illness-severity and the failure to respond are important patient-selection criteria, the severity of illness-criteria may take precedence in cases when waiting for treatment response may jeopardize safety or result in additional decline.

The terms "severe" and "failure to respond to adequate treatment" are fraught with controversy. However, both criteria should be taken into consideration for patient selection, whenever possible. An exception to these criteria would be a situation in which waiting for a treatment response would place an additional risk upon the youth and/or cause additional suffering. In these rare cases, where there are severe symptoms and/or there is imminent danger, the need for even one additional treatment trial may be waived. Such cases may include, although are not limited to, an imminently suicidal adolescent who carries additional risk factors for completed suicide (for example, positive family history of completed suicide, extreme risk-taking behaviors associated with an Axis I disorder) or severely compromised functions of daily living (food or fluid intake among others).

For the assessment of illness-severity, features may include not being able to function adequately, including inability to attend school, care for his or her activities of daily living (ADLs), engage socially, and care for any comorbid medical disorder. Food and fluid intake may be significantly reduced, and the teenager may be at imminent danger to self or others due to an Axis I psychiatric diagnosis. The second criteria, failure to respond adequately to prior treatment, should also take into consideration if there has been little or no response to two or three medication trials administered in adequate dosage (based on standard practice) and for an adequate duration (several weeks for most psychotropic agents), usually in combination with psychotherapy (if appropriate), such cases are unlikely to respond to yet another medication trial.

As previously stated, there are no controlled trials comparing ECT to continuing conventional treatment (pharmacotherapy combined with psychotherapy) in adolescents who have failed to respond to two or three previous psychotropic medication trials. However, case reports and case series published over the past two decades suggest that ECT may result in a robust response and is useful for alleviating severe symptoms, both in the short term (immediately following treatment) and in the medium long term, that is, months to 1–2 years following the treatment (10–19).

Adolescent-Adult Differences in Patient Selection

There is evidence to support that ECT is equally effective for the treatment of psychiatric disorders in adolescents as it is in adults (20). However, there are important age-related differences in practice and referral patterns. Probably the most significant age-related difference is that only a minority of patients treated with ECT are younger than 18 years. Studies in the United States and in Australia have found that minors constitute less than 1% of all patients treated with ECT (13, 21). Important diagnostic differences are found when adolescents who receive ECT are compared with adults; these differences indicate that the threshold for using ECT is much higher; that is, adolescents who receive ECT are likely to present with more severe forms of illness and may have failed many more medication trials, accompanied with long courses of psychotherapy. For instance, one study found that while adults are more likely to receive ECT for the lack of response to conventional treatment, adolescents are comparatively more likely to be treated for suicidality or for catatonia (22). Another study found that adolescents were more likely to receive ECT for psychotic spectrum disorders, while adults treated with ECT were more likely to be diagnosed with an affective spectrum disorder (20). In this author's (NG) experience, in adolescents who went on to receive ECT, the treatment was only administered after failure to respond to a larger number of medication trials (a mean number of 8 medication trials was noted [8.2 $\pm$ 4.2]) (19).

The current practice indicates that adolescents with severe psychiatric disorders are likely to be treated with ECT only when they fail to respond to multiple medication trials, are diagnosed with psychosis, display serious suicidality, or are diagnosed with catatonia in addition to overall severity of illness. It should be noted that this practice is neither supported by expected robust response following ECT or the relatively few, time-limited side effects noted in the literature.

Role of Psychologists and Allied Mental Health Professionals in Patient Selection

Psychologists and other mental health professionals involved in the care of adolescent patients have an important role in identifying treatment resistance and imminent risk, and requesting a timely referral for an ECT evaluation. Although psychologists and other allied mental health professionals in their typical role do not manage psychotropic medications, patients and their families who do not respond adequately to treatment may express their frustration or hopelessness to these professionals, especially because they are likely to have more frequent contact during the course of psychotherapy. Communicating this information to the treating psychiatrist can play an important role, if the clinician is knowledgeable about ECT. Following the start of ECT, the psychologist/allied professional may also contribute by promoting treatment engagement, preventing premature termination of treatment, identifying and assisting in overcoming patients' and their families' internal barriers (e.g., perceived dangerousness of ECT, side effects, stigma, shame; see Chapter 3, "ECT and Stigma") and external barriers (e.g., travel time for ECT, insurance-related issues, liaise with school, appropriate self-disclosure to family and friends) to pursuing an ECT recommendation.

There is a sparse literature from the nursing discipline about the use of ECT in adolescents or children. However, the discipline has made a rich and thoughtful contribution regarding ECT use in adults. As has been noted across disciplines, nurses are more likely to express positive attitudes when they have had greater contact and experience with patients who receive ECT (23). A recent publication had recognized the benefit of ECT, based on interviews conducted with nursing staff, but acknowledged that many patients, women in particular, had considered ECT a negative experience (24). Kavanagh and McLoughlin identified ECT as the most effective treatment for mood disorders and emphasized the role of education and training to assist nurses in making optimum, informed decisions, so that they may adequately support and care for patients receiving ECT (25). Lamont et al. published the development of an ECT service at a teaching hospital in Sydney, Australia, addressing important aspects such as credentialing, supervision, and coordination of care (26). Furthermore, in the experience of the author (NG), nursing staff play a critical role in the optimum use of ECT, such as during the decision-making process, and in treatment adherence, monitoring progress and giving support to the patient and his or her family throughout the treatment. It is, therefore, important that the primary-nurse of the young patient, while he or she is hospitalized, should be involved at every stage of the treatment.

A patient of one of the authors (PG), who was advised to receive ECT, expressed fear of being hospitalized during the ECT course. Though the psychologist attempted to answer all questions to help demystify the process, it became clear that the patient's concerns would be best addressed by a tour of the inpatient unit to allay his anxiety. The psychologist arranged a visit, which was very helpful. The psychologist later learned that none of the patient's fears about hospitalization could be explained by psychoeducation alone, and that an actual visit to the inpatient unit was essential to extinguish his fears.

INDICATIONS FOR ECT IN YOUTH

Indications for using ECT are:

1. Mood disorders: depressive or bipolar disorders;
2. Psychotic disorders, including schizophrenia;
3. Catatonia;
4. Neuroleptic malignant syndrome (NMS);
5. Severe self-injurious behavior (SIB).

Mood disorders are the main indication for ECT in youth and may include severe forms of major depressive disorder (MDD), dysthymia, depression not otherwise specified (NOS) or bipolar disorder (depressed, manic/hypomanic, or mixed phase). ECT can be helpful in the treatment of psychotic disorders, including schizoaffective disorder, schizophrenia or psychosis NOS when illness-severity or the criterion for failure to respond are met. Additionally, catatonia, NMS, and some forms of severe SIB are highly responsive to ECT. For further details, the reader is referred to Chapters 9–12 (respectively, "ECT for Adolescent Mood Disorders," "ECT for Schizophrenia Spectrum Disorders," "ECT for Catatonia in Autism," "ECT for Self-injurious Behavior").

CONTRAINDICATIONS FOR ECT

It is now widely accepted that the age of the patient or comorbid psychiatric conditions are not a contraindication for using ECT. While only a few medical disorders may be considered a relative contraindication, identifying all medical and psychiatric comorbid conditions, prior to ECT, should be a priority for effective and safe administration of the treatment.

Youth undergoing ECT in the presence of certain medical conditions should be worked up jointly with a specialist. Pheochromocytoma, although a rare condition, may be considered a contraindication for ECT, due to the elevation of blood pressure during treatment (27). An active respiratory infection should be treated prior to ECT. Although only rarely relevant to youth, a recent myocardial infarction (MI) may be a relative contraindication for ECT. Youth are considered at low risk for coronary artery disease and therefore do not require any specific cardiac tests except for a careful clinical evaluation and a non-invasive test such as an EKG. Based on experience from adults, ECT may be administered safely in the presence of many coexisting medical disorders, including brain tumors (28), cardiac pace maker (29), intracranial aneurysm (30, 31), and craniotomy with VP shunt—an adolescent female was successfully treated (32). It is mandatory that after identifying any medical disorder prior to ECT, the psychiatrist should work closely with the relevant specialist to make any treatment changes. (For additional details, readers are referred to Chapter 6, "ECT in Young People with Comorbid Medical and Neurological Disorders.")

Based on limited data from adolescents and more extensive experience in adult patients, certain comorbid psychiatric diagnoses or symptoms are associated with treatment resistance and possibly diminished response to ECT. These may include: prominent physical symptoms/ somatization disorders—a less robust response to ECT was noted in adults (33) and in adolescents (13); anxiety disorders—ECT is not indicated when the primary Axis I disorder is an anxiety disorder (34), but comorbid anxiety disorders are often diagnosed in adolescents who are treated with ECT (35); substance abuse/dependence disorders, which are known to coexist with treatment-resistant mood disorders, and some in this subgroup may benefit from ECT (36); and those with personality disorders, who appear to respond at rates lower than those without a personality disorder (37). A somewhat lower response has been shown in adolescents with MDD who were diagnosed with a comorbid personality disorder (13). Nevertheless, these adolescents should receive ECT, applying the same criteria that are used for patients who suffer from significant mood symptoms but without a personality disorder because of an elevated risk of completed suicide when the two conditions co-occur (37).

Remedial interventions, after identifying comorbid psychiatric and medical conditions,may include, a substance free period before ECT is initiated for adolescents diagnosed with substance use/abuse disorders; setting up realistic expectations regarding the treatment response when there are maladaptive problem-solving skills suggestive of a personality disorder; and, treating comorbid anxiety that may be a risk factor for recurrence in depression. In some cases, more intensive forms of psychotherapy may become possible after the adolescent has experienced symptom relief with ECT. Specific types of psychotherapy may be possible on completion of treatment and after recovery of short term memory. These may include dialectic behavior therapy for adolescents who have difficulty tolerating painful affect; CBT to address mood or other illness-related cognitive distortions; or behavior modification for specific phobias.

Most important, no comorbid psychiatric diagnoses should be considered as a contraindication for ECT, as long as other criteria necessary for treatment are met—that is, a diagnosis known to respond to ECT, lack of adequate treatment response of a severe Axis I disorder, or imminent risk conferred

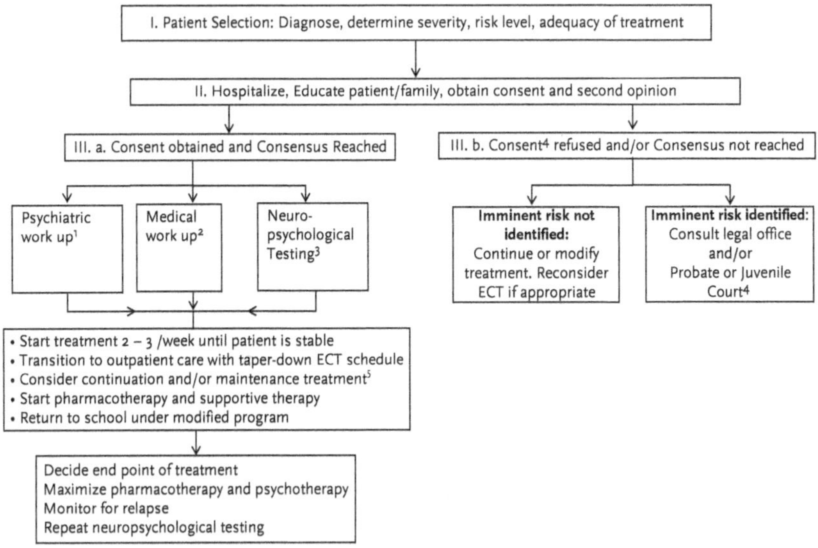

1-3: See section in text; 4: See chapter "Ethical aspects of Consent;" 5: See section in text

Figure 5.1:
Practical Tips and Steps when considering ECT in Children and Adolescents.

by waiting for treatment response with conventional treatments. Similarly, a comorbid medical disorder should be thoroughly investigated with the appropriate specialty input before making a final decision.

PROGNOSTIC FACTORS

Several prognostic factors are important in measuring outcomes in response to ECT. Treatment outcome may be based on the response rate—generally defined as a 50% improvement in symptoms, or the remission rate—defined as minimal or no symptoms. Factors that appear to influence outcome, including the primary psychiatric indication for ECT, are comorbid diagnoses, premorbid functioning, presence of prominent somatic symptoms, and possibly the age of initial psychiatric contact. See Figure 5.1 for suggested steps when ECT is considered for a child or an adolescent.

Primary Diagnosis

Axis I psychiatric disorders that manifest with prominent mood disturbance—unipolar or a bipolar disorders in pure or mixed forms—or, in which mood symptoms constitute a prominent part of another psychiatric syndrome (e.g., psychotic or schizoaffective disorders) are known to respond positively to ECT.

Some disorders, such as schizophrenia, schizoaffective, and psychotic disorder NOS are known to have lower response rates, however improvement is more likely when there are significant mood symptoms. Catatonia (agitated or retarded types), more often associated with mood disorders in adolescents (38), is also known to respond robustly to ECT. Rates of improvement reported for adolescents include 63% for depression, 80% for mania, 42% for schizophrenia, and 80% for catatonia (39). Realistic expectations can be best set following diagnostic clarification, which is essential prior to starting ECT for any adolescent.

Comorbid Diagnoses

Comorbid psychiatric conditions are commonly found in adolescents who are treated with ECT. While these conditions should not be used as a reason against using ECT, identifying these disorders is important for long-term treatment planning and for setting realistic treatment goals. These comorbid conditions may include anxiety disorders—generalized anxiety, social phobia and/or school-related phobia, post-traumatic stress disorder, and pervasive developmental disorders. The commonest comorbid conditions found among a group of adolescent patients with a primary diagnosis of MDD (n = 33) were 40% (n = 13) anxiety disorders and 20% (n = 7) with an autism spectrum disorder (19). Most adolescents with these and other comorbid disorders may respond well to ECT, but they often need a longer ECT course and ongoing pharmacotherapy and psychotherapy.

Premorbid Functioning

Premorbid functioning is an important factor in predicting treatment outcome. Patients with optimum social and emotional adjustment prior to illness-onset are more likely to achieve complete remission. However, a relatively large number of adolescents treated with ECT have long-standing symptoms, resulting in loss of normal development, and therefore have atypical premorbid functioning. Furthermore, many adolescents treated with ECT, who have been ill for a number of years, may have lost friends, have been unable to attend school, have experienced a decline in leisure activities, and have poor problem-solving skills. Therefore, while the assessment of premorbid functioning is important for setting up a realistic treatment outcome, the effect of a long-standing psychiatric disorder during an adolescent's key developmental period must not be ignored. Many adolescents require supportive psychotherapy, social skills training, or other interventions to make up for the time lost due to their long-standing psychiatric disorder.

Age of First Psychiatric Contact

The age at which the young patient first develops psychiatric problems, as suggested by the age of their first psychiatric contact, may have a prognostic implication. In the experience of one of the authors (NG), earlier age of first psychiatric contact (mean age 9.3 ± 4.7 years) predicted poorer treatment outcome compared to those with an older age at the time of their first psychiatric treatment/evaluation (12.2 ± 4.3 years) (19). Outcome in this study was defined on the basis of an estimate of global functioning. It may be hypothesized that earlier contact with psychiatric services is associated with treatment resistance because of a constellation of symptoms in this subgroup (possibly higher anxiety, impaired global function). However, an earlier age of psychiatric contact should by no means be regarded as a contraindication for ECT in youth who otherwise meet necessary criteria for the treatment.

Somatic Symptoms

Prominent physical symptoms, such as frequent or severe non-organic headaches, muscle or skeletal pain, and other somatic symptoms of anxiety, when associated with major depression, may predict a relatively poor outcome. Among adults treated with ECT, high levels of somatic anxiety have been found to predict a lower rate of sustained remission (33). Although studies in adolescents are lacking, adolescent patients with similar presentation appear to experience relapse, despite positive initial response to treatment, and may need a second or more treatment courses. In our unpublished case series of three adolescent patients, one male and two females (mean age = 16 years), all three patients were diagnosed with treatment-resistant depression and had a history of failure to respond to multiple and adequate medication trials, combined with psychotherapy. We found that two out of these three patients were receiving narcotic pain medications, prior to receiving ECT, due to the severe nature of their physical symptoms. On receiving ECT, all three experienced a positive response to the initial index ECT course. However, two of three patients relapsed upon follow-up. One male patient relapsed 3 to 4 months after the completion of the treatment; he subsequently decided to pursue non-traditional treatment (against medical advice, he decided to use medical marijuana). A female patient remained stable for approximately 9 months, stating that this was "the best that she had felt in years," but relapsed subsequently (she was receiving a repeat index course at the time of writing this case description). The third patient experienced improvement in her depression, although her somatic symptoms remained unchanged. We concluded that adolescents who suffer from prominent non-organic pain symptoms associated with major depression may not experience sustained remission and should be closely monitored for relapse, for up to a year after completing ECT. Continued pharmaco- and psychotherapy is recommended, while some may benefit from additional ECT.

In the absence of further data, prominent somatic symptoms associated with severe depression (or other Axis I diagnoses) in adolescents should not be regarded as a contraindication for ECT, but rather, as a clinical scenario with need for a comprehensive post-ECT treatment plan, including pharmacotherapy and psychotherapy and possibly additional ECT, if there is evidence for sufficient decline.

Intellectual and Other Developmental Disabilities

There is no evidence to suggest that intellectual disability or learning disability may compromise response to ECT. In a group of depressed adolescents diagnosed with MDD (n = 33), mental retardation was present in three cases, while six youth were in special education (including three youth with mental retardation). A 97% improvement rate with ECT was observed for the group as a whole (19).

Probably the most compelling data regarding the effectiveness of ECT in youth with mental retardation is based on its effective use for the treatment of severe self-injurious behaviors (SIB) (see Chapter 12, "ECT for Self-injurious Behavior"). Many of these patients who have been treated effectively are able to live at home, instead of being institutionalized, are able to attend educational or training programs, and are managed on relatively fewer psychotropic medications, which, unlike ECT, are commonly associated with serious metabolic and other side effects.

ASSESSMENT: PSYCHIATRY

A comprehensive psychiatric examination is an essential first step when considering treatment using ECT. The initial examination helps identify the primary diagnosis (whether the condition is known to respond to ECT), clarifies comorbid conditions, and elicits imminent risk, if present. This process also determines the target symptoms and provides the opportunity to delineate realistic treatment goals. Additionally, a thorough understanding of diagnoses helps with longer-term treatment planning. For instance, a youth with comorbid school phobia is likely to need extensive behavioral treatment, on completion of ECT, when his or her symptoms associated with the primary illness are better controlled. In addition to the diagnoses, assessment details should include family history (including suicide), past psychiatric history (history of suicide attempts, substance abuse, social functioning, coping skills), and past mental health treatment (the number, dosage, and duration of psychotropic medications and the type and duration of psychotherapy). These factors help to elucidate whether a patient meets criteria for treatment resistance or for imminent risk, as the case may be, and which medication and type of psychotherapy would be most appropriate upon completion of ECT. Information should be obtained from the parents and patients, past treatment providers, and potentially others, and from a thorough review of available medical charts.

The treatment-resistance criterion may be waived when illness-severity and/or safety concerns are paramount and waiting for response to additional treatments is likely to jeopardize the safety of the patient or prolong suffering (e.g., imminent suicidality, refusal to eat or drink, or inability to function). Similarly, prolonged waiting for treatment response in patients with catatonia, either when treating retarded or agitated forms, is generally not recommended, except when attempting a carefully monitored trial of a benzodiazepine. Symptoms such as inadequate fluid or nutritional intake, uncontrolled aggression (in agitated forms of illness), or signs and symptoms that suggest emergence of malignant catatonia (hemodynamic dysregulation, fever, rising levels of creatinine phosphokinase despite discontinuing any offending medication, altered consciousness) should all be regarded as evidence for an urgent evaluation for ECT. (For further details, refer to Chapter 11, "ECT for Catatonia in Autism.")

Objective documentation of symptom-severity must be included during the initial psychiatric evaluation to establish baseline-severity, during the ECT course and upon completion of treatment to document change in response to treatment. Commonly employed standardized rating scales for measuring depression may include the Children's Depression Rating Scale-Revised (CDRS-R, [40]) and the Hamilton Rating Scale (HRSD, [41]); to measure psychotic symptoms, depression, anxiety, and behavior, the Brief Psychiatric Rating Scale-Child (BPRS-C, [42]); for measuring cognition, Mini Mental Status Examination (MMSE, [43], or the Montreal Cognitive Assessment (MoCA, [44]); and to measure signs and symptoms of catatonia, the Bush Francis Catatonia Rating Scale (BFCRS, [45]). These measures should be repeated at regular intervals, possibly every one to two weeks over the treatment course. Most scales require no longer than a few minutes and may be completed using observation and information gathered from the patient and parents.

ASSESSMENT FOR ANESTHESIA

The medical assessment has a twofold purpose. The first is to identify any medical disorders that may impact the psychiatric diagnosis, and the second is to detect any medical condition that may interfere with the administration of ECT or anesthesia. The medical assessment should include a careful history, reviewing past documentation, a physical examination, and laboratory work up. Laboratory tests generally include complete blood counts (CBC), urine analysis (UA), toxicology studies, pregnancy test in females, thyroid function tests, EKG, EEG, and an MRI. Brain imaging is recommended to rule out any brain pathology that may increase the intracranial pressure during treatment. Although, in the past a brain tumor was considered an absolute contraindication for ECT, this is no longer the case, and successful treatment may be possible in some carefully selected cases, despite the presence of a brain tumor (46). (For additional details, see Chapter 6, "ECT in Young People with Comorbid Medical and Neurological Disorders.")

The oral cavity should be examined to identify any loose teeth or prostheses and to prevent the risk of aspiration. Most institutions require that every youth must be evaluated by an anesthesiologist to identify anesthesia-related risks and for any additional laboratory studies that may be recommended. Consultation with other specialties should be decided on a case-by-case basis.

NEUROPSYCHOLOGICAL ASSESSMENT

Knowledge about neuropsychological side effects associated with ECT in treatment refractory depression (TRD) in children is limited. However, there are studies of adults that have examined the potential neuropsychological side effects. It should be noted that the extent to which adult outcomes apply to children is unclear. In a recent meta-analysis of adult ECT patients, Semkovska et al. examined 24 neuropsychological outcomes from 84 studies (n = 2,981) across varying time frames relative to ECT initiation or completion (47). In order to better understand immediate, short-term, and long-term outcomes, the assessment periods were divided into three groups, based on the time-point of the assessments: within 0–3 days of final treatment (sub-acute), within 4–15 days of final treatment (short-term), and greater than 15 days after final treatment (long-term). The authors identified 22 tests that were commonly used across all studies, assessing domains of neuropsychological functioning that included attention and working memory, processing speed, short-term and long-term memory. In the sub-acute period, deficits in processing speed, attention/working memory, verbal memory, visual memory, and spatial problem solving were observed; however, recovery of function to baseline in all studies was observed by the short-term (4–15 day) evaluation period. For studies examining outcomes in the long term, recovery of function and performance were improved. With regard to outcomes in adolescents, Ghaziuddin et al. examined a sample of adolescents ranging in age from 13 to 18 years who were treated with ECT (48). Neuropsychological test performance was compared at three points in time: prior to ECT, within three weeks after ECT treatment was completed, and finally several months after final treatment. Comparison of pre-ECT to post-ECT testing within the first three weeks showed deficits in attention, verbal- and visual-delayed recall, and verbal fluency. However, complete recovery was observed during the second post-ECT testing. Similar to the adult studies cited above, there were no deficits in problem-solving ability, comparing the pre- and post-ECT testing sessions. More recently, Ghaziuddin, Dumas, and Hodges examined pre- and post-ECT cognitive functioning in a case-series of six subjects who underwent ECT treatment (35). In all but one subject, follow-up testing showed improved performance across domains, including an almost 1-standard deviation improvement in delayed verbal memory.

NEUROPSYCHOLOGICAL TEST BATTERY

Neuropsychological testing should be included as a part of a patient's routine clinical care in ECT treatment. Based on the above findings, pre-treatment testing should be completed shortly before treatment initiation. Follow-up testing should also occur within at least 6 months, and ideally again at 12 months. Neuropsychological findings can be used to assist with academic planning for adolescents and to determine if school curriculum should be modified to best meet the needs of the child. Unfortunately, many patients may not have insurance coverage for more than one evaluation within a 12-month period. In such cases, testing should be completed within the year, and a shorter-screening measure is recommended during follow-up appointments with his or her treating psychiatrist.

The neuropsychological battery should include measures related to general intellect, academic skills, attention, and working memory. Memory testing should include short-term and long-term recall, as well as delayed recognition. Mood and personality measures that specifically address depression should be administered, and a thorough clinical interview should be conducted. Autobiographical memory (AM) tests may be used to assess personal memories of events that occurred prior to ECT treatments. These tests are designed to measure autobiographical information related to personal events and to measure retrograde amnesia. However, it is noteworthy that there is increasing controversy regarding the use and interpretation of these measures in ECT protocols. AM testing has been controversial because instruments that have been developed to assess this type of memory were primarily developed for depressed patients undergoing ECT. Thus, there is no normative information on other populations, and it is unclear how AM may function in a heterogeneous sample. In addition, some have pointed out that depression in and of itself may contribute to variability to encode events efficiently for later recall (49). Although AM measures can be included in ECT batteries, interpretation should be approached cautiously.

Psychotropic Medications Administered During and on Completion of ECT

The Practice Parameters for the use of ECT in adolescents (American Academy of Child and Adolescent Psychiatry (AACAP) (50), the American Psychiatric Association (51), and clinicians who treat youth with ECT recommend that psychotropic medications, especially antidepressants, antipsychotic agents, and anti-epileptic drugs (AED) should be discontinued, whenever possible, during ECT (11). Frequently cited reasons are, first, that there is no rationale for continuing one or more agents that have failed to improve the symptoms, and second, that children may have a higher susceptibility for prolonged seizures during ECT. It should be noted, however, that the frequency of prolonged seizures during ECT have varied from rates as low as 0.4% (42 minors who were given 450 treatments (13) to a higher rate of 9.5% (11 minors who were given 135 treatments (11).

Findings from studies involving adults have also yielded mixed results about the outcome when ECT is combined with antidepressants. For instance, one adult study found that there was no effect on seizure duration, during the first ECT treatment, in a group that was treated with an SSRI (selective serotonin reuptake inhibitor) or a TCA (tricyclic antidepressant), compared to those who had not received these agents (52). On the other hand, another large adult study found evidence for prolonged seizures when SSRIs were combined with ECT and lower postictal suppression when SSRIs or mirtazapine were combined with ECT (53).

Based on the seizure-lowering properties of antipsychotic agents, it is generally recommended that this group of agents should be discontinued during ECT. Outside of ECT, a two- to fourfold higher rate of seizures have been reported in patients receiving these agents (54). Furthermore, antipsychotics may have a deleterious effect in patients with catatonia and/or SIB and may increase the risk for developing neuroleptic malignant syndrome (NMS) (see Chapters 11 and 12). Another potential risk of antipsychotic agents is the prolongation of the QTc interval (atrio-ventrical conduction) although, one adult study found that co-administration of these agents may be safe, at least in respect to the QTc interval (55).

Regarding lithium, earlier reports had suggested that concurrent use of lithium with ECT may increase the risk of delirium and prolonged seizures (56). However, more recent data indicate that lithium may be safely administered during ECT, although it may be beneficial to keep the serum level at the lower end of the therapeutic range (57). Holding the dose of lithium for approximately 12 to 18 hours prior to administering ECT may be an additional useful strategy. The same strategy may be used for antiepileptic mood stabilizers, which may either be discontinued during ECT, or be withheld for several hours prior to ECT.

Benzodiazepines can be safely used during the ECT course because these agents can be reversed using intravenous benzodiazepine receptor antagonist, flumazenil (also known as flumazepil), which has a rapid onset of action and can be administered during anesthesia. Additionally, benzodiazepines may have an additive therapeutic benefit (58) when administered to youth being treated for catatonia.

In addition to psychiatric medications, attention should be paid to the sedative agents used during anesthesia. One study found that the anticonvulsive properties of narcotic agents used (usually barbiturates) during anesthesia may interfere with treatment response, and lighter anesthesia may be associated with faster remission (59). (see Chapter 7, "Anesthesia," for additional details about the role of anesthesia in ECT.)

Psychotropic medication should be initiated to maintain clinical improvement. Although there are no data to guide the timing of this intervention, in the experience of the author (NG), medications can be introduced when the frequency of ECT has been titrated down from three times a week to twice or once a week.

PSYCHOTHERAPY DURING AND FOLLOWING ECT

There are no systematic data regarding the use of psychotherapy during ECT or on completion of the treatment. However, there is anecdotal evidence that supportive therapy is helpful during the treatment, and more intensive psychotherapy may be possible following the completion of ECT, when the adolescent may feel well enough to address additional symptoms or maladaptive behaviors (self-injury for emotional relief, school refusal, or specific phobias).

Given the absence of any data about the use of psychotherapy during ECT, the author (PG) has included the following excerpts from her experience in treating a young male.

CASE VIGNETTE

John (fictitious identifier) is a 13-year-old Caucasian male with a significant psychiatric history of two major depressive episodes, generalized anxiety and obsessive-compulsive disorders, accompanied by suicidal ideation and NSSI (non-suicidal self-injurious behaviors). Family history was remarkable for anxiety/mood disorders, suicidal attempts, and psychiatric hospitalizations. Following the unexpected death of a pet, John's functioning deteriorated. He was noted to improve somewhat in response to ongoing treatment, but he did not ever fully experience remission, spanning a 3-year period. Numerous medication trials were attempted (>30; including various agents/combinations). Per parental report, John had received antidepressants, mood stabilizers, antipsychotics, benzodiazepines, anticonvulsants, and psychosocial interventions (individual and family cognitive behavioral therapy) to no avail. Consequently, it was evident to John and his parents that both pharmacological and psychosocial interventions (the gold standard) had been unsuccessful in returning John to his baseline level of functioning.

Per parental report, 1½ years prior to initiating ECT, this treatment had been recommended by his psychiatrist. However, John and his parents did not accept the recommendation, and instead opted to focus on readjusting his medication regimen. When ECT was recommended for the second time, John's family was able to overcome their reservations and decided to proceed with this treatment. Factors that likely helped them accept ECT were that John was chronically suicidal, his depression accompanied by anxiety was severe, and he was significantly impaired across multiple settings, including home and school; his inability to attend school had resulted in home schooling for the past year and he had progressively withdrawn from family and friends. Altogether, John's unrelenting emotional distress became too much for the family, and they felt that they could no longer continue with conventional treatments.

As part of promoting engagement in treatment and rapport building, the psychotherapist (PG), inquired about his past treatment history. This identified that John had experienced difficulty in establishing rapport with previous treatment providers and in setting treatment goals. It was evident to the therapist that John was motivated to reengage in the public school system, indicating that he was ready to do whatever was necessary to overcome his depression and anxiety. It was also apparent that the symptoms had contributed to his downward spiral, impacting academic performance. It was noteworthy that despite being motivated initially, his motivation appeared to wax and wane over time, but his mother's presence and participation in therapy sessions appeared to energize him toward his treatment goals. To that end, the treatment approach was modified from an individual to a family CBT approach. Although John was able to adhere to psychotherapy homework assignments, his functioning continued to deteriorate. External reinforcements were used, such as a home based reward system contingent upon John's active engagement during and outside the psychotherapy session; however, there was only limited benefit. While therapy was being modified, his psychiatrist continued to make medication adjustments, also with no success. Finally, these factors, combined with the patient's past history of failure to respond to treatment over a 3-year period, resulted in John becoming a candidate for ECT.

Family CBT-focused cognitive restructuring was continued until ECT was initiated. Notably, at the first psychotherapy session, following his initial course of ECT, John appeared to be irritable and agitated. Also, John's mother expressed concern about his persistent sense of hopelessness. Psychosocial interventions implemented during the ECT course were modified from a more active to a supportive form of psychotherapy, and included strategies to improve behavioral activation and increase supportive networks.

As the treatment progressed, additional treatment goals were conceptualized, which included (1) medication adherence; (2) supportive family-based psychotherapy that included asking John to bring his favorite game to the therapy session (this strategy was used to focus on behavioral activation around social and physical activities); (3) re-engagement in the public-school setting; (4) and increasing social support, primarily via his extended family while maximizing existing peer relationships. However, this plan was revised once it became evident that John would not be able to attend school while undergoing ECT. Therefore, John returned to being homeschooled while the psychotherapist continued to work with school officials and the family to initiate an Individualized Education Plan (IEP). The IEP allowed John to qualify under the special education services available for children and adolescents who experience educational problems secondary to a health condition.

By the end of his ECT course, John was able to transition back to the public school system, with special accommodations that permitted him a reduced class schedule (i.e., a shorter day at school) and reduced expectations for class and homework assignments. Additionally, John was excused for a temporary period from any course work that would require memorizing large amounts of information.

John had an excellent overall response to ECT (14 bilateral treatments), pharmacotherapy (sertraline, lithium, and lamotrigine) and psychotherapy. He was euthymic at his last recorded follow-up appointment at 17 months after the completion of ECT. However, school-related anxiety persisted. As a result, he was enrolled in a combined educational program, which included a combination of home-based (academic classes) and additional in-school classes (non-academic classes).

ECT DEVICES

The commonly used devices in United States are the Thymatron and MECTA. Both devices deliver a brief-pulse electrical stimulus via electrodes placed on the patient's head to induce a generalized brain seizure. The electrodes may be placed bilaterally (BL) or unilaterally (UL). The electrodes are applied to opposing temporal fossae during bilateral temporal placement (BL) or to the forehead region in bifrontal BL application. During UL placement, both electrodes are placed on the non-dominant side of the head (non-dominant for language), which corresponds to the right side of the brain in the majority of patients; one electrode is placed in the right temporal fossa, while a second electrode is placed on the right parietal prominence.

The devices deliver a brief-pulse electrical output that can be adjusted using several parameters (duration, frequency, pulse-width, and the amplitude of the current) and have the provision for EEG recording. The capability of adjusting multiple electrical parameters is considered an important feature of each device. Additionally, the ability to record EEG is a considerable advancement, as it allows the exact duration of the seizure to be determined, thereby avoiding unnecessarily high electrical dosages and terminating a prolonged seizure in a timely manner.

THE PROCEDURE

The recommended standard of care is that youth who receive ECT should be hospitalized prior to the procedure. This allows for completion of the required pre-ECT workup and initiation of the index course. However, treatment may be initiated on an outpatient basis under exceptional circumstances, where the risk of withholding the treatment may outweigh the risks of outpatient treatment.

On the night prior to treatment, the child remains nil per os (NPO) following dinner. Medications may be administered until the time for treatment, but only a sip of water may be permitted. Early next morning, the patient is transported with the help of a nurse to a surgical suite (an area where patients undergo minor surgical procedures); parents may accompany, if they so wish, but are not allowed to witness the actual procedure (this is a common institutional policy in the majority of hospitals and applies to surgical and other medical procedures). An intravenous line is placed by an anesthesiology staff member, and the child is wheeled into the treatment room. The treatment team comprises one or two psychiatrists (one staff psychiatrist and one resident/ fellow) and nurse anesthetists, who are supervised by an anesthesiologist. The patient is oxygenated, vital signs are continuously monitored, and medications used for the induction of anesthesia are injected in rapid succession via the IV line, keeping in mind that all agents used have a short half-life and therefore there is a time constraint (see Chapter 7, "Anesthesia"). Electrical parameters are adjusted based on age, gender, and previous treatments. BL electrode placement, where electrodes are symmetrically placed in the two temporal fossae, is preferred over other types of electrode placement because of greater predictability of response, and it is considered the standard against which other types of electrode placements are assessed (60). There is evidence, albeit in older patients, that time to relapse and rehospitalization may be longer in patients treated with BL placement compared with other types of electrode placement (61). After the completion of the treatment, usually completed within 20 minutes or so, the patient is moved to the recovery area, where he or she is closely supervised for vital signs, signs of agitation, nausea, or vomiting. Children who are hospitalized for their index course return to the ward, whereas patients on a taper-down treatment schedule, who are usually outpatients, are discharged to the care of their family with a schedule given for their next appointment.

OBSERVATION OF THE PROCEDURE: A PSYCHOLOGIST'S PERSONAL EXPERIENCE (AUTHOR PG)

"As a child psychologist who had no prior experience of ECT, observing the procedure was educational and allayed many unfounded misconceptions.

Prior to this opportunity, I had envisioned that the patient would experience violent and unpredictable movements. I wondered to myself whether I would ever be comfortable enough to refer a patient for ECT, let alone a child. I soon realized that my concerns were not based on any real knowledge about ECT or whether this treatment could actually help my patient. My patient, John, who is described in an earlier section of this chapter, was being considered for this treatment at the time. As I saw the first patient being wheeled in for treatment, I felt my heart race. The treating psychiatrist (NG) provided a commentary to help me learn about the procedure, the rationale of each step, and the treatment safeguards. To my relief, I quickly overcame my initial unease, especially when it became clear that the patient was asleep, looked comfortable, and did not experience any severe or distressing movements. In fact, my sense of ease turned to surprise when an imperceptible flicker of the patient's foot was referred to as the *seizure*. I subsequently observed numerous treatments (10 in all) and felt that I was amply prepared to help John and his family accept this treatment and would be able to answer their questions."

MAINTENANCE AND CONTINUATION ECT

Continuation ECT (C-ECT) is defined as ECT administered during a 6-month period after the completion of an index course, while maintenance treatment (M-ECT) is ECT given beyond the 6-month period. One major limitation of ECT is that, despite being a highly effective treatment for an acute illness episode, it does not appear to prevent relapse. C-ECT, on the other hand, has been shown to achieve and prolong remission and does not have significant adverse effects on cognition, probably due to the longer intervals between treatments (62).

Although there are limited data about the use of C-ECT and M-ECT in minors, these data suggest that C-ECT and/or M-ECT may be helpful in the treatment of SIB/catatonia (63) and in the treatment of schizophrenia (64) (see Chapter 12, "ECT for Self-injurious Behavior," and Chapter 10, "ECT for Schizophrenia Spectrum Disorders"). In regards with treatment resistant depression, Ghaziuddin and colleagues (2011) found that five out of a group of six adolescents (age range = 14–17 years) were able to achieve their premorbid functioning using C-ECT and/or M-ECT combined with pharmacotherapy and psychotherapy. Based on comparison of pre and post-ECT neuropsychological testing, no significant cognitive or other adverse effects were detected. In fact, a trend toward improved auditory and verbal memory was noted, which was hypothesized as being secondary to the absence of mood symptoms (35).

FOLLOW-UP

Adolescents who are treated with ECT should receive careful follow-up, both during hospitalization and during the outpatient treatment. The frequency of outpatient visits are generally based on the frequency of ECT; a patient who receives weekly ECT would likely need to be seen once every other week, while more frequent visits would be necessary if the treatments were more frequent. Key components of a follow-up visit should include close monitoring of symptoms, including the target symptoms identified prior to ECT (subjective and objective measures; information gathered from the youth and an adult caregiver), using standardized rating scales to measure mood, anxiety, suicidality, cognition, or any other symptom; record side effects of ECT or of the psychotropic agent; and identify any evidence of treatment emergent-hypomania. Although frank hypomania is rare, irritability and disinhibition are frequently seen. ECT should be continued until remission or until the symptoms have plateaued. Neuropsychological testing should be repeated after the completion of ECT. Ideally, testing is recommended immediately upon completion of the index course (for making educational adjustments) and repeated between 3 and 6 months after completion of the course (50). Treatment adjustments should be made promptly to prevent relapse. Some adolescents may benefit from an additional course of ECT, depending on the severity of their past illness and current symptomatology.

CONCLUSION

ECT can be used safely and effectively for a selected group of pre pubertal children and adolescents who meet the diagnostic criteria for severe Axis I disorders. It is essential that physicians and allied mental health professionals have adequate training and experience for the optimum use of this powerful treatment modality.

QUESTIONS AND ANSWERS

1. *What are the steps after the decision to treat with ECT has been made?*

   The patient will be seen by two or three child psychiatrists. The number of additional consults is based on state and/or institutional guidelines. The parents/legal guardian will be asked to sign a consent document, while the minor patient will give assent (see Chapter 4, "Ethical and Consent Aspects"). The patient will also receive laboratory tests, including brain imaging in most cases.

2. *Must every child be hospitalized when ECT is initiated?*

   This is generally desirable for both medical reasons (e.g., laboratory tests and consultation with other specialists may be needed) and psychiatric reasons (these patients are generally severely ill and require careful monitoring). However, there may be exceptions when the need for ECT may supersede the need for hospitalization.

3. *Will the child return to his or her pre-illness baseline after completion of ECT?*

   There is a great deal of variability in outcome among different patients. However, the majority of patients appear to improve. Many continue to improve after completion of ECT, usually while receiving psychotherapy and medications. Some experts believe that patients treated with ECT often become more responsive to previously tried medications.

DISCLOSURES

Dr. Neera Ghaziuddin has no conflicts to disclose. She is funded, for unrelated studies, by the Centers for Disease Control (CDC) and receives institutional funding from the University of Michigan.

Dr. Elise Hodges has no conflicts to disclose. She is funded by the National Institutes of Health (NIH). Grant support includes the following:

1. National Institutes of Health, NIDDKS (5U01DK066174). "Chronic Kidney Disease in Children Study (CKiD)." Co-Investigator 9/2003-7/2013 ($47,900 direct costs annually).
2. National Institutes of Health (R01 HL105999). "Sleep-disordered Breathing and CPAP after Adenotonsillectomy in Children." Co-Investigator 12/2011-12-2016 ($411,459 direct cost annually).

Dr. Polly Gipson has no conflicts of interest to disclose. She is funded by a Centers for Disease Control (CDC), Prevention grant and a Substance Abuse and Mental Health Services Administration (SAMHSA) grant (start date July 1, 2013); all funding is unrelated to this chapter.

REFERENCES

1. Ghaziuddin N, Kaza M, Ghazi N, King C, Walter G, Rey JM. Electroconvulsive therapy for minors: experiences and attitudes of child psychiatrists and psychologists. *J ECT*. 2001 Jun;17(2):109.
2. Walter G, Rey JM, Starling J. Experience, knowledge and attitudes of child psychiatrists regarding electroconvulsive therapy in the young. *AustNZ J Psychiat*. 1997 Oct;31(5):676.

3. Walter G, Rey JM. How fixed are child psychiatrists' views about ECT in the young? *J ECT*. 2003 Jun;19(2):88.
4. Dinwiddie SH, Spitz D. Resident education in electroconvulsive therapy. *J ECT*. 2010 Dec;26(4):310–6.
5. Pandya M, Pozuelo L, Malone D. Electroconvulsive therapy: what the internist needs to know. *Cleveland Clin J Med*. [Research Support, Non-U.S. Gov't Review]. 2007 Sep;74(9):679–85.
6. Oldewening K, Lange RT, Willan S, Strangway C, Kang N, Iverson GL. Effects of an education training program on attitudes to electroconvulsive therapy. *J ECT*. 2007 Jun;23(2):82–8.
7. Dolenc TJ, Philbrick KL. Achieving competency in electroconvulsive therapy: a model curriculum. *Acad Psychiatr*. 2007 Jan-Feb;31(1):65–7.
8. Parmar R. Attitudes of child psychiatrists to electroconvulsive therapy. *Psychiat Bull*. 1993;17:12–3.
9. Sutker PB, Adams HE, eds. Mood disorders: Unipolar and bipolar. *Comprehensive Handbook of Psychopathology*. Springer-Verlag New York, LLC; 2001:277–308.
10. Paillere-Martinot ML, Zivi A, Basquin M. [Use of electroconvulsive therapy in adolescence]. *Encephale*.[English Abstract Review]. 1990 Sep-Oct;16(5):399–404.
11. Ghaziuddin N, King CA, Naylor MW, Ghaziuddin M, Chaudhary N, Giordani B, et al. Electroconvulsive treatment in adolescents with pharmacotherapy-refractory depression. *J Child Adol Psychop*. [Clinical Trial]. 1996;6(4):259–71.
12. Moise FN, Petrides G. Case study: electroconvulsive therapy in adolescents. *J Am Acad Child Adol Psychiat*. 1996 Mar;35(3):312–8.
13. Walter G, Rey JM. An epidemiological study of the use of ECT in adolescents. *J Am Acad Child Adol Psychiat*. [Research Support, Non-U.S. Gov't]. 1997 Jun;36(6):809–15.
14. Cohen D, Paillere-Martinot ML, Basquin M. Use of electroconvulsive therapy in adolescents. *Convulsive Therapy*. 1997 Mar;13(1):25–31.
15. Willoughby CL, Hradek EA, Richards NR. Use of electroconvulsive therapy with children: an overview and case report. *J Child Adol Psychiat Nurs*.[Case Reports Review]. 1997 Jul-Sep;10(3):11–7.
16. Taieb O, Flament MF, Chevret S, Jeammet P, Allilaire JF, Mazet P, et al. Clinical relevance of electroconvulsive therapy (ECT) in adolescents with severe mood disorder: evidence from a follow-up study. *Eur Psychiatry*.[Research Support, Non-U.S. Gov't Validation Studies]. 2002 Jul;17(4):206–12.
17. Hegeman JM, Doesborgh SJC, van Niel MC, van Megen HJGM. [The efficacy of electroconvulsive therapy in adolescents. A restrospective study]. *Tijdschrift voor Psychiatrie*. [English Abstract]. 2008;50(1):23–31.
18. Shoirah H, Hamoda HM. Electroconvulsive therapy in children and adolescents. *Expert Rev Neurother*. [Research Support, Non-U.S. Gov't Review]. 2011 Jan;11(1):127–37.
19. Ghaziuddin N. Treatment Resistant Depression in Adolescents in Symposium, Treatment Resistant Depression: A Roadmap for Effective Care (Chair: Greden JF). American Psychiatric Association; 2011; Honolulu, Hawaii.
20. Bloch Y, Levcovitch Y, Bloch AM, Mendlovic S, Ratzoni G. Electroconvulsive therapy in adolescents: similarities to and differences from adults. *J Am Acad Child Adol Psychiat*. [Comparative Study Evaluation Studies]. 2001 Nov;40(11):1332–6.

21. Bertagnoli MW, Borchardt CM. A review of ECT for children and adolescents. *J Am Acad Child Adol Psychiat.* [Case Reports Review]. 1990 Mar;29(2):302–7.
22. Bloch Y, Sobol D, Levkovitz Y, Kron S, Ratzoni G. Reasons for referral for electroconvulsive therapy: a comparison between adolescents and adults. *Australas Psychiatry.* [Comparative Study Research Support, Non-U.S. Gov't]. 2008 Jun;16(3):191–4.
23. Wood JH, Chambers M, White SJ. Nurses' knowledge of and attitude to electroconvulsive therapy. *J ECT.* 2007 Dec;23(4):251–4.
24. Leslie van Daalen-Smith C. Waiting for oblivion: women's experiences with electroshock. *Iss Ment Health Nu.* 2011;32(7):457–72.
25. Kavanagh A, McLoughlin DM. Electroconvulsive therapy and nursing care. *Brit J Nursing.* [Review]. 1372 1374-7, 2009 Dec 10-2010 Jan 13;18(22):1370.
26. Lamont S, Brunero S, Barclay C, Wijeratne C. Evaluation of an electroconvulsive therapy service in a general hospital. *Int J Ment Health Nu.* 2011 Jun;20(3):223–9.
27. Carr ME, Jr., Woods JW. Electroconvulsive therapy in a patient with unsuspected pheochromocytoma. *Southern Med J.*[Case Reports]. 1985 May;78(5):613–5.
28. Dressler DM, Folk J. The treatment of depression with ECT in the presence of brain tumor. *Am J Psychiat.* [Case Reports]. 1975 Dec;132(12):1320–1.
29. Giltay EJ, Kho KH, Keijzer LTM, Leijenaar M, van Schaick HW, Blansjaar BA. Electroconvulsive therapy (ECT) in a patient with a dual-chamber sensing, VDDR pacemaker. *J ECT.* [Case Reports]. 2005 Mar;21(1):35–8.
30. Bader GM, Silk KR, Dequardo JR, Tandon R. Electroconvulsive therapy and intracranial aneurysm. *Convulsive Therapy.* [Case Reports]. 1995 Jun;11(2):139–43.
31. Maltbie AA, Wingfield MS, Volow MR, Weiner RD, Sullivan JL, Cavenar JO, Jr. Electroconvulsive therapy in the presence of brain tumor. Case reports and an evaluation of risk. *J Nerv Ment Dis.* [Case Reports]. 1980 Jul;168(7):400–5.
32. Ghaziuddin N, DeQuardo JR, Ghaziuddin M, King CA. Electroconvulsive treatment of a bipolar adolescent postcraniotomy for brain stem astrocytoma. *J Child Adol Psychop.* [Case Reports]. 1999;9(1):63–9.
33. Rasmussen KG, Snyder KA, Knapp RG, Mueller M, Yim E, Husain MM, et al. Relationship between somatization and remission with ECT. *Psychiat Res.* [Research Support, U.S. Gov't, P.H.S.]. 2004 Dec 30;129(3):293–5.
34. Fink M. ECT in anxiety: an appraisal. *Am J Psychother.* 1982 Jul;36(3):371–8.
35. Ghaziuddin N, Dumas S, Hodges E. Use of continuation or maintenance electroconvulsive therapy in adolescents with severe treatment-resistant depression. *J ECT.* 2011 Jun;27(2):168–74.
36. Nunes EV, Deliyannides D, Donovan S, McGrath PJ. The management of treatment resistance in depressed patients with substance use disorders. *Psychiat Clin N Am.* [Case Reports Research Support, U.S. Gov't, P.H.S. Review]. 1996 Jun;19(2):311–27.
37. Flint V, Hill-Johnes S. How effective is ECT for those with borderline personality disorder? *Nursing NZ.* [Case Reports Review]. 2008 Sep;14(9):12–4.
38. Thakur A, Jagadheesan K, Dutta S, Sinha VK. Incidence of catatonia in children and adolescents in a paediatric psychiatric clinic. *Aust NZ J Psychiat.* 2003 Apr;37(2):200–3.

39. Rey JM, Walter G. Half a century of ECT use in young people. *Am JPsychiat.* [Review]. 1997 May;154(5):595–602.
40. Poznanski EO, Grossman JA, Buchsbaum Y, Banegas M, Freeman L, Gibbons R. Preliminary studies of the reliability and validity of the children's depression rating scale. *J Am Acad Child Psychiat.* [Research Support, U.S. Gov't, P.H.S.]. 1984 Mar;23(2):191–7.
41. Hamilton M. A rating scale for depression. *J Neurol Neurosur Ps.* 1960;23:56–62.
42. Overall JE, Pfefferbaum B. The Brief Psychiatric Rating Scale for Children. *Psychopharmacol Bull.* [Research Support, U.S. Gov't, P.H.S.]. 1982 Apr;18(2):10–6.
43. Folstein M, Folstien S, McHugh P. "Mini-mental state": a practical method for grading the cognitive state of patients for the clinician. *J Psychiat Res.* 1975;12(3):189–98.
44. Nasreddine Z, Phillips N, Bedirian V, Charbonneau S, Whitehead V, Collin I, et al. The Montreal Cognitive Assessment, MoCA: a brief screening tool for mild cognitive impairment. *J Am Geriatric Soc.* 2005;53(4):695–9.
45. Bush G, Fink M, Petrides G, Dowling A. Catatonia. I. Rating scale and standardized examination. *Acta Psychiatrica Scandinavica.* 1996;93(2):129–36.
46. Patkar AA, Hill KP, Weinstein SP, Schwartz SL. ECT in the presence of brain tumor and increased intracranial pressure: evaluation and reduction of risk. *J ECT.* [Case Reports]. 2000 Jun;16(2):189–97.
47. Semkovska M, McLoughlin DM. Objective cognitive performance associated with electroconvulsive therapy for depression: a systematic review and meta-analysis. *Biol Psychiat.* 2010;68(6):568–77.
48. Ghaziuddin N, Laughrin D, Giordani B. Cognitive side effects of electroconvulsive therapy in adolescents. *J Child Adolt Psychop.* 2000;10(4):269.
49. Semkovska M, Noone M, et al. Measuring consistency of autobiographical memory recall in depression. *Psychiat Res.* 2012;197(1–2):41–48.
50. Ghaziuddin N, Kutcher SP, Knapp P, American Academy of C, Adolescent Psychiatry Work Group on Quality I. Summary of the practice parameter for the use of electroconvulsive therapy with adolescents. *J Am Acad Child Adol Psychiat.* 2004 Jan;43(1):119–22.
51. Coffey CE, Weiner RD, eds. *The Practice of Electroconvulsive Therapy: Recommendations for Treatment, Training and Privileging: A Task Force Report of The American Psychiatric Association.* 2nd ed. American Psychiatric Association; 2002; Washington, DC: 117–354.
52. Dursun SM, Patel JK, Drybala T, Shinkwin R, Drybala G, Reveley MA. Effects of antidepressant treatments on first-ECT seizure duration in depression. *Prog Neuro-Psychoph.* [Clinical Trial Comparative Study Controlled Clinical Trial Research Support, Non-U.S. Gov't]. 2001 Feb;25(2):437–43.
53. Baghai TC, Marcuse A, Brosch M, Schule C, Eser D, Nothdurfter C, et al. The influence of concomitant antidepressant medication on safety, tolerability and clinical effectiveness of electroconvulsive therapy. *World J Biol Psychiat.* 2006;7(2):82–90.
54. Steinert T, Baier H, Froscher W, Jandl M. [Epileptic seizures during treatment with antidepressants and neuroleptics]. *Fortschritte der Neurologie-Psychiatrie.* [English Abstract Review]. 2011 Mar;79(3):138–43.
55. Oulis P, Florakis A, Markatou M, Tzanoulinos G, Masdrakis VG. Corrected QT interval changes during electroconvulsive therapy-antidepressants-atypical

antipsychotics coadministration: safety issues. *J ECT*. [Case Reports]. 2011 Mar;27(1):e4–6.

56. Sartorius A, Wolf J, Henn FA. Lithium and ECT—concurrent use still demands attention: three case reports. *World J Biol Psychiat*. [Case Reports]. 2005;6(2):121–4.
57. Thirthalli J, Harish T, Gangadhar BN. A prospective comparative study of interaction between lithium and modified electroconvulsive therapy. *World J Biol Psychiat*. [Comparative Study]. 2011 Mar;12(2):149–55.
58. Petrides G, Divadeenam KM, Bush G, Francis A. Synergism of lorazepam and electroconvulsive therapy in the treatment of catatonia. *Biol Psychiat*. [Case Reports Clinical Trial]. 1997 Sep 1;42(5):375–81.
59. Bundy BD, Hewer W, Andres F-J, Gass P, Sartorius A. Influence of anesthetic drugs and concurrent psychiatric medication on seizure adequacy during electroconvulsive therapy. *J Clin Psychiat*. [Comparative Study]. 2010 Jun;71(6):775–7.
60. Kellner CH, Tobias KG, Wiegand J. Electrode placement in electroconvulsive therapy (ECT): A review of the literature. *J ECT*. [Review]. 2010 Sep;26(3):175–80.
61. Little JD, Munday J, Atkins MR, Khalid A. Does electrode placement predict time to rehospitalization? *J ECT*. 2004 Dec;20(4):213–8.
62. Trevino K, McClintock SM, Husain MM. A review of continuation electroconvulsive therapy: application, safety, and efficacy. *J ECT*. [Review]. 2010 Sep;26(3):186–95.
63. Wachtel LE, Hermida A, Dhossche DM. Maintenance electroconvulsive therapy in autistic catatonia: a case series review. *Progress in Neuro Psychopharmacology & Biological Psychiatry*. 2010;34(4):581–7.
64. Consoli A, Boulicot V, Cornic F, Fossati P, Barbeau M, Cohen D. Moderate clinical improvement with maintenance ECT in a 17-year-old boy with intractable catatonic schizophrenia. *Eur Child Adoles Psy*. [Case Reports]. 2009 Apr;18(4):250–4.

CHAPTER 6

ECT in Youth with Comorbid Medical and Neurological Disorders

DANIEL F. MAIXNER

KEY POINTS

- ECT is a safe and an effective in numerous medical and neurological conditions.
- There are no absolute medical or neurological contraindications to ECT.
- Risk factors should be thoroughly assessed prior to initiating treatment and documented in the patient record.
- Pre-ECT physical examinations should focus particularly on the cardiovascular, neurological, and pulmonary systems.
- Routine laboratory tests prior to ECT typically include complete blood count (CBC), metabolic profile, thyroid and liver functions, pregnancy test, and toxicology screen for substance abuse. EEG, brain scan, and any additional tests should be ordered based on the medical history and physical examination.
- Collaboration with medical, anesthesiology, and neurology specialists is important in managing the complex ECT patient.
- During ECT, most psychotropic agents are typically reduced or discontinued. Some medications may have utility during ECT when severe acute symptoms of mania, psychosis, or agitation are present.
- Non-psychotropic medications for comorbid medical conditions or agents used to manage ECT side effects may be continued during an ECT course.

OVERVIEW

In general, there are no *absolute* contraindications to administer electroconvulsive therapy (ECT). ECT is deemed extremely safe, and in studies involving adults, the estimated mortality is as low as 2 deaths per 100,000 treatments (1, 2). This mortality rate is comparable to estimated mortality rates of 1.3 to 3.7 deaths per 100,000 general anesthesia inductions (3, 4). However, it is important to manage medical and neurological comorbidities during an ECT course, and this is most effectively done when the diagnoses are made prior to initiating treatment. These comorbid conditions impact the safe administration of ECT and allow the treatment team to adjust, add, taper, or discontinue any psychiatric or medical medications before or during an ECT course. In addition, medical conditions may require special anesthesia considerations (covered in Chapter 7, "Anesthesia"), medical assessments, and collaboration with other specialists prior to ECT.

This chapter includes a discussion of the pre-ECT medical evaluation and the essential components of obtaining a thorough medical and family medical history for any patient being considered for treatment. Also included is the literature about known neurological and medical conditions in patients treated with ECT. Knowledge of complex medical patients who have been successfully treated with ECT is primarily derived from case reports and case series. Nevertheless, these reports are an important source of data regarding the safe administration of ECT in the presence of medical disorders. Finally, the chapter includes a section on the management of medical and psychiatric medications during a course of ECT. [It should be noted that terms such as "children," "youth," and "minors" are used interchangeably and refer to patients younger than 18 years. "Adolescents" refers to individuals who range in age from 12 to 18 years, whereas pre-pubertal children are those below age 12. Due to paucity of data in pre-pubertal children, the majority of the information presented in this chapter is based on experience with adolescents.]

PRE-ECT EVALUATION

General Considerations

The first step during the pre-ECT assessment should focus on identifying any known medical disorders and determining if ECT treatment is optimum and can be safely administered. The medical record should fully document the history and medical decision-making. To ensure thoroughness, medical record templates can be developed to include critical checklists of important comorbidities that should be routinely reviewed, such as history of a seizure disorder, head trauma, and so on. Other pediatric specialists should be consulted to strategize and assist in managing medical disorders and to reduce the risks of the procedure.

Physical Examination

A complete physical examination is necessary with an emphasis on systems that are most critical for ECT treatment. Due to the administration of anesthesia, the induction of a seizure, and the cardiovascular effects of ECT, special attention should be given to the neurological, cardiovascular, and pulmonary systems (5).

Laboratory Testing

Laboratory tests should be completed prior to ECT and are ordered based on active medical problems and any suspected diagnoses that may arise after obtaining a thorough medical history. Typically, a complete blood count (CBC), basic metabolic panel, and electrocardiogram should be completed (6). Other tests are optional and include thyroid-stimulating hormone, chest X-ray, drug levels (e.g., lithium), liver function tests, neuropsychological tests, and neuroimaging. Spinal X-rays are no longer considered mandatory and should be reserved for those with significant musculoskeletal disease or injury. Youth with mental retardation or autism referred for ECT may have a markedly higher prevalence of seizures (7). In these cases, screening for seizures with an electroencephalogram (EEG) is appropriate.

ECT USE WITH COMORBID MEDICAL CONDITIONS

There is very limited literature about the use of ECT in children or adolescents with comorbid medical or a neurological disorders. The majority of the data are derived from the use of ECT in comorbid conditions in adult patients. However, these data are an important source of information and provide vital guidance to child and adolescent psychiatrists in managing younger patients.

Pulmonary Disease

Common pulmonary conditions that may add risk to respiratory depression include asthma, obstructive sleep apnea, chronic obstructive pulmonary disease, and pneumonia.

The most common pulmonary condition in youth is asthma. With anesthesia during ECT, breathing is assisted and monitored closely. ECT appears to be safe in this situation, as evidenced by a retrospective study of 34 adult patients in which only 12% (four patients) experienced exacerbations of their asthma on a total of five occasions (8). These episodes responded to standard treatment medications and all patients were able to successfully complete their course of ECT.

Diabetes

Psychiatric patients who have diabetes are often treated with ECT. In a study of type II diabetic patients pre- and post-ECT, glycemic control showed no major change (9). Typically, recommendations for type I diabetic patients include checking blood glucose prior to treatment and treating patients first or early during the ECT schedule since they are not allowed food or drink overnight. In addition, insulin can either be held until after ECT or can be administered with a split dosage schedule. Since hypoglycemia contributes to risk of seizures, an intravenous glucose solution can be used instead of saline. For extremely brittle diabetic patients, collaboration with a pediatric or endocrine specialist may be warranted.

Cardiovascular Disease

Given the stress on the cardiovascular system during ECT, history-taking should screen for hypertension, coronary artery disease, heart failure, arrhythmias, and use of pacemaker. Physiological changes during ECT include a sharp parasympathetic vagal outflow with the ECT stimulation that can induce bradycardia and a brief asystole. Anticholinergic agents such as glycopyrrolate or atropine are given pre-ECT, to prevent or limit this response. A sympathetic surge during the seizure is associated with tachycardia and elevations in blood pressure. Post-ictal heart rate and blood pressure then drop rapidly (10). Patients with hypertension have a more pronounced blood pressure elevation than normotensive patients (11). Although hypertension was believed to be rare in children and adolescents, evidence now suggests that the prevalence of high blood pressure in this age group is on the rise (12, 13). Thus, preexisting hypertension, irrespective of age, will be adversely affected by elevated blood pressure due to the physiological responses of ECT.

Generally, patients with known cardiac conditions have a higher cardiovascular risk with ECT (14). However, patients with significant cardiovascular conditions and hypertension can be safely treated, while carefully monitoring their blood pressure and by controlling elevated blood pressure before and during ECT. Commonly, patients should receive their antihypertensive medications before ECT. Despite the known physiological burden on the cardiovascular system, ECT has been safely administered post-myocardial infarction (15, 16). Adult patients with known cardiac and abdominal aortic aneurysms have also been treated successfully with ECT, following perioperative administration of antihypertensive agents for tachycardia and for elevated blood pressure. Mueller et al. (17) had reviewed 10 patients with aortic valve stenosis treated with ECT who did not experience any complications.

ECT may be safely administered to patients with implanted cardiac devices, such as pacemakers and cardioverter defibrillators (18–20). In the largest retrospective study of adult ECT patients, 26 patients with a pacemaker and three with implantable defibrillators were treated successfully. Complications included one patient with a pacemaker who experienced an episode of supraventricular tachycardia without severe hemodynamic instability. This patient required acute treatment with amiodarone and esmolol and was monitored for 24 hours in a coronary care unit. However, he went on to receive 24 more ECTs without complications. Inhibition or activation of pacemakers in demand mode could theoretically occur in reaction to myopotentials from skeletal muscle activity, such as fasciculations during anesthesia-induction with succinylcholine. If there is inhibition of the pacemaker during ECT, a magnet may be placed over the generator to switch to asynchronous mode (19). However, in another retrospective study of 10 adults with pacemakers, it was found that ECT could be administered safely without any additional precautions, other than routine ECG monitoring (21). With cardioverter defibrillators, deactivation of the device pre-ECT treatment is the most common practice to avoid risk of inappropriate discharges, resulting in discomfort to the patient or a ventricular dysrhythmia during normal rhythm. Consultation with a cardiologist to review the type of device and management strategies is recommended (19).

Pregnancy

Pregnant adolescent girls and adult women with severe psychiatric disorders face daunting treatment choices. The main consideration for an adolescent who is pregnant and needs to be treated with ECT is the safety of both mother and baby. Collaboration with obstetric specialists is strongly recommended. Among several challenges faced by pregnant patients, complications may include exposure to psychotropic agents and the risk of teratogenic complications, neonatal toxicity, and postnatal behavioral problems (22). Given these issues with medications, ECT may be a reasonable treatment option. However, the experience with treating pregnant adolescents with ECT is limited to one reported case in a 16-year-old with history of depression, psychosis, and dangerous behaviors; she was successfully treated with ECT (23). However, there is considerably more adult literature, spanning 65 years with a total of 339 cases, where ECT was safely administered during pregnancy. In a literature review of ECT in pregnancy from 1941 to 2007, 78% of the reported cases resulted in at least partial remission of symptoms. There were 25 fetal or neonatal complications. In many cases, the abnormality likely arose months after ECT, and the events included bradycardia and/or decelerations, periotonitis, club foot, prematurity, congential pulmonary cysts, congenital blindness, great vessel transposition, aorta coarctation, cortical infarcts, anencephaly, VATER syndrome, mental retardation, and death. In eleven cases of reported neonatal or fetal death, only one was felt to be a direct result of ECT. This death occurred in the context of status epilepticus in the mother secondary to ECT (24). Due to the efficacy and safety of ECT, the APA ECT Task Force (2001) (6) has recommended that ECT can be administered in all three trimesters for severe pre-partum psychiatric disorders.

Management of the pregnant ECT patient may include the need to intubate in late pregnancy due to the risk of aspiration by an expanding uterus, causing upward pressure on the stomach. Elevation of the right hip may avoid aortocaval compression and hypotension. After 14 weeks gestational age, non-invasive fetal heart monitoring and collaboration with an obstetric specialist are routinely recommended at each treatment, at both pre- and post-ECT.

NEUROLOGICAL COMORBIDITY

Some neurological conditions can either mimic or contribute to psychiatric illness, while others may add to the risk of complications during ECT. Thus, potential ECT patients should be screened for epilepsy, space-occupying lesions, stroke, arteriovenous malformations, aneurysms, migraines, and ventricular shunts; special care is necessary when considering ECT in patients with these conditions. Physiological change during ECT includes an increased intracranial pressure during the procedure, which places the patient at an added risk for herniation of the brain stem if there is a space-occupying lesion, or may result in a bleed if there is a susceptible lesion.

Epilepsy

Seizure disorders require careful management. Although it is not a reason to deny ECT, a child or the adolescent patient may be receiving an anticonvulsant, which in turn may interfere with a therapeutic seizure. With proper planning and precautions, ECT can be administered effectively and safely in these youth with seizure disorders.

Based on the literature, albeit limited, patients with psychiatric disorders comorbid with epilepsy may be safely treated with ECT. In the largest published report, Lunde et al. (25) reviewed their experience in treating 43 epilepsy patients with ECT. They found that the majority of patients had adequate seizures despite receiving anticonvulsant medications, although a few required dose reduction. Seven patients had spontaneous episodes suggestive of seizures during the ECT course, but the possibility of pseudoseizures or nonictal events seemed likely in several cases. Overall, the clinical management of patients with epilepsy during an ECT course is based on limited available data. However, common recommendations include reducing the anticonvulsant agents to obtain an adequate ECT seizure and withholding the morning dose of the anticonvulsant agent. Patients should be monitored between treatments for any unusual episodic motor or behavioral changes, as these may represent the emergence of seizure activity.

Not only can ECT be used for the treatment of psychiatric syndromes in patients with epilepsy, but ECT has been considered as a possible treatment for intractable seizures due to its anticonvulsant properties and propensity to elevate the seizure threshold during the treatment course (26). There are only a few case reports describing ECT for the treatment of intractable seizures. For instance, Griesemer et al. reported two cases of severe refractory epilepsy in a 10-year-old girl with microcephaly and a 13-year-old boy with microgyria. The boy also suffered from intermittent bouts of non-convulsive status epilepticus. Both children were treated with brief courses of three ECT on several occasions to curtail status epilepticus and to reduce the severity and frequency of the episodes in the short term (27). In another case, Shin et al. employed ECT to treat non-convulsive status in a 7-year-old girl with cerebral palsy, microgyria, and developmental delay (28); consecutive treatments over two days were administered twice, a week apart. After the second pair of sessions, status epilepticus ceased, allowing reduction in anticonvulsant medications and a better quality of life. Since the anticonvulsant benefits of ECT are believed to be short-lived, Shah et al. described the use of maintenance ECT over 20 months in treating an 18-year-old man with mental retardation and refractory epilepsy. Seizure frequency was dramatically reduced with ECT from 24 to 6 seizures per week, followed by reduction to 1 to 2 per week; ECT was administered on an average of once every 12 days (29). Clearly, more studies are necessary to better understand the role of ECT in patients with refractory epilepsy, although ECT may be a treatment option when other conventional strategies have failed.

CASE VIGNETTE

The following case is a 16-year-old adolescent male with mental retardation, autism, and catatonia who was treated with ECT. Despite a normal pre-ECT assessment, this patient developed seizures during the course of ECT. This case highlights the complexity of managing a seizure disorder during ECT and underscores that clinicians should be vigilant in monitoring for potential seizures and obtain appropriate diagnostic tests and/or implement empirical medication trials, when appropriate.

A 16 year-old adolescent boy presented for psychiatric admission with a history of moderate to severe mental retardation and autism. His development history revealed that he had experienced regression of milestones at 20 months and had developed limited speech. The main presenting symptoms were severe episodes of aggression, self-injurious behaviors, and stereotypies. Significant behavioral disturbances had been prominent since age 13, but had worsened only recently. In addition, exposure to a number of atypical and older generation antipsychotic agents appeared to worsen his agitation. His parents reported that the patient would "freeze" and have staring spells. Suspicions for an occult seizure disorder resulted in extensive neurological and metabolic workup; his MRI of the brain showed mild volume loss. However, his EEG was normal prior to starting ECT, as was a 48-hour EEG, which did not detect seizure activity even during episodes of agitation and aggression. Given a number of motor signs, the patient was diagnosed with an atypical presentation of catatonia and ECT was recommended. During an initial long course of 29 ECT, the patient improved with a dramatic reduction of aggression and catatonic signs and was noted to have increased speech. He was able to return to his special education classroom. However, he relapsed over the subsequent 2–3 years, and received two additional courses of ECT followed by prolonged, taper-down maintenance ECT. Tapering down the ECT resulted in the return of episodes of mood and behavioral disturbances that were similar to his presentation prior to ECT. This resulted in additional investigations to detect a seizure disorder, while empirical trials of anticonvulsant agents were complicated because the patient was unable to tolerate phenytoin, and carbamazepine resulted in thrombocytopenia. Following consultation with neurology colleagues and a 72-hour EEG, bilateral temporal lobe abnormalities were found, which were also associated with behavior disregulation (screaming, agitation). Cessation of ECT at that point resulted in relapse with return in agitation and aggression; therefore, ECT had to be resumed due to serious risk of injury to others and self. At the time of writing this chapter, the patient is receiving valproic acid and phenobarbital, which are being titrated up slowly, while carefully tapering down the ECT. He has remained stable on ECT for the past 5 years with current treatment frequency at 10 to 14 day intervals.

Space-Occupying Lesions

There is sparse literature about the use of ECT in youth with brain tumors. Tumors that cause the greatest concern are those accompanied by a prominent mass effect or edema. Many cases described in the literature may not have been particularly high-risk lesions, and it is difficult to make generalizations. The quality of life in patients with tumors with depression or other kinds of psychiatric morbidity is an important consideration when choosing ECT. Given the somewhat sparse literature involving this age group, a thorough discussion of the risks and benefits is necessary, involving both the patient and his or her family.

Ghaziuddin et al. described ECT in a 16-year-old female with a history of brain stem glioma who was post-craniotomy. The patient had presented with severe suicidal ideation, labile mood, insomnia, agitation, and psychosis, which had been resistant to numerous medications. The patient's mood was significantly improved and there was remission in psychosis noted after ECT (30).

In the last three decades, there have been numerous successful reports of using ECT in adult patients with brain tumors including meningioma, astrocytoma, and metastatic cancer (31–34). Consultation with a neurologist or a neurosurgical specialist is strongly recommended, if a tumor with a mass effect and/or edema is detected, to consider pre-medication with steroids, diuretics, and intraoperative antihypertensive agents (34). Furthermore, patients with a brain mass who have undergone craniotomy may have skull defects or metallic skull plates, which may create a path of low resistance for the electrical stimulation. In such cases, improvised placements of electrodes is recommended, such as unique unilateral positions to avoid placement of the electrodes over a skull deformity (35).

Ventricular Shunts and Idiopathic Intracranial Hypertension

Congenital hydrocephalus is a relatively common condition affecting an estimated 1 in 500 children. Furthermore, hydrocephalus may occur secondary to several conditions of the central nervous system, including an infection, stroke/hemorrhage, or head injury (36). However, there is limited experience regarding the use of ECT in patients with hydrocephalus. Among the few cases reported, ECT was successfully used in a 17-year-old boy with a ventricular shunt, seizures, history of meningomyelocele, and depression (37); no complications were noted in this case. Another adolescent, a 13-year-old boy with congenital hydrocephalus, multiple shunt revisions, a stable arachnoid cyst, and catatonia, was successfully treated with ECT, followed by considerable improvement in his condition (38). Other published reports include adult patients with shunts, who were successfully treated with ECT (39, 40).

Idiopathic intracranial hypertension ("pseudotumor cerebri") is a condition associated with elevated intracranial pressure, but without a space-occupying lesion. There are two reported cases of successful ECT treatment in depressed adult patients with idiopathic intracranial hypertension (41, 42).

CASE VIGNETTE

This case highlights the safe administration of ECT in a patient with idiopathic intracranial hypertension, which was administered in close collaboration with neurology specialists. This patient had an excellent outcome and is looking forward to attending college.

A 17-year-old girl with a four-year history of depression had experienced worsening symptoms, including a serious plan to suicide. Past psychiatric history was significant for failing to respond to numerous antidepressants. She was also placed on lithium for antidepressant augmentation and mood stabilization. She had rapidly gained 30 to 50 pounds over the previous year, which was attributed to depression and to her medications. A few months prior to the acute psychiatric crisis, she had experienced severe headaches and peripheral vision changes. Consultation with ophthalmology found bilateral papilledema, and she was diagnosed with idiopathic intracranial hypertension; her weight gain and lithium were believed to be contributing factors. Pediatric neurology and ophthalmology colleagues revisted her diagnostic tests, including an MRI/MRA of brain showing mildly irregular and narrowed bilateral transverse sinuses suggestive of idiopathic intracranial hyptertension. An opening pressure during lumbar puncture was borderline abnormal/high. Recommendations during the ECT course included intermittent fundoscopic exams, the use of acetazolamide, and discontinuation of lithium. Her papilledema was found to improve, despite receiving ECT, and she achieved remission in depression after 15 index ECT and a brief continuation course.

Cerebral Aneurysms

Patients with cerebral aneurysms are theoretically at risk of a bleed due to a surge in intracranial pressure during the ECT seizure. The published literature includes 15 cases of ECT in patients with such aneurysms. In all cases, ECT was administered without complication and with positive outcomes. In most cases, blood pressure was lowered prior to ECT to reduce the risk of bleeding. Medications administered pre-ECT included oral or intravenous beta-blocking agents. Often intravenous nitroprusside or other vasodilating medications were used with the beta-blocker to maximize blood pressure control (43).

Other Neurological Conditions

Psychiatric syndromes may occur in patients with several other neurological disorders. Cases described in the literature include the safe and effective use of ECT in patients with intracranial cysts, subdural hematomas, cerebral palsy, traumatic brain injury, stroke, Huntington's chorea, myasthenia gravis, and CNS systemic lupus erythematosus (44–47).

GASTROINTESTINAL

There is a potential risk of aspirating gastric contents due to the use of muscle relaxants during ECT. Poorly controlled gastroesophageal reflux disease can increase the risk of aspirating the gastric contents during anesthesia, despite the patient being "nil per os" (NPO) overnight prior to ECT. Patients should be advised to continue antacid medications, such as H2 blockers or proton pump inhibitors, which may be given with a sip of water 30–60 minutes pre-ECT. Alternatively, oral sodium citrate liquid may be given just prior to ECT. For severe, uncontrolled gastroesophageal reflux disease, the anesthesiology consultant may choose to intubate the patient during ECT, to prevent aspiration.

METABOLIC

Diabetes and electrolyte imbalances pose clinical challenges and could contribute to complications such as prolonged seizures or arrhythmias. Any metabolic disturbance should be identified prior to ECT and treated with adequate hydration and electrolytes. Consultation with an endocrinologist is recommended to adjust the dose of insulin in youth with insulin-dependent diabetes mellitus.

MUSCULOSKELETAL

Modern anesthesia has virtually eliminated the risk of fractures with ECT. However, screening for musculoskeletal or spinal abnormalities is important so that the dose of the muscle relaxant used during ECT may be adjusted accordingly.

DENTAL

During ECT, patients experience vigorous clenching of the jaw due to the direct stimulation of the masseter muscle. Even with proper safeguards and a bite guard in place, poorly maintained teeth are at risk for fracture, posing a serious risk of aspiration. Patients with poor oral hygiene, in particular, may have loose or chipped teeth. Therefore, the oral cavity should be routinely examined for any loose teeth, and consultation with a dentist for an extraction is highly recommended if a loose tooth is identified.

OCULAR

ECT induces elevated intracranial and intraocular pressures. Children and adolescents should be asked about any history of retinal detachment or glaucoma. Ophthalmology consultation may be necessary to review the medications that may be required before proceeding with ECT.

CONCURRENT USE OF PSYCHOTROPIC AND OTHER MEDICATIONS DURING ECT

Psychotropic Medications and ECT

Psychiatric medications are often tapered during the pre-ECT period (see Table 6.1). The utility of continuing medications during ECT must be weighed against side effects or other risks associated with the combination of ECT and concurrent medications. In some patients, it may not be feasible to taper the medications due to severity of symptoms (e.g. symptoms of psychosis, mania, or severe agitation).

Antidepressants

There is no clear evidence from the literature that antidepressant use with ECT is unsafe. Most concerns stem from isolated case reports and known side effects. Specifically, some reports describe prolonged seizures in patients on fluoxetine, while other reports do not. Buproprion has a known association with seizures in certain patients, and status epilepticus during ECT has been described in one case report (48). Tricyclic antidepressants and monoamine oxidase inhibitors have been administered with ECT with no contraindication for use, but theoretically could contribute to hypertension or hypotension during ECT.

Older literature had indicated that tricyclic antidepressants may enhance the effect of ECT. One large recent study also suggested that both venlafaxine and nortriptyline improve outcomes in ECT. However, a greater negative effect on cognition was found in the group that was given venlafaxine, when compared with those on placebo (49). Therefore, additional studies are necessary to confirm these findings of added benefit when combining antidepressants and ECT.

In children and adolescent patients, tapering down antidepressants is usually appropriate because of the potential risk of additive side effects during ECT. Also, discontinuing antidepressants is appropriate when patients have been unresponsive to the current medication regimen; in this situation, a switch to another agent following ECT is generally recommended.

Lithium

The potential risks of administering lithium concurrently with ECT include prolonged muscle relaxation, delirium, and seizures. Management options, when continuing lithium is indicated, include tapering the dose of lithium during the acute/index ECT course. For some patients who may benefit from lithium during the maintenance phase of treatment, lithium may be withheld the night before ECT, which likely reduces the blood level during the treatment (50).

Anticonvulsants

These agents are known to elevate the seizure threshold and may, therefore, interfere with the full expression of an ECT seizure. Further potential complications of these medications may include a greater cardiovascular risk due to subthreshold electrical stimulation and confusion following ECT, both linked to repeated attempts to elicit an adequate seizure. Among the autonomic changes during ECT, the initial electrical stimulation elicits a parasympathetic response. Secondly, the seizure itself induces a sympathetic surge (tachycardia, elevated blood pressure), which counteracts the initial parasympathetic flow. When there is failure to induce a successful seizure and consequent lack of sympathetic stimulation, there is an increased accompanying risk of bradycardia and asystole due to unopposed parasympathetic flow. In such instances, restimulation using a higher electrical dosage may be necessary (in order to elicit an adequate seizure). This in turn may contribute to increased post-treatment confusion or agitation. In a review of anticonvulsant use in ECT, Sienaert and Peuskens (2007) found no evidence to support the combined use of anticonvulsants with ECT to enhance the latter's efficacy (51). Therefore, for the reasons outlined, the usual recommendation is to taper down or discontinue anticonvulsants for patients who are receiving these medications for mood stabilization.

Benzodiazepines

These agents are powerful anticonvulsants; therefore, tapering the benzodiazepines pre-ECT in most cases is an appropriate step to lower the anticonvulsant burden. However, exceptions include some anxious, agitated, or catatonic patients, for whom tapering benzodiazepines may not be safe or may result in significant discomfort. In these situations, flumazenil, a benzodiazepine receptor antagonist, is used to reverse the effect of benzodiazepines and can be administered intravenously, just seconds after the infusion of the anesthetic agent (52, 53).

Antipsychotics

Evidence in the literature supports the use of antipsychotic medications with ECT for selected patients with difficult to treat psychotic illness; in some cases

Table 6.1. SUGGESTED MANAGEMENT OF PSYCHIATRIC MEDICATIONS FOR CHILDREN AND ADOLESCENTS DURING ECT

Medication Class	Risks	Adjustments/Options
Antidepressants (SSRI, SNRI, TCA, MAOI, others)	• Confusion/delirium • Lower seizure threshold • Hypotension/hypertension	• Taper or discontinue
Lithium	• Possible postoperative delirium • Possible prolonged muscle relaxation	• Discontinue • Hold night/day before ECT
Anticonvulsants	• Raise seizure threshold • May elevate cardiovascular risk • May increase post-ECT confusion	• Taper, discontinue, or hold for 12 hours
Benzodiazepines	• Raise seizure threshold • Sedation • Risk during pregnancy	• Taper or discontinue • Reverse with flumazenil 0.5–1 mg pre-ECT
Antipsychotics	• Lower seizure threshold • Additive sedation • Cardiac problems (hypotension, arrhythmia, QT prolongation)	• Reduce/limit • Avoid/taper when signs of catatonia • Possible synergistic benefit (may use for severe agitation, mania, or psychosis)

the combination may, in fact, enhance the efficacy (54). As described with antidepressants, the reasons to taper these agents pre-ECT are potential complications during the procedure, such as hypotension or additive sedation beyond what might be secondary due to the anesthetic agents. Some antipsychotics, clozapine in particular, have been associated with spontaneous seizures (55) and could theoretically contribute to prolonged ECT seizures. In addition, antipsychotics should be tapered in cases of neuroleptic malignant syndrome (NMS) or catatonia, as these agents may worsen these syndromes (see Chapter 11, "ECT for Catatonia in Autism"). Furthermore, ECT alone is usually effective for both NMS and catatonia. Rarely, for patients with severe agitation, mania, or psychosis, antipsychotic medications may be used carefully with ECT, although it may be best to discontinue antipsychotics when treating depression.

Non-psychotropic Medications and ECT

Medications for general medical conditions in patients receiving ECT may be continued and are not contraindicated. Often, medications can be safely administered pre-ECT on the morning of treatment and may help reduce potential risks of ECT or prevent ECT side effects in some cases. Table 6.2

Table 6.2. SUGGESTED MANAGEMENT OF NON-PSYCHOTROPIC MEDICATIONS DURING ECT

Medication Class	Risks	Adjustments/Options
Antihypertensives	• Hypertension during ECT if not given	• Give with sip of water 30–60 min. pre-ECT • Hold diuretics to avoid enuresis
Reflux medications (H2 blocker, Proton pump inhibitors)	• Aspiration with poorly controlled reflux	• Give with sip of water 30–60 min pre-ECT • Citric acid/sodium citrate 30cc pre-ECT
Pain medications (NSAIDS, migraine medications)	• If not given, risk of post-ECT headache or migraine exacerbation	• Acetaminophen 500–1000 pre-ECT • Other NSAIDs pre- and post-ECT • Serotonin agonist (SQ or Intranasal) pre/post ECT
Pulmonary (asthma medications)	• If not given, asthma exacerbation, difficult airway management	• Continue inhalers pre-ECT
Ophthalmic (glaucoma medications)	• Risk of elevated • Intraocular pressure • Retinal detachment	• Continue glaucoma medications
Hypoglycemic/diabetes medications (oral hypoglycemic agents and insulin)	• Risk of hypoglycemia if administered while NPO	• Treat diabetic patient first on the schedule • Hold oral hypoglycemic agents • Hold or administer partial dose of insulin • Consult with endocrinologist

highlights commonly prescribed medications in patients receiving ECT and the associated risks and side effects.

CONCLUSION

ECT may be used safely and effectively in youth who have medical or neurological conditions, and indeed there are no absolute medical or neurological contraindications to the treatment in this age group. At the same time, it is always important to thoroughly assess risk factors prior to commencing ECT, to conduct pre-ECT physical examination focusing on the cardiovascular, neurological, and pulmonary systems, to perform necessary laboratory tests and scans, and to collaborate with medical specialists in other fields as appropriate. Careful attention also needs to be given to both psychotropic and non-psychotropic medication-use during the ECT course.

QUESTIONS AND ANSWERS

1. *Is ECT a safe procedure?*

   ECT is extremely safe. For patients who are otherwise healthy, the risk of severe complications such as a cardiac arrest or death is exceptionally low and generally no different from other procedures using anesthesia.

2. *What should parents expect for the medical workup for a child or adolescent referred for ECT?*

   A thorough physical exam is completed for any patient receiving ECT. Patients may undergo routine blood tests and electrocardiogram (ECG) as part of the assessment. Other specialized tests such as brain scans or an electroencephalogram (EEG) may not be mandatory but are nevertheless common, especially if symptoms or behaviors are suggestive of a neurological problem.

3. *Can a child or adolescent be treated with ECT in the presence of a heart problem?*

   During ECT, heart rate and blood pressure are briefly elevated. Patients with cardiac illnesses are thus at a greater risk of complications with ECT. However, with input from internal medicine, anesthesiology, and/or cardiology specialists, ECT can be safetly admininistered to most patients, even those with cardiac conditions.

4. *Does epilepsy preclude a child or an adolescent from receiving ECT?*

   There is a complex association between seizures, certain psychiatric disorders, and the effect of ECT-induced seizures during treatment. Interestingly, ECT is known to have anticonvulsant properties. Therefore, the risk of worsening epilepsy during ECT is very low. Also, epileptic seizures may contribute to or mimic psychiatric symptoms. Overall, patients with epilepsy may benefit from ECT.

5. *Should antidepressants be stopped during ECT?*

   It is common practice to withdraw psychiatric medications that do not have clear utility during the ECT course. ECT is a potent and a rapidly acting treatment, and combining ECT with antidepressants for added benefit is not well established. In addition, since patients who receive ECT are likely to be resistant to their current medications, clinicians often remove antidepressants during ECT with a plan to start a different antidepressant following ECT.

6. *Can medications used for a general medical disorder be continued during ECT?*

   Most medications for medical conditions can be continued while a patient is receiving ECT. In fact, many medications can be administered even in the morning before ECT. Medication may be given for conditions such as diabetes, heartburn, headaches/migraines, asthma, or high blood pressure.

DISCLOSURES

Dr. Daniel Maixner, MD, has no direct conflicts of interest pertinent to the work completed for this book. He has current funding for deep brain stimulation research by St. Jude Medical, Inc. and transcranial magnetic stimulation by Neuronetics, Inc. He has no other compensation or consultation work for any pharmaceutical companies.

REFERENCES

1. Kramer BA. Use of ECT in California, 1977–1983. *Am J Psychiatry.* 1985;142(10):1190–2.
2. Shiwach RS, Reid WH, Carmody TJ. An analysis of reported deaths following electroconvulsive therapy in Texas, 1993-1998. *Psychiatr Serv.* 2001;52(8):1095–7.
3. Jenkins K, Baker AB. Consent and anaesthetic risk. *Anaesthesia.* 2003; 58(10):962–84.
4. J. H. Eichorn RCM, ed. *Patient Safety in Anesthetic Practice.* St. Louis, MO: Churchill Livingstone; 1997.
5. Tess AV, Smetana GW. Medical evaluation of patients undergoing electroconvulsive therapy. *N Engl J Med.* 2009;360(14):1437–44.
6. Therapy APACoE, ed. *The Practice of Electroconvulsive Therapy: Recommendations for Treatment, Training, and Privileging.* 2nd ed. Washington, DC: American Psychiatric Association; 2001.
7. Schieve LA, Gonzalez V, Boulet SL, Visser SN, Rice CE, Braun KV, et al. Concurrent medical conditions and health care use and needs among children with learning and behavioral developmental disabilities, National Health Interview Survey, 2006–2010. *Res Dev Disabil.* 2012;33(2):467–76.
8. Mueller PS, Schak KM, Barnes RD, Rasmussen KG. Safety of electroconvulsive therapy in patients with asthma. *Neth J Med.* 2006;64(11):417–21.
9. Rasmussen KG, Ryan DA, Mueller PS. Blood glucose before and after ECT treatments in Type 2 diabetic patients. *J ECT.* 2006;22(2):124–6.
10. Abrams R. *Electroconvulsive Therapy.* 4th ed. New York, NY: Oxford University Press; 2002.
11. Prudic J, Sackeim HA, Decina P, Hopkins N, Ross FR, Malitz S. Acute effects of ECT on cardiovascular functioning: relations to patient and treatment variables. *Acta Psychiatr Scand.* 1987;75(4):344–51.

12. Din-Dzietham R, Liu Y, Bielo MV, Shamsa F. High blood pressure trends in children and adolescents in national surveys, 1963 to 2002. *Circulation*. 2007;116(13):1488–96.
13. Feber J, Ahmed M. Hypertension in children: new trends and challenges. *Clin Sci (Lond)*. 2010;119(4):151–61.
14. Zielinski RJ, Roose SP, Devanand DP, Woodring S, Sackeim HA. Cardiovascular complications of ECT in depressed patients with cardiac disease. *Am J Psychiatry*. 1993;150(6):904–9.
15. Aloysi AS, Maloutas E, Gomes A, Kellner CH. Safe resumption of electroconvulsive therapy after non-ST segment elevation myocardial infarction. *J ECT*. 2011;27(1):e39–41.
16. Magid M, Lapid MI, Sampson SM, Mueller PS. Use of electroconvulsive therapy in a patient 10 days after myocardial infarction. *J ECT*. 2005;21(3):182–5.
17. Mueller PS, Barnes RD, Varghese R, Nishimura RA, Rasmussen KG. The safety of electroconvulsive therapy in patients with severe aortic stenosis. *Mayo Clin Proc*. 2007;82(11):1360–3.
18. Davis A, Zisselman M, Simmons T, McCall WV, McCafferty J, Rosenquist PB. Electroconvulsive therapy in the setting of implantable cardioverter-defibrillators. *J ECT*. 2009;25(3):198–201.
19. Dolenc TJ, Barnes RD, Hayes DL, Rasmussen KG. Electroconvulsive therapy in patients with cardiac pacemakers and implantable cardioverter defibrillators. *Pacing Clin Electrophysiol*. 2004;27(9):1257–63.
20. Lapid MI, Rummans TA, Hofmann VE, Olney BA. ECT and automatic internal cardioverter-defibrillator. *J ECT*. 2001;17(2):146–8.
21. MacPherson RD, Loo CK, Barrett N. Electroconvulsive therapy in patients with cardiac pacemakers. Anaesth Intensive *Care*. 2006;34(4):470–4.
22. Altshuler LL, Cohen L, Szuba MP, Burt VK, Gitlin M, Mintz J. Pharmacologic management of psychiatric illness during pregnancy: dilemmas and guidelines. *Am J Psychiatry*. 1996;153(5):592–606.
23. Serim B, Ulas H, Ozerdem A, Alkin T. Electroconvulsive therapy in an adolescent pregnant patient. *Prog Neuropsychopharmacol Biol Psychiatry*. 2010;34(3):546–7.
24. Anderson EL, Reti IM. ECT in pregnancy: a review of the literature from 1941 to 2007. *Psychosom Med*. 2009;71(2):235–42.
25. Lunde ME, Lee EK, Rasmussen KG. Electroconvulsive therapy in patients with epilepsy. *Epilepsy Behav*. 2006;9(2):355–9.
26. Sackeim HA, Decina P, Prohovnik I, Malitz S, Resor SR. Anticonvulsant and antidepressant properties of electroconvulsive therapy: a proposed mechanism of action. *Biol Psychiatry*. 1983;18(11):1301–10.
27. Griesemer DA, Kellner CH, Beale MD, Smith GM. Electroconvulsive therapy for treatment of intractable seizures. Initial findings in two children. *Neurology*. 1997;49(5):1389–92.
28. Shin HW, O'Donovan CA, Boggs JG, Grefe A, Harper A, Bell WL, et al. Successful ECT treatment for medically refractory nonconvulsive status epilepticus in pediatric patient. *Seizure*. 2011;20(5):433–6.
29. Shah N, Pande N, Bhat T, Murke M, Andrade C. Maintenance ECT as a therapeutic approach to medication-refractory epilepsy in an adult with mental retardation: case report and review of literature. *J ECT*. 2012;28(2):136–40.
30. Ghaziuddin N, DeQuardo JR, Ghaziuddin M, King CA. Electroconvulsive treatment of a bipolar adolescent postcraniotomy for brain stem astrocytoma. *J Child Adolesc Psychopharmacol*. 1999;9(1):63–9.

31. Gursky JT, Rummans TA, Black JL. ECT administration in a patient after craniotomy and gamma knife surgery: a case report and review. *J ECT*. 2000; 16(3):295–9.
32. Kohler CG, Burock M. ECT for psychotic depression associated with a brain tumor. *Am J Psychiatry*. 2001;158(12):2089.
33. Patkar AA, Hill KP, Weinstein SP, Schwartz SL. ECT in the presence of brain tumor and increased intracranial pressure: evaluation and reduction of risk. *J ECT*. 2000;16(2):189–97.
34. Rasmussen KG, Perry CL, Sutor B, Moore KM. ECT in patients with intracranial masses. *J Neuropsychiatry Clin Neurosci*. 2007;19(2):191–3.
35. Ling T, 3rd, Manepalli J, Grossberg G. Electroconvulsive therapy in the presence of a metallic skull plate after meningioma resection. *J ECT*. 2010;26(2):136–8.
36. Stroke NIoNDa. Hydrocephalus Fact Sheet. 2011; Available from: http://www.ninds.nih.gov/disorders/hydrocephalus/detail_hydrocephalus.htm.
37. Mansheim P. ECT in the treatment of a depressed adolescent with meningomyelocele, hydrocephalus, and seizures. *J Clin Psychiatry*. 1983;44(10):385–6.
38. Wachtel LE, Baranano K, Reti IM. Electroconvulsive therapy for catatonia in a boy with hydrocephalus and an arachnoid cyst. *Pediatr Neurol*. 2010; 43(1):73–5.
39. Coffey CE, Hoffman G, Weiner RD, Moossy JJ. Electroconvulsive therapy in a depressed patient with a functioning ventriculoatrial shunt. *Convuls Ther*. 1987;3(4):302–6.
40. Hanretta AT, Malek-Ahmadi P. Successful ECT in a patient with hydrocephalus, shunt, hypopituitarism, and paraplegia. *J ECT*. 2001;17(1):71–4.
41. Adam LA, Crowe RR. Use of ECT in idiopathic intracranial hypertension. *J ECT*. 2003;19(4):234–7.
42. Moreno MV, Cruz MR, Rieder CR, Fleck MP. Successful electroconvulsive therapy in a drug-refractory depressed patient with idiopathic intracranial hypertension. *J ECT*. 2011;27(1):e29–31.
43. van Herck E, Sienaert P, Hagon A. [Electroconvulsive therapy for patients with intracranial aneurysms: a case study and literature review]. *Tijdschr Psychiatr*. 2009;51(1):43–51.
44. Fam J, Lee TS, Lee HY, Ng BY. Electroconvulsive therapy for catatonia in neuropsychiatric systemic lupus erythematosus. *J ECT*. 2010;26(2):143–4.
45. Krystal AD, Coffey CE. Neuropsychiatric considerations in the use of electroconvulsive therapy. *J Neuropsychiatry Clin Neurosci*. 1997;9(2):283–92.
46. Perry CL, Lindell EP, Rasmussen KG. ECT in patients with arachnoid cysts. *J ECT*. 2007;23(1):36–7.
47. Rasmussen KG, Keegan BM. Electroconvulsive therapy in patients with multiple sclerosis. *J ECT*. 2007;23(3):179–80.
48. Dersch R, Zwernemann S, Voderholzer U. Partial status epilepticus after electroconvulsive therapy and medical treatment with bupropion. *Pharmacopsychiatry*. 2011;44(7):344–6.
49. Sackeim HA, Dillingham EM, Prudic J, Cooper T, McCall WV, Rosenquist P, et al. Effect of concomitant pharmacotherapy on electroconvulsive therapy outcomes: short-term efficacy and adverse effects. *Arch Gen Psychiatry*. 2009;66(7):729–37.

50. Thirthalli J, Harish T, Gangadhar BN. A prospective comparative study of interaction between lithium and modified electroconvulsive therapy. *World J Biol Psychiatry*. 2011;12(2):149–55.
51. Sienaert P, Peuskens J. Anticonvulsants during electroconvulsive therapy: review and recommendations. *J ECT*. 2007;23(2):120–3.
52. Bailine SH, Safferman A, Vital-Herne J, Bernstein S. Flumazenil reversal of benzodiazepine-induced sedation for a patient with severe pre-ECT anxiety. *Convuls Ther*. 1994;10(1):65–8.
53. Krystal AD, Watts BV, Weiner RD, Moore S, Steffens DC, Lindahl V. The use of flumazenil in the anxious and benzodiazepine-dependent ECT patient. *J ECT*. 1998;14(1):5–14.
54. Haskett RF, Loo C. Adjunctive psychotropic medications during electroconvulsive therapy in the treatment of depression, mania, and schizophrenia. *J ECT*. 2010;26(3):196–201.
55. Fitzsimons J, Berk M, Lambert T, Bourin M, Dodd S. A review of clozapine safety. *Expert Opin Drug Saf*. 2005;4(4):731–44.

CHAPTER 7

Anesthesia

DANIEL E. GIH, EMMA TAYLOR,
AND BERNARD BIERMANN

KEY POINTS

- Modern anesthesia administered during ECT is safe and effective, has a short duration of action, and has rendered the treatment free of major discomfort or injury.
- There are no data to suggest that anesthesia administered to younger patients is riskier than in adult patients.
- In addition to removing discomfort during treatment, anesthesia may change the characteristics of the seizure, such as seizure threshold or duration, which may enhance treatment.
- Three main classes of medications employed during anesthesia are a sedative, a muscle relaxant, and an anticholinergic agent.
- Anesthesiologists and psychiatrists involved with ECT should have specialized knowledge about the principles of treatment and the procedures involved.
- A liaison anesthesiologist for ECT, with direct clinical involvement and allocated sessional time, should be identified.
- ECT commonly takes place in a specially designated setting, with anesthesia provided by a small cohort of regularly assigned anesthesiologists.
- Written guidelines should be available at the site regarding the practice of anesthesia for ECT and standards of monitoring. A comprehensive record detailing the patient pathway, incorporating equipment checks, pre-assessment details, drug dosages, and responses should be kept.
- There should be provision for adequate supervision for patients treated on an outpatient basis, with careful monitoring until the patient is fully awake. Contingency plans should include arrangements for overnight admission if needed.

OVERVIEW

This chapter describes modern anesthesia techniques currently used for administering electroconvulsive therapy (ECT) to adolescents, and very rarely to younger children. Considerable advances in anesthesiology have rendered ECT a procedure with minimal discomfort or pain. Serious physical injury or death due to ECT in children or adolescents has not been reported. In this chapter, we describe the selection of the most appropriate sedative agent, muscle relaxant, and anticholinergic agent, the role of the anesthesiologist-starting with pre-ECT assessment of the patient, administering and monitoring the patient during and following the treatment, and the role and safety of other medications that the patient may be taking for a medical or psychiatric condition. Special measures for allaying anxiety in younger patients, including involvement of the parent/caregiver and the need for privacy, are discussed. [It should be noted that terms such as "children," "youth," and "minors" are used interchangeably and refer to patients younger than 18 years. "Adolescents" refers to individuals who range in age from 12 to 18 years, whereas pre-pubertal children are those below age 12. Due to paucity of data in pre-pubertal children, the majority of the information presented in this chapter is based on experience with adolescents.]

HISTORICAL PERSPECTIVE ON ANESTHESIA

ECT treatment was first described in the 1940s, and became popular throughout the 1950s and 1960s, leading to further investigation to better understand its mechanism of action. The main drawback of the literature in youth, pertaining both to ECT and anesthesia for the treatment, is the absence of large-scale or prospective studies. However, anecdotal reports and retrospective studies support the position that modern anesthesia administered during ECT is safe and devoid of lasting side effects. The currently available expertise with anesthetic agents was not known in the 1930s and 1940s, when ECT was initially described among children and adolescents. It is very likely that this gap in knowledge was one of several reasons that ECT became increasingly unpopular for this age group, until its revival in the late 1980s. (For additional details, see Chapter 1, "The History of Pediatric ECT.")

It is feasible that the ongoing and the widespread reluctance to use ECT in children stems in part from the unpleasant notion of ECT without anesthesia (or unmodified ECT). Likewise, the portrayal of unmodified ECT in movies probably contributed to a ban of ECT in some states of the United States for certain age groups. Although unmodified treatment continues to be used in some developing countries, its use is declining. It should be noted that, in contrast with historical use of the term implying no anesthesia, today the term "unmodified" has come to mean "use of benzodiazepine alone" rather than "without anesthesia" (1).

Despite concerns over its use, the efficacy and safety of ECT are borne out by increasing use without adverse event (2, 3). However, there is much more experience of ECT in adolescents than in prepubertal children. While the reports of use in prepubertal children are few, existing cases described in the literature favor its use (4–11), especially in cases of severe mood disorders and catatonia (12, 13).

AIMS OF MODERN ANESTHETIC AGENTS

Induction Agents

A variety of induction agents, medications that bring about a state of general anesthesia, may be used during anesthesia for ECT. Commonly used agents include propofol, methohexital, thiopentone, ketamine, and etomidate. Among these, propofol is the most commonly utilized agent. Typically, intravenous (IV) induction is utilized and, as such, ECT requires establishing IV access for each treatment. If IV access is especially difficult to obtain, a peripherally inserted central catheter (PICC) line or a port may be placed in order to proceed with a course of ECT. Ideal characteristics of an induction agent include rapid onset and recovery, suitability for repeated use, and no interference with seizure duration or the seizure threshold. Furthermore, since ECT results in activation of the sympathetic nervous system and ensuing catecholamine release, hemodynamic and cardiovascular effects of various induction agents should be considered (14). A careful balance will need to be struck between the clinical characteristics of the patient and the induction agent utilized. In some cases, the anesthetic agent may be changed to a different agent over the course of ECT treatment.

Barbiturates, such as methohexital (0.8–1 mg/kg), are classic induction agents and are frequently employed in practice. Methohexital is preferred over thiopental for faster recovery due to its more rapid pharmacokinetic profile. Thiopental (2–5 mg/kg) was used until quite recently in some countries; however, its use has declined due to the less favorable recovery time. Owing to the anticonvulsant properties of methohexital and thiopental, these agents may interfere with ECT in patients who have a higher seizure threshold at baseline. However, because of the known association between younger age and lower seizure threshold, this property of methohexital is relatively less concerning in children and adolescents. Another drawback of methohexital is mild pain experienced upon injection by some patients.

Propofol (0.75–2.5 mg/kg) is universally becoming the induction agent of choice, and is the most commonly used parenteral anesthetic in some parts of the United States. Its half-life is shorter than the aforementioned barbiturates, making it ideal for short procedures such as ECT. It has the additional advantage of greater cardiovascular stability over thiopental (15). One relative disadvantage of propofol is that it reduces seizure duration significantly (16). The addition of a short-acting opioid to methohexital or propofol has been suggested to enhance seizure length (14). However, it is unclear whether the duration of motor seizures is related to the overall efficacy of ECT (17).

Etomidate (0.15–0.3 mg/kg) as the inductive agent has the advantage of increasing the seizure duration and promoting seizure activity in those for whom seizures have been previously difficult to elicit. It has the least negative effect of all the agents on both motor and electroencephalogram (EEG) seizures, followed in order by methohexital, thiopental, and propofol. Moreover, patients at risk for hypotension during anesthesia may benefit from etomidate, as it is more likely to maintain the cardiovascular stability after induction. Another agent-, ketamine, an N-methyl-d-aspartate (NMDA) receptor antagonist, may not be an appropriate agent due to the potential for hypertension, and prolonged emergence phenomenon (restoration of spontaneous respiration and consciousness) or "wake-up" profile. It also has the undesirable sequela of confusion or agitation upon emergence from anesthesia (18). However, use of ketamine is associated with a lower seizure threshold and increased seizure duration when compared with thiopental (19). Another advantage of ketamine is its usefulness in patients at high risk for bronchospasm. Increased salivation associated with ketamine infusion can be prevented by glycopyrrolate and other anticholinergic agents.

Inhalational Agents

In children, especially those in the younger age groups, establishing IV access for induction of anesthesia can present a challenge, and an inhalational induction may be considered, although this is not a standard practice.

Sevoflurane is the only agent in widespread use for inhalational induction of anesthesia. There are at present conflicting views on the effect of this agent on seizure threshold and duration (20), although most evidence points to a favorable effect (21). In more general terms, sevoflurane produces a slower induction but a more rapid recovery, with a lower incidence of apnea. There may also be a higher incidence of postoperative nausea and vomiting with inhalational anesthesia in certain patient groups. Risk factors for nausea and vomiting associated with anesthesia include females over the pubertal age, history of nausea and vomiting with surgery and anesthesia, and strong history of travel sickness.

Muscle Relaxants

Muscle relaxants have played an important role in the safe administration of ECT, by virtually eliminating skeletal or soft tissue injuries that were commonly reported 50 years ago.

The aim of the muscle relaxant is to attenuate the musculoskeletal activity due to the seizure and, therefore, to reduce iatrogenic injury. This is most often achieved with the use of the short-acting depolarizing muscle relaxant suxamethonium (0.5–1 mg/kg), also known as succinylcholine. Contraindications to the use of suxamethonium include a history of malignant hyperpyrexia, pseudocholinesterase deficiency, neuromuscular disorders, and major burns, which may necessitate use of a non-depolarizing muscle relaxant such as atracurium (0.3–0.4 mg/kg) or rocuronium (0.6–0.9 mg/kg). Prior to administering the muscle relaxant, blood flow to an extremity (usually the right foot) is restricted through the use of a blood pressure cuff. This "isolated limb" method allows safe observation and measurement of motor seizure activity (14).

Anticholinergic Agents

Anticholinergic agents, such as atropine or glycopyrrolate, are traditionally administered prior to ECT. Although, there is ongoing debate regarding the necessity of routinely administering these agents, this practice is to protect against the vagal stimulation induced by ECT, which may result in bradycardia or asystole. In event of successful seizure induced during ECT, the vagal response is counteracted by accompanying sympathetic stimulation, and thus the vagal effects are avoided. However, most practitioners choose to use an anticholinergic routinely, to prevent complications of vagal stimulation, especially when there is inadequate sympathetic flow. Anticholinergic agents may be particularly useful in patients who are receiving sympathetic blocking agents, such as beta-blockers. The other group of patients who should routinely receive anticholinergic agents is those in whom a seizure threshold has not yet been established (i.e., for those undergoing their first ECT session).

Medications for Pain, Nausea, and Vomiting

Agents used to relieve pain, nausea or vomiting have a key role in reducing discomfort and the frequency and severity of side effects associated with ECT. Common side effects are headache, body aches, or nausea secondary to the anesthetic. Based on the experience of the authors, most agents can be administered prior to ECT or soon afterward, especially in a patient who may have reported excessive post-treatment discomfort during a prior treatment.

Headache is the most commonly reported complaint after ECT, occurring in approximately half of all patients; it is usually mild and transient, and responds to simple over-the-counter medications such as acetaminophen or ibuprofen. Some patients who suffer from severe headache may require prophylactic treatment with, for example, intravenous ketorolac. Similarly, oral acetaminophen in the morning prior to ECT may also ward off headaches.

Ondansetron is a clinically effective antiemetic agent used in children for the prevention of post-operative vomiting. There is a dose-related response, with the optimal dose being 0.15 mg/kg. The addition of dexamethasone at a dose of 0.1 mg/kg is helpful in groups at higher risk (past history of nausea secondary to anesthesia, severe motion sickness, post-pubertal females) and should be used in combination with ondansetron (0.1 mg/kg). Dexamethasone should be administered under anesthesia as its administration may cause perineal discomfort; a slow push, even under general anesthesia should be used because of this known side effect (22). Older style antihistamine anti-nausea agents such as diphenhydramine, prochlorperazine, and cyclizine should be reserved for rare cases where ondansetron and dexamethasone are ineffective alone.

SEIZURE ACTIVITY

The series of events observed after the electrical stimulation include short-lived tonic activity, followed by a period of observable clonic motor seizure activity. These observable effects are followed by generalized seizure activity in the brain, which is monitored by EEG recording. Oxygen saturation, measured using pulse oximetry on a finger probe, should not be allowed to fall below 90%. A ventilation mask for oxygenation should thus be used throughout the course of the treatment. A missed seizure or an inadequate seizure may be caused by inadequate intensity or duration of the electrical stimulus, hypercarbia, dehydration, electrolyte abnormalities, use of other medications such as benzodiazepines, or the anesthetic agent itself. Relative overdose of the anesthetic agent may also cause a missed or a focal seizure. For best results, there should be a delay of approximately 60 seconds prior to re-stimulation, while atropine or glycopyrrolate should be immediately available in case bradycardia ensues. Prolonged or tardive seizures, lasting over 2 minutes, can complicate recovery and require airway maintenance. Termination of such seizures can be accomplished by the use of a benzodiazepine, administered by the intravenous route.

The initial contraction of the masseter muscles necessitates placement of a soft bite block (for example, a taped roll of swabs) to protect dentition. Care should be taken to remove this promptly before the patient emerges from anesthesia.

CHANGES IN VITAL SIGNS DURING ECT

Vital signs are continually monitored throughout the course of ECT. As the stimulus is administered and during the seizure, there is an initial parasympathetic stimulation that results in transient bradycardia, lasting approximately 10–15 seconds. This is followed by a more prominent and prolonged sympathetic response with tachycardia and hypertension. The usual magnitude rise in systolic blood pressure is 30–40%, whereas there is a 20% rise in the heart rate. The combined effect of these changes is a significant increase in myocardial oxygen consumption and release of catecholamine, which may result in occasional short-lived tachyarrythmias. As such, it is important to monitor vital signs before, during, and after the treatment. Typically, vital signs return to baseline within several minutes. Patients who remain tachycardic or hypertensive in the postictal period will sometimes require pharmacologic management,which may include beta-blockers (labetolol). This is more of a concern in patients with underlying cardiovascular conditions, such as essential hypertension; this is rarely encountered in children or adolescents receiving ECT.

MEDICAL WORKUP PRIOR TO ANESTHESIA

The initial pre-procedure assessment by an anesthesiologist may be performed immediately prior to the treatment. Therefore, it is helpful to utilize a checklist, so that potential problems may be highlighted and communicated in a timely manner to the anesthesiologist performing the procedure. Conditions of particular interest include currently prescribed medicines, diabetes, hiatus hernia, obesity, dental problems, problems with anesthetic agents used previously, and known drug allergies. Preoperative examination should include measurement of weight, blood pressure, heart rate, and oxygen saturation. General physical examination should include chest auscultation and airway examination. It would be prudent for the lead anesthesiologist involved with ECT to provide guidelines regarding acceptable vital signs and when a finding should prompt a referral for a more detailed anesthetic assessment.

A list of relative and absolute contraindications for anesthesia should be included in the anesthetic guidelines. An obvious and a prudent approach must take into consideration when ECT is deemed to be lifesaving. In such a case, there may be no absolute contraindications. Readers are referred to Chapter 5, "A Practical Guide to Using ECT in Minors," for additional details. It should be noted that implantable pacemakers are not a contraindication, and implantable defibrillators should have their functions disabled prior to the procedure (23). Additional details are noted in Chapter 6, "ECT in Youth with Comorbid Medical and Neurological Disorders."

Due to the acute cognitive effects of ECT, patients and their families may welcome a reminder phone call or notification from the clinical staff to remain "nil per os" (NPO) or "nil by mouth" (NBM) on evenings prior to the procedure. The patient must have no solid food 6 hours prior to the time of treatment, although a sip or two of water to take oral medications is permitted.

CASE VIGNETTE

A is a 13-year-old female who often forgot that she was NPO. She would wake up in the middle of the night and have a drink, which resulted in canceling her treatment on multiple occasions. A suggested strategy was that a parent would post a sign in bold lettering, reminding the patient not to drink after a certain time during the night. Additionally, the parents were advised to place drinks in a relatively inaccessible place at night. These strategies worked and the patient was then able to consistently maintain her NPO status.

PATIENT MEDICATIONS

Most regularly received medications have a beneficial effect on anesthesia. For example, antihypertensives and antacids, respectively, improve the management of hypertension and reflux symptoms in patients. Agents that are regularly used by the patient should be given preoperatively, with the common exception of angiotensin converting enzyme inhibitors, which should be omitted on the day of surgery or the day before, if administered in the evening, because of the propensity for severe hypotension when combined with anesthetic agents (24).

Concurrent psychiatric medications are more likely to interfere with ECT than with the anesthetic agents. All psychotropics should be discontinued, whenever possible. However, the detrimental consequences of abruptly terminating these medications should be carefully balanced in tandem with the psychiatric team.

Anticonvulsants and hypnotics are likely to raise the seizure threshold. However, benzodiazepines can be reversed with relative ease, using a benzodiazepine receptor antagonist such as flumazenil, while anticonvulsants are often withheld for 12 hours or longer prior to ECT.

Tricyclic antidepressants have limited value in children or younger adolescents with mood disorders due to lack of efficacy (25) and should be discontinued. However, these agents are occasionally prescribed for other reasons, such as for migraine headaches. For patients on lithium, the serum level should be carefully monitored and kept within the range of 0.4–1 mmol/l. One 2005 review had indicated that lithium may lower the seizure threshold and enhance the risk of post-ECT delirium (26). However, this potential complication can be managed by withholding lithium prior to ECT (for at least 12 hours) and resuming the agent upon recovery from anesthesia.

Antipsychotic medications are known to lower the seizure threshold, with clozapine considered as the most likely agent for inducing this effect. An additional risk of antipsychotic agents is inducing or worsening neuroleptic malignant syndrome (NMS) and catatonia. Therefore, it is advisable that neuroleptic or antipsychotic medications should be discontinued during the ECT course. Anti-emetics, such as metoclopramide or prochlorperazine, may exacerbate catatonia or NMS, due to dopamine blockade as the mechanism of action (27). Similarly, there are reports of NMS associated with the use of other agents, such as hyoscine, which may cause reduced dopamine activity in the central nervous system (28).

DAY OF SURGERY

Documentation of previous anesthetic and ECT, if any, should be available and reviewed. Consent and confirmation of NPO status should also be verified. Usual NPO precautions should be taken. Clear fluids and oral medications, administered with a sip of water, may be permitted for up to 2 hours prior to treatment. The most common reason for treatment cancellation is the failure to comply with NPO instructions. It is, therefore, necessary to emphasize these and verify that the patient is compliant. Written reminders given to the patient and the caregiver following recovery can be helpful. In addition, a review of medications conducted on the day of the treatment provides an opportunity for the family to be made aware of any changes prior to the next treatment.

PRE- AND POST-TREATMENT CARE FACILITY

ECT is generally administered in a specially designated area where there is adequate physical space for pre- and post-treatment observation, skilled nursing care, and the safe administration of the treatment. Adequate privacy and access should be provided for parents and other caregivers, so that they are able to remain with their child for as long as it is safely possible. Staff should be readily available to answer questions and offer reassurance to the young patient and his or her family.

Equipment in the ECT Suite Reception Area

Suggested items in the reception area include:

- weighing scales;
- non-invasive blood pressure (NIBP) monitor;
- sphygmomanometer and stethoscope;

- pulse oximeter;
- thermometer;
- blood glucose testing kit;
- clock with a second hand;
- disposables (gloves, syringes, needles);
- electocardiogram (ECG) electrodes.

Anesthetic Equipment

A full range of equipment for the provision of anesthesia as well as emergency and resuscitation equipment should be available. The lead staff member responsible for the anesthesia team should create a checklist that should be kept in the area. Suggested items may include:

- Laryngoscopes, endotracheal tubes, laryngeal mask airways, face masks;
- Pipeline gas supply (ideally); if not possible, adequate O_2 cylinder supply;
- Anesthetic machine and disposables (circuits/CO_2 sampling tubing);
- Suction wall supply and disposables (tubing/Yankauer);
- Breathing circuit (Jackson Rees);
- Soft bite block.

Emergency/Resuscitation Equipment

Suggested items include:

- Equipment for a "difficult airway"; specifics should be decided by the treatment team and guided by familiarity and availability;
- IV fluids, giving sets (fluid administration apparatus), IV cannulas;
- Emergency drugs;
- Defibrillator;
- Self-inflating bag-valve-mask (e.g., Ambu bag).

All equipment should be periodically checked, at agreed-upon intervals, for example daily or weekly, which is likely guided by the volume of work. Clear guidelines for the management of any anesthetic emergency should be established and posted in the ECT area.

Record Keeping and Organization

Patient records containing details of the preoperative examination, anesthesia and recovery phase should be signed, dated, and kept in a secure cabinet.

Recovery Area

This should be a designated space close to the treatment area, with staff trained in the recovery of patients from anesthesia. Monitors for ECG, non-invasive blood pressure and oxygen saturation should be available, as well as an oxygen supply and suction equipment. The emergency equipment should be easily accessible for both the treatment and the recovery areas. One important consideration for ECT recovery entails the management of post-anesthesia and post-ictal cognitive and behavioral sequelae. Not uncommonly, patients experience a brief period of confusion or mild agitation during post-ictal emergence from anesthesia. Strategies for managing behaviors include reassurance, verbal redirection, and medication, such as a benzodiazepine. In rare cases, it may be necessary to use restraints for a brief period, to prevent injury to the patient or to the staff members.

SPECIAL STRATEGIES DURING ECT

Hyperventilation

This strategy is often used to maximize the seizure duration, although there is no consensus on whether hyperventilation extends the seizure duration, or indeed if the extended seizure activity is associated with greater efficacy of ECT (29). However, this strategy may be a useful adjunct to augment seizure duration prior to administering the electrical stimulus (30). Moderate hyperventilation to achieve an end tidal carbon dioxide of around 30mm Hg is generally considered safe. An additional advantage of hyperventilation, given immediately prior to ECT, is more rapid orientation following the treatment (31).

Theophylline has been used to facilitate seizure activity in patients with seizure inhibition. In adults, the drug is infused 30 minutes prior to therapy, as a slow infusion over a few minutes (32). There are no reported studies of its use in children. There are, however, concerns over its safety, such as status epilepticus in adults, resulting in neurological damage; therefore, caution is warranted when administering ECT in children who are taking a preparation that contains theophylline (33).

Caffeine has also been used to lower seizure threshold and to augment the duration of the seizure. Although there are anecdotal reports of its safe use, systematic data regarding use or safety in children are lacking. Nevertheless, because of its effect on the seizure threshold, caffeine intake is a pertinent part of the history-taking in a youth who is being worked up to receive ECT (34).

PATIENTS WITH SPECIAL NEEDS

Owing to the types of disorder that are treated with ECT, it is not infrequent that anxiety and aggression will complicate management. Often, it will be desirable that a parent or a caregiver is present before the patient is taken into the treatment room in order to allay anxiety and help in the management of any aggressive behavior. The ECT team should discuss each patient on a case-by-case basis to address potential issues and the utility of having a family member present.

It is important that expectations and questions about the process of anesthesia are addressed prior to ECT. The team should be unified with a full and unequivocal explanation given to families regarding the expectations around contact with their child pre- and post-treatment. Safety dictates that the treatment team has unobstructed access to patients at all times. Consequently, families must depart the clinical area when asked to do so.

RISKS ASSOCIATED WITH ANESTHESIA DURING ECT

There are concerns about the effect of ECT on a developing brain; however, these concerns remain unfounded and should be weighed against the risks of a prolonged, severe psychiatric disorder or a medical condition. For example, poorer long-term outcome has been shown in patients who did not receive an antipsychotic agent during their first-break psychotic illness, while improved outcomes are more likely with treatment (35). Similarly, poorer long-term outcome has been shown in patients with long-standing, untreated mood disorders.

Anesthesia-related mortality is estimated to be 1.1 per 10,000 anesthesia procedures. A report by the US Department of Health and Human Services purported such risks to be similar in children as in adults (36). There is no evidence that ECT in children or adults is associated with higher rates of anesthesia-related mortality, when compared with anesthesia given for another equivalent procedure.

Prompt management of prolonged seizures is necessary to prevent a greater degree of amnesia, greater post-ictal confusion, and complications of secondary hypoxia. Children have a lower seizure threshold, and although there is no clear evidence that children or adolescents experience a higher frequency of prolonged seizures, any seizure lasting longer than 2 minutes should be promptly terminated with intravenous benzodiazepine or with propofol. It is also essential to control prolonged seizures in order to prevent progression to status epilepticus and to prevent any associated morbidity (37).

CONCLUSION

Modern anesthesia for ECT is very different from the anesthesia that was used when ECT was first administered to young people in the early 1940s. Contemporary anesthesia for ECT is safe, effective, and short-acting, and has rendered the treatment free of major discomfort or injury. Further, there are no data to suggest that anesthesia administered to young patients is riskier than in adults. It is essential that due attention is given to a range of processes and factors, including key personnel involved in the treatment, medical workup, anesthetic agents, anesthetic equipment, pre- and post-treatment care facility and patient supervision and monitoring. Attention to factors which influence the ECTseizure quality, have helped ensure that ECT in young persons is performed safely and with optimal benefit.

QUESTIONS AND ANSWERS

1. *Is repeated anesthesia dangerous for a child or an adolescent?*

   There is evidence to suggest that anesthesia and surgery before the age of 2 to 3 years is an independent risk factor for ongoing learning difficulty (38). However, youth who receive this treatment are invariably much older. Very young age may render greater vulnerability to the neurotoxic effects of anesthesia, which has been shown in rodents and in non-human primates (38). However, this evidence is limited due to being retrospective and lacking in standardized outcome measures. Unrelated to ECT, the safety of anesthesia in children is being studied in two ongoing prospective studies: the PANDA project (Pediatric Anesthesia and Neurodevelopmental Assessment), which is investigating effects on children under the age of 36 months undergoing inguinal hernia surgery, and the GAS (General Anesthesia Spinal study), which is examining a similar cohort of patients comparing regional anesthesia with general anesthesia. Nevertheless, at this time there is no evidence to support that repeated anesthesia is dangerous to children or to adolescents.

2. *Is anesthesia always administered by an anesthesiologist?*

   Anesthesia may be administered by a physician anesthesiologist, or a certified registered nurse anesthetist (CRNA) working under the supervision of a physician anesthesiologist.

3. *When does a child have to stop eating and drinking prior to anesthesia?*

   Nothing should be eaten within 6 hours of the start of the procedure: 6 hours before the scheduled time the child can have a light meal, a glass of milk, or a fizzy drink. Children can become more rapidly dehydrated than adults; therefore, it is advisable that fluid is given promptly following the procedure, whenever it is safe to do so.

4. *What side effects should a parent or a caregiver look for on the day of the treatment?*

   Common side effects are headache, body ache, nausea, confusion, and memory loss. The hospital staff always ensures that the patient is sent home with suitable analgesia (see below). Occasionally, children feel or are sick after an anesthetic, and this may occur in the car on the way home (1 in 10). There are medicines that can be given to prevent this effect; if the child is prone to travel sickness, a medication for nausea may be requested at the hospital. All patients and families should be advised to contact the hospital, in case of concerns.

5. *What measures can be used to alleviate or prevent progression to a severe headache in a child or an adolescent who has experienced a severe headache after treatment, despite receiving pre-treatment ibuprofen or acetaminophen?*

   Pre-treatment is usually not offered prior to the first ECT session. If headache occurs after the first treatment, then simple analgesics such as acetaminophen or ibuprofen may be administered. IV ketorolac may be used if the pain is more severe in conjunction with IV hydration. In cases of severe headache, requiring ketorolac, the patient may receive prophylactic ketorolac during subsequent treatment sessions. Both ibuprofen and ketorolac belong to the NSAID group of medication and are contraindicated in patients with sensitivity to this group of agents. If headache is not controlled with this regimen, anti-migraine medication may be effective; sumatriptan can be used in children over the age of 12 years but should be avoided in patients with congenital heart disease.

6. *How should anxiety be managed in a child or an adolescent who is anxious about ECT on the night prior to the procedure?*

   Transparency is a key issue. All children should be told that they are going to the hospital for treatment, and the procedure should be explained in age-appropriate language. In most cases, verbal reassurance may be sufficient. However, a low dose benzodiazepine may be helpful in more severe cases of anxiety.

DISCLOSURES

Dr. Daniel Gih has no conflicts to disclose.

Dr. Emma Louise Taylor has no conflicts of interest, financial or otherwise, including direct or indirect financial or personal relationships, interests, and affiliations, whether or not directly related to the subject of the chapter.

Dr. Bernard Biermann has no conflicts of interest to report. He has no affiliation with industry and is not receiving any grant funding at present.

REFERENCES

1. Shah N, Mahadeshwar S, Bhakta S, Bhirud M, Fernandes P, Andrade C. The safety and efficacy of benzodiazepine-modified treatments as a special form of unmodified ECT. *J ECT*. Mar 2010;26(1):23–9.
2. Schneekloth TD, Rummans TA, Logan KM. Electroconvulsive therapy in adolescents. *Convuls Ther*. 1993;9(3):158–66.
3. Moise FN, Petrides G. Case study: electroconvulsive therapy in adolescents. *J Am Acad Child Adolesc Psychiatry*. Mar 1996;35(3):312–8.
4. Russell PS, Tharyan P, Arun Kumar K, Cherian A. Electro convulsive therapy in a pre-pubertal child with severe depression. *J Postgrad Med*. Oct-Dec 2002;48(4):290–1.
5. Black DW, Winokur G, Nasrallah A. Treatment of mania: a naturalistic study of electroconvulsive therapy versus lithium in 438 patients. *J Clin Psychiatry*. Apr 1987;48(4):132–9.
6. Carr V, Dorrington C, Schrader G, Wale J. The use of ECT for mania in childhood bipolar disorder. *Br J Psychiatry*. Oct 1983;143:411–5.
7. Cizadlo BC, Wheaton A. Case study: ECT treatment of a young girl with catatonia. *J Am Acad Child Adolesc Psychiatry*. Mar 1995;34(3):332–5.
8. Clardy ER, Rumpf EM. The effect of electric shock treatment on children having schizophrenic manifestations. *Psychiatr Q*. 1954;28(4):616–23.
9. Gurevitz S, Helme WH. Effects of electroconvulsive therapy on personality and intellectual functioning of the schizophrenic child. *J Nerv Ment Dis*. Sep-Oct 1954;120(3-4):213–26.
10. Guttmacher LB, Cretella H. Electroconvulsive therapy in one child and three adolescents. *J Clin Psychiatry*. Jan 1988;49(1):20–3.
11. Powell JC, Silveira WR, Lindsay R. Pre-pubertal depressive stupor: a case report. *Br J Psychiatry*. Nov 1988;153:689–92.
12. Fink M, Klein D. An ethical dilemma in child psychiatry. *Psychiat Bull*. 1995; 19:650–1.
13. Fink M, Carlson GA. ECT and prepubertal children. *J Am Acad Child Adolesc Psychiatry*. Oct 1995;34(10):1256–7.
14. Hooten WM, Rasmussen KG, Jr. Effects of general anesthetic agents in adults receiving electroconvulsive therapy: a systematic review. *J ECT*. Sep 2008;24(3):208–23.
15. Kadoi Y, Saito S, Ide M, Toda H, Sekimoto K, Seki S, et al. The comparative effects of propofol versus thiopentone on left ventricular function during electroconvulsive therapy. *Anaesth Intensive Care*. Apr 2003;31(2):172–5.
16. Walter G, Rey JM. An epidemiological study of the use of ECT in adolescents. *J Am Acad Child Adolesc Psychiatry*. 1997 Jun;36(6):809–15.
17. Fear CF, Littlejohns CS, Rouse E, McQuail P. Propofol anaesthesia in electroconvulsive therapy. Reduced seizure duration may not be relevant. *Br J Psychiatry*. Oct 1994;165(4):506–9.
18. Rasmussen KG, Jarvis MR, Zorumski CF. Ketamine anesthesia in electroconvulsive therapy. *Convuls Ther*. Dec 1996;12(4):217–23.
19. Kranaster L, Kammerer-Ciernioch J, Hoyer C, Sartorius A. Clinically favourable effects of ketamine as an anaesthetic for electroconvulsive therapy: a retrospective study. *Eur Arch Psychiatry Clin Neurosci*. Dec 2011;261(8):575–82.
20. Palmer J, Khalil M, Meagher D. Inhalation induction with sevoflurane for electroconvulsive therapy: a case series. *Psychiat Bull*. 2004;28:326–8.

21. Rasmussen KG, Laurila DR, Brady BM, Lewis CL, Niemeyer KD, Sun NM, et al. Anesthesia outcomes in a randomized double-blind trial of sevoflurane and thiopental for induction of general anesthesia in electroconvulsive therapy. *J ECT.* Dec 2007;23(4):236–8.
22. Carr AS, Courtman S, Holtby H, Morton N, Jacobson S, Brennan L, et al. *Guidelines on the Prevention of Post-operative Vomiting in Children.* London: The Association of Paediatric Anaesthetists of Great Britain & Ireland; 2009.
23. Diprose P, Pierce J. CEPD reviews. *Br J Anaesth.* 2001;1:166–70.
24. Whinney C. Perioperative medication management: general principles and practical applications. *Cleve Clin J Med.* Nov 2009;76 Suppl 4:S126–32.
25. Hazell P, O'Connell D, Heathcote D, Henry D. Tricyclic drugs for depression in children and adolescents. *Cochrane Database Syst Rev.* 2002(2):CD002317.
26. Dolenc TJ, Rasmussen KG. The safety of electroconvulsive therapy and lithium in combination: a case series and review of the literature. *J ECT.* Sep 2005;21(3):165–70.
27. Rodgers C. Extrapyramidal side effects of antiemetics presenting as psychiatric illness. *Gen Hosp Psychiatry.* 1992 May;14(3):192–5.
28. Kashyap GL, Patel AG. Neuroleptic Malignant syndrome (NMS): a rare presentation induced by an antiemetic—case report. *Psychiatr Danub.* Sep 2011;23 Suppl 1:S43–5.
29. Loo CK, Kaill A, Paton P, Simpson B. The difficult-to-treat electroconvulsive therapy patient—Strategies for augmenting outcomes. *J Affect Disord.* 2010 Aug;124(3):219–27.
30. Sawayama E, Takahashi M, Inoue A, Nakajima K, Kano A, Sawayama T, et al. Moderate hyperventilation prolongs electroencephalogram seizure duration of the first electroconvulsive therapy. *J ECT.* Sep 2008;24(3):195–8.
31. Mayur P, Bray A, Fernandes J, Bythe K, Gilbett D. Impact of hyperventilation on stimulus efficiency during the early phase of an electroconvulsive therapy course: a randomized double-blind study. *J ECT.* 2010 Jun;26(2):91–4.
32. Leentjens AF, van den Broek WW, Kusuma A, Bruijn JA. Facilitation of ECT by intravenous administration of theophylline. Convuls Ther. Dec 1996;12(4):232–7.
33. Rasmussen KG, Zorumski CF. Electroconvulsive therapy in patients taking theophylline. *J Clin Psychiatry.* Nov 1993;54(11):427–31.
34. Coffey CE, Figiel GS, Weiner RD, Saunders WB. Caffeine augmentation of ECT. *Am J Psychiatry.* May 1990;147(5):579–85.
35. Wyatt RJ. Neuroleptics and the natural course of schizophrenia. *Schizophr Bull.* 1991;17(2):325–51.
36. U.S. Department of Health and Human Services. *Mental Health: A Report of the Surgeon General.* Rockville, MD: U.S. Department of Health and Human Services, Substance Abuse and Mental Health Services Administration, Center for Mental Health Services, National Institutes of Health, National Institute of Mental Health, 1999:259–60.
37. Cristancho MA, Alici Y, Augoustides JG, O'Reardon JP. Uncommon but serious complications associated with electroconvulsive therapy: recognition and management for the clinician. *Curr Psychiatry Rep.* Dec 2008;10(6):474–80.
38. Sun L. Early childhood general anaesthesia exposure and neurocognitive development. *Br J Anaesth.* Dec 2010;105 Suppl 1:i61–8.

CHAPTER 8

Side Effects of ECT

ANGÈLE CONSOLI, WILLIAM DE CARVALHO,
AND DAVID COHEN

KEY POINTS

- Electroconvulsive therapy (ECT) is a low-risk procedure.
- In adults, the risk of death is the same as in anesthesia for ambulatory surgery and lower than that reported for normal childbirth.
- No deaths have been reported in adolescents to date.
- Minor side effects are generally benign and transient, occur hours or days following the ECT session, and include headache, nausea, vomiting, and confusion.
- Anterograde amnesia is temporary and disappears in the weeks or months following ECT, in adolescents and adults.
- Regarding retrograde memory impairment, some periods of lacunar amnesia involving events close to ECT sessions can be permanent.
- Prolonged seizures and headaches are more frequent in adolescents compared to older adults.
- Confusional states seem to be more frequent in older adults compared to adolescents and young adults.

OVERVIEW

In this chapter, we describe the short- and long-term side effects of electroconvulsive therapy (ECT). It should be acknowledged, however, that there are no controlled studies of ECT in adolescents. Based on the available data, albeit scant, in adolescents and extensive data in adults, the side effects of ECT appear to have a favorable risk-benefit ratio for the treatment of severe psychiatric disorders in young persons.

Numerous myths and fear exist among the general population regarding ECT. These largely unfounded beliefs include that ECT induces permanent memory loss, causes brain damage and is not compatible with the practice of psychotherapy. Existing data indicate that the treatment is effective in treating severe psychiatric disorders in both adults and adolescents; it is a safe procedure and can be lifesaving in some cases. However, systematic research exploring short- and long-term side effects of ECT, especially in young people, are essential.

REVIEW OF ADULT LITERATURE

In adults, the mortality rate of ECT is currently estimated at about 2 deaths per 100,000 treatments (1). This is equivalent to the mortality rate attributed to anesthesia for ambulatory surgery (2) and is below that reported for normal childbirth (1). The cause of death during ECT is essentially from cardiovascular disorder—most often, a previous anomaly that has not been taken into account (for example, cardiac rhythm disorder or hypertension). Mortality associated with ECT has markedly decreased with improvement in anesthesia and medical monitoring during a session. Currently, ECT can be considered a low-risk procedure, even among older patients with cardiac disorders (3). Four non-randomized cohort studies compared mortality rates in depressed patients receiving ECT with patients who had not been treated with ECT. This study found no differences in patients who had received ECT (4–7). Furthermore, it has been suggested that the mortality rate attributed to ECT is below that among patients treated with tricyclic antidepressants (8). Even cerebral-vascular complications, despite a two- or threefold increase in cerebral blood pressure during the procedure, are very rare (9). Other side effects may occur in association with the anesthesia and may include disturbance in cardiac rhythm, variations in blood pressure, respiratory incidents, and allergic reactions. These require careful monitoring and are better managed using current technology, compared to two or three decades ago. Prolonged apnea is rare and mainly involves patients with an enzyme deficiency (pseudocholinesterase deficiency, affecting less than 1% of the population) (10–12). Post-ECT agitation may affect up to 7% of patients (13). The responsible factors are thought to include disorientation and abnormally high concentrations of plasma lactate due to insufficient curarization.

To understand memory impairment in ECT, it is necessary to review the cognitive architecture of memory, which includes diverse subtypes. Anterograde memory enables retaining newly learned information, and retrograde memory concerns the recall of information acquired before a specific event, while long-term memory concerns the recall of events after storage. Long-term memory includes two distinct systems: explicit and implicit memories. Explicit memory concerns naming and describing conscious memories and includes episodic (or autobiographic) memory and semantic memory.

Autobiographical memory (also known as episodic memory) involves the storage of all personal information and memories, whereas semantic memory concerns the storage of world knowledge. Implicit memory includes memory that is expressed otherwise than with words and includes procedural memory (enabling the acquisition of skills), associative memory (involved in data recovery process), and visuo-spatial memory (memory of positioning of objects in the space).

Although memory is altered in the period immediately following ECT (1, 14–17), permanent memory loss is uncommon, even after numerous ECT sessions (1, 6, 18). Memory disturbance following ECT is known to result in temporary anterograde and retrograde amnesia (19–23). Anterograde amnesia disappears most often within a few months following the end of the ECT course (6, 24). However, a cumulative effect on memory exists during an ECT course, and severity of the impairment may increase with the number of treatments. Retrograde amnesia can last for some time (6, 25) and may vary from a few hours to two years before the ECT session (19, 26). Deficits in retrograde memory may involve public events and autobiographical memory (such as vacations, family gatherings). Amnestic effects seem greatest and most persistent for knowledge about the world ("impersonal memory") compared with knowledge about the self ("personal memory") (21). These deficits, more often partial, mostly concern events that occurred in the period close to the treatment. Some periods of lacunar amnesia, defined by loss of memory of a specific event, can be permanent for events close to the ECT sessions (27).

The degree of memory impairment depends on several factors (1, 6): the number of ECT sessions (28), whether or not the seizure threshold is exceeded (29), the nature of the current (brief pulsed or sinusoidal) (30), the lateralization of the electrodes, and the presence of persistent depressive symptoms prior to ECT (31). Explicit memory, associative memory and visuo-spatial memory are also modified by ECT (14, 32, 33). Implicit memory, procedural memory, and semantic memory are not modified by ECT (28, 34).

There is no consensus regarding the extent of memory impairment or time to recovery, but most authors assert that there is no detectable deficit 3 to 6 months after ECT (14). Recovery time can vary according to age, position of electrodes, lateralization, and electrical dosage in relation to the seizure threshold (33). Calev. reported absence of anterograde memory impairment one month after the last ECT session (bilateral ECT, intensity moderately above the threshold). Six months later, the same authors reported total recovery and a better level of acquisition than before ECT (35). Several years after ECT, patients who received ECT do not differ in their cognitive functions from those who did not receive ECT (18, 36). Another study, in which cognitive impairment was assessed 6 months after ECT, found no significant difference in a group of patients who had received real ECT compared to a group of patients who had received simulated ECT for subjective memory impairment, new learning, and remote memory (37). Similarly, a controlled trial found no significant difference in memory impairment measured at the end of the course of ECT in patients who had received ECT compared to those who had received pharmacotherapy (38). However, another study found that a greater number of patients who had been treated with ECT complained of loss of memory, compared with patients treated with medication (39). Studies using bilateral versus unilateral ECT showed longer time to recovery of orientation and greater anterograde memory impairment within 7 days of the end of the randomized phase of treatment. Nevertheless, in relation to longer term cognitive outcomes, two studies found a lack of significant difference between unilateral and bilateral electrode placement on short- and long-term memory functions (30, 40). Other relevant findings include that more frequent ECT is more likely to lead to greater cognitive impairment, and higher dose ECT is also associated with greater anterograde memory impairment and longer time to regain orientation (6). However, bilateral ECT is moderately more effective than unilateral ECT, and high-dose ECT is more effective than low dose. Hence, different clinical situations will probably require a different approach for the optimum administration of ECT.

Regarding side effects of maintenance ECT, a case-control study found impaired verbal fluency (41, 42). A long-term study in adults who were receiving maintenance ECT found lower memory scores and impaired verbal learning in comparison to a control group (43). However, another study found no significant difference between patients receiving maintenance ECT and a control group (44).

Variability in results based on these studies is partly due to the difficulty in assessing memory functions. Assessment of memory function depends upon the time between learning and recall and on the nature of recall used (free or cued—subject is given cues at the time of recall). It is noteworthy that other cognitive functions are not modified by ECT, except for verbal fluency (45). Indeed, intelligence, language, perceptual reasoning, visuo-spatial, motor functions, manual dexterity, and attention do not appear to be modified hours or days following the last ECT treatment session (14). Only verbal fluency seems to be modified by ECT, via altered semantic memory (46, 47). Finally, Calev. reported that non-memory functions assessed from one week to seven months after the last ECT treatment had improved, compared with the non-memory functions assessed prior to ECT (33). This improvement is probably due to improvement in cognitive functions that were affected by depressive symptoms and thus improved by ECT. Some studies have reported differences in relation to electrical variables during ECT, such as the wave form and the pulse type (brief pulse versus sine wave form) (6).

The data are sparse regarding the frequency of prolonged seizures during ECT. It is possible that many cases of prolonged seizures are unreported, and thus the under-reporting may have resulted in inaccurate estimation (48).

Table 8.1. SIDE EFFECTS OF ECT IN YOUTH

Studies	Number of subjects	Major side effects					Minor side effects
		Death	Objective memory impairment	Subjective memory impairment	Prolonged seizures	Tardive seizures	
Guttmacher and Cretella, 1988	4	No	No assessment	Not reported	n=3	None	Not reported
Schneekloth et al., 1993	20	No	No assessment	Not reported	n=2 (during first ECT session)	n=1 (after first ECT session)	Not reported
Kutcher and Robertson, 1995	16	No	No assessment	≤5% just after ECT	None	None	Mild symptoms: headache (54%), confusion (18%), vomiting (2%), agitation, hypomanic symptoms (9%)
Moise and Petrides, 1996	13	No	No assessment	None 8 months to 3 years after last ECT (phone interview; n= 8)	n=3 (seizure duration >180 seconds)	None	Not reported
Walter and Rey, 1997	42	No	No assessment	N=9 (22%)	0.4% of all ECT sessions	None	Minor and transient: headaches (65%), confusion (18%), nausea/vomiting (14%), muscular aches (12%), manic switch (4%)

Ghaziuddin et al., 2000	16	No	Attention, concentration deficits and long term memory impairment were noted one week after, but not after an average of 8 months		n=7		/
Cohen et al., 2000	10	No	No difference with control group for antero-grade memory (mean follow-up 5 years after ECT)	Memory impairment just after ECT (50%) Memory impairment 5 years after ECT (10%)	n=1	n=1 *(the same patient who had prolonged seizure)*	Benign and transient
Ghaziuddin et al., 2011	6	No	No decline in intellectual functioning, short-term memory, or verbal learning. Improvement on long-term delayed memory recall.	Not reported	n = 4 (duration >120 seconds)	None	Not reported
De la Serna et al., 2011	9	No	No difference with control group for cogni-tive variables two years after ECT	Not reported	None	None	Mild and transient: headache (5.9%), agitation (0.5%)

Generally, a prolonged seizure is defined as one that exceeds 120 seconds. The mechanisms behind prolonged seizures are thought to include electrolyte imbalance, concomitant use of medication (e.g., theophylline, lithium) modifying the seizure threshold, repeated electrical stimulation, and withdrawal symptoms from anticonvulsant medication (49). According to some authors, the prevalence rate of prolonged seizures is about 1% of ECT sessions (50). The risk of spontaneous seizures that are distant from the treatment (also known as tardive seizures) is about the same as in the general population (51). Finally, there is no credible evidence of structural brain damage as a result of ECT (52). One study reported an association between older age and severity of white matter lesions in patients who received ECT, but no association with past treatment with ECT (53).

In relation to psychiatric consequences, ECT-induced hypomania and mania are reported in the literature (54), but they do not appear to be frequent; when these side effects do occur, this is generally during the first few ECT sessions. However, most ECT experts recommend that treatment with ECT should be continued when there is treatment induced hypomania.

Minor side effects in adults include headache, confusional states, nausea, vomiting, and muscular pain. Headache affects about 45% of patients (55–57). Headache may be more common among young adults than in older subjects and could be due to differences in the seizure threshold, which increases with age (58). Mechanisms generating headache include contraction of the temporal and masseter muscles, vascular modifications, and disturbance of the serotoninergic system. The frequency of nausea is variable across studies and may range from 2% to 24% of patients (59, 60). Nausea may appear at any time in the treatment and it is not necessarily associated with headache.

Confusional states are frequent, indeed almost routine, during the two hours following the ECT session. This is an immediate effect of ECT treatment and is correlated with the number of ECT sessions (61), the intensity of the current in relation to seizure threshold (35, 61), and the nature of the current used (may last a few minutes with use of brief pulse current, or several hours with sinusoidal current) (30). Complete temporal-spatial disorientation can lead to behavioral disorders (62). In case of longer-lasting confusion, seizures should be suspected (63). Confusional states are more frequent among older adults compared to younger subjects because of frequently associated comorbid conditions and concurrent pharmacological treatment, which can modify the seizure threshold and increase the blood pressure. If confusion commences several hours after the ECT session, further investigation is necessary.

In the past, fracture, luxation, and broken teeth were sometimes reported with ECT. However, these are extremely rare with modern ECT, which prevents such problems with the use of curarization and close monitoring during each ECT session.

REVIEW OF CHILD AND ADOLESCENT LITERATURE

It is noteworthy that no deaths have been reported to date in children or adolescents. However, there is theoretical risk of death, which is similar to the risk associated with brief general anesthesia in young people (64). The side effects of ECT described in adolescents include transient memory impairments, prolonged seizures (more frequent in adolescents than in adults), tardive seizures, and other benign and transitory effects (e.g., headache, confusional states, nausea, muscular pains) (65–70). See Table 8.1 for a summary of side effects reported in youth and Table 8.2 for a comparison of side effects between adults and adolescents.

Table 8.2. ECT AND SIDE EFFECTS: COMPARISON BETWEEN ADULTS AND YOUNG PEOPLE

Side effects	Adolescents	Adults
Side effects due to anesthesia		
Death	No case reports to date	2 deaths /100,000 treatments
Prolonged apnea	Unreported to date	Rare
Post-ECT agitation	Rare	Up to 7% of patients
Other *(variations in cardiac rhythm, blood pressure . . .)*	Unreported to date	Benign and transient
Major side effects		
Prolonged seizure	0.4% of treatments / few case reports *More frequent in young people than older adults*	1% of treatments
Spontaneous seizure	Few case reports	Same risk as in general population
Anterograde and retrograde memory impairment	Anterograde memory impairment: after ECT and disappears in the weeks following/ permanent lacunar amnesia for events close to ECT or related to autobiographical memory	Anterogarde memory impairment: after ECT and disappears in the weeks following/ permanent lacunar amnesia for events close to ECT or related to autobiographical memory
Cerebro-vascular complications	Unreported to date	Rare
ECT-induced hypomania/ mania	Few cases reported	Yes
Minor side effects		
Confusional state	Frequent (18% of the patients)	Frequent in the 2 hours following ECT/*more frequent in older adults than young people*
Headaches	Very frequent (54-65% of the patients)	Frequent (about 45%). *More frequent in young people than older* people
Nausea	Frequent (2-14%)	From 2 to 24% of the patients

Memory Disturbance

There are sparse objective data regarding cognitive side effects relating to ECT in young people. However, three studies have reported no residual memory impairment a few months after the last session of ECT (66, 69, 71). Ghaziuddin et al. (72) compared pre- and post-ECT cognitive functions in a small group of adolescents (n = 6) 4 to 81 weeks after the initiation of ECT; participants had been treated with an index course of ECT, followed by a continuation course (6 months after the end of the index course) and/or maintenance ECT (additional treatment that extended beyond 6 months after the end of the index course). Paired comparison (within subject, pre- and post-testing results) found a significant gain in delayed memory, whereas other functions (intellectual function, verbal fluency, and motor speed) were not significantly affected. In another study, Ghaziuddin et al. retrospectively assessed cognitive functions in 16 adolescents prior to ECT, approximately one week after and 8 months after ECT (66, 73). Some dysfunction, including attention and concentration deficits and long-term memory impairment, was reported one week after the ECT course; however, no dysfunction was observed several months afterward.

The only study assessing long-term memory after ECT comprised 10 adolescents (71), with mean age 17.6 years, who received bilateral ECT for severe mood disorder with psychotic features (five with major depressive disorder with melancholic characteristics, three with manic episode, two with mixed episode). Cognitive functions were assessed on an average 5.2 years after ECT (+/- 2.6 years), using the California Verbal Learning Test, Squire's Subjective Memory Questionnaire, and the attention-concentration index from the Weschler Scale. Two patients in this group were treated a second time, and the mean time-lapsed after ECT was 3.5 years (+/- 1.7 years). The adolescents were randomly matched according to age, sex, school level, current psychiatric diagnosis, and the place where they were hospitalized. No significant difference was found regarding long-term anterograde memory, between subjects receiving ECT and controls and the reference values reported in the general population. Six of 10 patients reported memory impairment just after ECT, but only one reported subjective memory impairment at the time of the assessment. All subjects (the patients receiving ECT and the control group) were assessed for diagnosis, symptoms, social adaptation, and educational attainment (74). No significant difference was found on these variables, except for educational attainment which might be due to the severity of the disorder rather than due to ECT (74). Similarly, another study involving adolescents did not find any cognitive deficits between controls and adolescents with schizophrenia, when tested two years after completion of ECT (69).

A wide range of impairments involving subjective memory have been reported in adolescents who had been treated with ECT (67, 71, 75, 76). For instance, subjective memory complaints reported just after ECT were found by Kutcher and Robertson to be less than 5% (75), 22% by Walter and Rey (67), and approximately 50% by Cohen et al. (65). In one study, among eight adolescents interviewed by telephone after the last ECT session, none reported subjective memory impairment at 8 months to 3 years after the final ECT session (76). In a study by Cohen et al., one patient continued to complain of subjective memory impairment two years after ECT (71). More recently, nine adolescents diagnosed with a psychosis spectrum disorder were assessed just before ECT and at 2-year follow-up; there was no significant difference in cognitive variables between adolescents receiving ECT and controls at the 2-year follow-up (69).

Prolonged and Tardive Seizures

Prolonged seizures and tardive seizures among adolescent ECT recipients have been reported in a few, but not all studies (77–80). Some believe that there is a higher frequency of prolonged seizures in adolescents compared with older adults, probably due to the lower seizure threshold among the young. Thus, it is crucial to follow guidelines for administering ECT and be attentive to appropriate threshold of stimulation and to the duration of seizures in adolescents. Guttmacher and Cretella had reported prolonged seizures in three adolescent cases despite using electrical stimuli that were lower than those used for adults (77). In another study, 2 patients out of 20 experienced a prolonged seizure during the first ECT session, and one had a tardive seizure after the first ECT session (78). However, other studies have reported no association with age, duration of seizures, and response to treatment (76, 78). Studies that have found a positive association with young age include that by Ghaziuddin et al., who had reported seven out of 11 adolescents having at least one prolonged seizure during ECT, and one adolescent had a tardive seizure several hours after the end of the ECT session (73). Similarly, Moise and Petrides reported that 3 out of 13 patients had prolonged seizures (76) and Cohen et al. described one adolescent with a prolonged seizure during an ECT session, who developed a seizure disorder 6 months later (65). Unlike these studies, Walter and Rey found that prolonged seizures are relatively rare and were noted in only 0.4% of all ECT sessions (67).

MANAGEMENT OF MINOR SIDE EFFECTS

Minor, transient side effects are often reported in adolescents treated with ECT and include confusional states, headache, nausea, vomiting, and muscular pain (65, 67, 73).

Headache

Headache is often noted upon waking up after the treatment and may persist over several hours. Therefore, it is important to ascertain headache in all adolescents, keeping in mind that an obtunded patient may not report this side effect. The initial recommendation may include having the patient lie down and rest in darkness, and this could be followed by administering analgesic medications, such as salicylic acid, acetaminophen, or other NSAIDs. Some clinicians prefer to administer analgesic treatment prior to the start of the headache, including prior to the ECT sessions. In case of severe or intractable headaches, sumatriptan (6 mg sub-cutaneously or 100 mg orally) or ketorolac (15 to 30 mg intravenously) can be useful.

Nausea

Nausea can occur at any time and may be independent of headache. Medications generally used are metoclopramide or injectable ondasetron (4 to 8 mg), which may be given alone or in combination with diphenhydramine (25 to 50 mg). Vomiting is less frequent and does not preclude continuing with ECT treatment; however, it may become necessary to medicate the patient prior to the ECT session. Some cases of nausea or vomiting may be associated with the anesthetic agent used, which could be changed if necessary after discussion with the anesthesiologist.

Confusional States

As noted earlier, confusional states are frequent. If a confusional state persists for several hours after ECT, it is important to suspect a subclinical seizure. Another relevant factor is the use of certain pharmacological agents, particularly lithium salts, which are known to increase confusion (1). Withholding the dose of lithium for approximately 12 to 18 hours prior to ECT is known to reduce the likelihood of confusion. There is no clear preventive treatment for confusional states, but careful attention to pharmacological agents being used, the ECT technique and the electrical parameters can be helpful (6). Some advocate the use of unilateral positioning of the electrodes; however, others suggest that patients treated with high-dose unilateral ECT may take longer to regain orientation than those who were treated with a lower dose (81–83). Other useful strategies include ensuring the presence of auxiliary nursing staff and the patient's family, so that the patient may feel reassured and orientation can be restored.

Fear

Fear of ECT is common and, as noted in Chapter 1 ("The History of Pediatric ECT") and Chapter 3 ("ECT and Stigma"), is partly related to negative depictions of ECT in the popular media that extend back over several decades. Addressing fears and myths about ECT and presenting appropriately positive information in the presence of the patient and his or her family is often helpful. Sometimes, fear can be a reason for refusing ECT or ceasing a course once ECT has been commenced. Some patients express apprehension and fear about the potential experience of being paralyzed while not being fully sedated. Adequate sedation before the muscle relaxant is administered, and a small dose of oral lorazepam (1 to 2 mg) given with a sip of water, 1 to 2 hours prior to ECT, can be helpful. It should be noted that the altered seizure threshold following lorazepam can be easily reversed during treatment with intravenously administered benzodiazepine antagonist, flumazenil.

Other Side Effects

Fractures were a known side effect prior to modern anesthesia. However, modern practice with adequate curarization has virtually eliminated this risk. In any patient with osteoporosis, curarization should be maximized to prevent fractures. Fortunately, fractures associated with osteoporosis are an unlikely occurrence in children or adolescents. However, congenital disorders that increase susceptibility to fractures should be borne in mind.

MANAGEMENT OF MAJOR SIDE EFFECTS

Side Effects Associated with Anesthesia and the Electrical Current

Several physiological changes are known to occur during anesthesia. These are mostly benign in nature and, with careful monitoring, more serious problems can be avoided (1). The changes may include variations in cardiac rhythm observed during anesthesia or curarization, including, in rare cases, vagal shock. Therefore, it is essential that ECT should be administered in a suitable medical setting, with trained staff, medications, and a cardiac defibrillator. During the administering of the electrical current, two types of incident are known to occur: a sub-threshold electrical stimulus (when no seizure is elicited) may induce bradycardia, while a supra-threshold stimulus often results in tachycardia. These events are mostly physiological responses and should disappear spontaneously. In some cases, there may be risk factors for a cardiac rhythm disorder, where defibrillation may become necessary. Variation in blood pressure is also known to occur when the electrical current is delivered, and complications attributable to preexisting medical conditions (such as an aneurysm) may arise. Thus, a complete pre-ECT medical examination and laboratory tests, such as a brain scan, are often necessary, although the decision to complete brain imaging may be decided on a case-by-case basis.

Hypertension, mainly relevant to older adults, may be managed by administering ganglion-blocking drugs, such as trimetaphan, which prevents any additional elevation of the blood pressure; there are some data that support an association between memory impairment and blood pressure (84). Although the use of this medication in adults has been shown to have a beneficial effect in the management of blood pressure, there has been no similar study in adolescents (85).

In relation to respiratory effects, hypocapnia may be induced by hyperventilation, which may result from anxiety. In some cases, anxiolytics may be necessary for this problem. Bronchial inhalation of vomitus is a potential risk and may require suction equipment to prevent aspiration and its complications. Prolonged apnea is rare, but oxygenation may be necessary after treatment. A prolonged apnea is particularly relevant in patients with pseudocholinesterase deficiency, who may exhibit a delayed recovery from muscle relaxants.

Allergic reactions to curare or medications that are used for anesthesia are also possible. Allergic reactions to succinylcholine may occur in theory but are rarely seen. In case of an allergic reaction, treatment with sympatho-mimetic agents effectively improves the symptoms of shock. In pediatric patients, succinylcholine—which is used for neuromuscular blockade during ECT—poses a theoretical risk of malignant hyperthermia and, to this effect, the Food and Drug Administration (FDA) has issued a "black box" warning for pediatric usage in the United States.

Post-ECT agitation following ECT may affect some patients, and physical restraint and/or additional sedation (including a small dose of the anesthetic agent used) are usually necessary in these cases. Post-ECT agitation constitutes a real problem, which can lead to discontinuing treatment if the problem is not promptly addressed (86). This may occur during an ECT treatment session, and is not always limited to the early stage of a treatment course.

It should be emphasized that careful medical monitoring (EKG, pulse oxymetery, continuous monitoring of heart rate and blood pressure, availability of a defibrillator and suction equipment) is essential for the safe management of these side effects, which may be associated with either the anesthesia or the electrical current used during ECT.

Memory Impairment

Cognitive impairment associated with ECT may be minimized using measures that include the electrical parameters selected for ECT (6, 45, 87), lateralization and positioning of the electrodes (22, 88–94), electrical dosage in relation to the seizure threshold (81, 82, 95), nature of the current (brief or ultra-brief pulsed or sinusoidal) (30, 89, 94), and frequency of ECT sessions (twice or three times weekly) (47, 96). Some pharmacological treatments have been used in an attempt to reduce cognitive side effects of ECT. However, except for modest benefit when ECT was administered concurrently with triiodothyronin or caffeine (97–99), these attempts have been largely unsuccessful. The proposed mechanism of benefit for triiodothyronin may be through a reduction in the number of ECT sessions needed to elicit an antidepressant effect (98), while caffeine may confer benefit via increasing the seizure duration, without lowering the seizure threshold. Nevertheless, caffeine has been used less frequently since the introduction of pre- and post-seizure electroencephalogram (EEG) monitoring, which allows for better management of the duration and the quality of the convulsion (100). Given that blood pressure also plays a role in cognitive impairment, some authors recommend medications to block the hypertensive peak and thus reduce cognitive deficit (85, 101). However, it is worth keeping in mind that increased blood pressure during ECT is also associated with an efficient convulsion (84).

Based on adult data, bilateral ECT appears to be associated with greater impairment than unilateral ECT, three times a week treatment appears to cause greater impairment than twice a week, and high-dose ECT seems to produce greater impairment than low-dose ECT. There is little evidence from randomized studies that sine wave electrical stimulus causes more memory impairment than brief pulse (6, 94). Given the limited amount of data in adolescents, one should be cautious about generalizing these results. Memory impairment following ECT should also be considered in the context of illness severity and the effect of untreated psychiatric disorders on cognition.

Prolonged Seizures

A seizure is considered prolonged when it exceeds 120 seconds (1). In case of a prolonged seizure, the patient should be oxygenated and given an anticonvulsive medication (midazolam, hypnovel). Prolonged seizures are not a contraindication to ECT, but rather their occurrence suggests that any underlying cause or contributing factor, such as the concurrent use of medication that lowers seizure threshold, electrolytic imbalance, or inadequate hydration, should be ascertained, and electrical parameters should be examined and modified if necessary. In young people, the frequency of prolonged seizures appears to be higher than in adults, presumably because of the lower seizure threshold in the young. Particular attention should be given in adolescents to the stimulation threshold and to the duration of the seizure (15, 64), and in some cases the use of propofol may prevent prolonged seizures (67).

ECT-Induced Hypomania or Mania

Mania or hypomania may be induced by ECT. Symptoms of hypomania may include subclinical manifestations such as irritability, disinhibition, or other behaviors that may be out of character for the patient. Most clinicians recommend continuing the ECT course in the presence of mania or hypomania. However, appropriate precautions to maintain safety should be contemplated (e.g., continued hospitalization, initiation of an antipsychotic agent for irritability), and a mood stabilizer at the conclusion of the ECT course (102) may be considered.

CONCLUSION

It will be reassuring to young patients, families, and clinicians that the side effects of ECT in young persons are generally mild and transient, as in the adult population. Both young ECT recipients and their parents describe the treatment favourably and as well tolerated, despite pretreatment apprehension (103, 104). It will also be comforting to know that there have been no ECT-related deaths in young people. It is nevertheless important to be mindful of the range of side effects of ECT in young people and, for clinicians, the measures that can be taken to reduce the likelihood and to treat promptly.

QUESTIONS AND ANSWERS

1. *Can ECT be fatal?*

   In theory, this is possible. However, no deaths have been ever reported in an adolescent or a child directly due to ECT. Even in adults, the risk of death during ECT is believed to be lower than that reported during normal child birth. Nevertheless, ECT should be administered in a carefully monitored medical setting with staff members who are trained in the care of unconscious patients.

2. *How does ECT affect the heart and the cardiovascular system?*

   Passage of an electrical current is known to result in bradycardia (slowed heart rate). This is followed by tachyarcardia (accelerated heart rate). Certain medications (atropine or atropine like agents) are administered prior to ECT to minimize these side effects.

3. *Is there significant memory loss after ECT?*

   Memory impairment is commonly noted during and following ECT. Ability to learn new information, or what is termed “short term memory,” is most affected. However, most data suggest that there is a complete recovery of memory by 3 to 6 months following ECT.

4. *What other intellectual functions may be affected by ECT?*
   The overall intellectual capacity is not adversely affected by ECT. Other deficits noted during and following ECT may include impairments in verbal fluency, attention and concentration. However, these deficits usually resolve completely within six months of the treatment.

5. *What are the less serious side effects of ECT?*
   The less serious side effects of ECT may include headache and muscle pain, nausea (with or without vomiting), confusion following treatment, and fears about ECT. These side effects are usually limited to the day of the treatment and are ameliorated with support, with over the counter medications and certain commonly prescribed agents.

6. *What do patients who receive ECT think about this treatment?*
   Despite fear being expressed by many adolescents, ECT is usually well tolerated, based on information gathered from patients who have received this treatment and their parents. In addition, studies indicate that most former adolescent recipients report a positive experience and attitude toward ECT, despite initial apprehension.

DISCLOSURES

Dr. Angèle Consoli received travel support from BMS in 2010. Dr. William de Carvalho received support from Bristol Myers Squibb, Janssen Cilag, Astra-Zeneca and Otsuka, variously as a lecturer, researcher and study board Member. Prof. David Cohen reported past consultation and receipt of honoraria from Schering-Plough, Bristol-Myers-Squibb, Otsuka, Shire, Lundbeck, Janssen, Sanofi-Aventis, and IntegraGen.

REFERENCES

1. Abrams R. *Electroconvulsive Therapy*. 4th ed. New York: Oxford University Press; 2002.
2. Reid WH, Keller S, Leatherman M, Mason M. ECT in Texas: 19 months of mandatory reporting. *J Clin Psychiatry*. 1998;59:8–13.
3. Abrams R. The mortality rate with ECT. *Convuls Ther*. 1997;13:125–7.
4. Avery D, Winokur G. Mortality in depressed patients treated with electroconvulsive therapy and antidepressants. *Arch Gen Psychiatry*. 1976;33:1029–37.

5. Babigian HM, Guttmacher LB. Epidemiologic considerations in electroconvulsive therapy. *Arch Gen Psychiatry*. 1984;41:246–53.
6. The UK ECT Review Group. Efficacy and safety of electroconvulsive therapy in depressive disorders: a systematic review and meta-analysis. *Lancet*. 2003;361:799–808.
7. Philibert RA, Richards L, Lynch CF, Winokur G. Effect of ECT on mortality and clinical outcome in geriatric unipolar depression. *J Clin Psychiatry*. 1995;56:390–4.
8. Abrams R. *Electroconvulsive Therapy*. 2nd ed. New York: Oxford University Press; 1992.
9. Hsiao JK, Messenheimer JA, Evans DL. ECT and Neurological Disorders. *Convuls Ther*. 1987;3:121–36.
10. Packman PM, Meyer DA, Verdun RM. Hazards of succinylcholine administration during electrotherapy. *Arch Gen Psychiatry*. 1978;35:1137–41.
11. Reti IM, Torres J, Morad A, Jayaram G. Pseudocholinesterase deficiency in an ECT patient: a case report. *Psychosomatics*. 2011;52:392–3.
12. Williams J, Rosenquist P, Arias L, McCall WV. Pseudocholinesterase deficiency and electroconvulsive therapy. *J ECT*. 2007;23:198–200.
13. Auriacombe M, Grabot D, Lincheneau PM, Zeiter D, Tignol J. Use of midazolam for ECT anesthesia: effects on antidepressive efficacy and seizure duration. Preliminary findings. *Eur Psychiatry*. 1995;10:312–6.
14. Calev A, Pass H, Shapira B. ECT and memory. In: Coffey, CE, ed. *The Clinical Science of Electroconvulsive Therapy*. Washington DC: American Psychiatric Press; 1993, pp. 125–209.
15. Fink M, Coffey CE. Electroconvulsive therapy. In: Coffey CE, Brumback R, editors. *Texbook of Pediatric Neuropsychiatry*. Washington DC: American Psychiatric Press; 1998; 1389–1408.
16. Price TR. Short- and long-term cognitive effects of ECT: Part I—Effects on memory. *Psychopharmacol Bull*. 1982;18:81–91.
17. Sackeim H. *The Cognitive Effects of Electroconvulsive Therapy. Cognitive Disorders: Pathophysiology and Treatment*. New York: Marcel Dekker; 1992, pp. 183–228.
18. Devanand DP, Verma AK, Tirumalasetti F, Sackeim HA. Absence of cognitive impairment after more than 100 lifetime ECT treatments. *Am J Psychiatry*. 1991;148:929–32.
19. Squire LR, Slater PC. Electroconvulsive therapy and complaints of memory dysfunction: a prospective three-year follow-up study. *Br J Psychiatry*. 1983;142:1–8.
20. Ingram A, Saling MM, Schweitzer I. Cognitive side effects of brief pulse electroconvulsive therapy: a review. *J ECT*. 2008;24:3–9.
21. Lisanby SH, Maddox JH, Prudic J, Devanand DP, Sackeim HA. The effects of electroconvulsive therapy on memory of autobiographical and public events. *Arch Gen Psychiatry*. 2000;57:581–90.
22. Squire LR, Chace PM. Memory functions six to nine months after electroconvulsive therapy. 1975. *Convuls Ther*. 1996;12:239–56; discussion 8.
23. Rami-Gonzalez L, Bernardo M, Boget T, Salamero M, Gil-Verona JA, Junque C. Subtypes of memory dysfunction associated with ECT: characteristics and neurobiological bases. *J ECT*. 2001;17:129–35.
24. Smith GE, Rasmussen KG, Jr., Cullum CM, Felmlee-Devine MD, Petrides G, Rummans TA, et al. A randomized controlled trial comparing the memory effects of continuation electroconvulsive therapy versus continuation pharmacotherapy: results from the Consortium for Research in ECT (CORE) study. *J Clin Psychiatry*. 2010;71:185–93.

25. Meeter M, Murre JM, Janssen SM, Birkenhager T, van den Broek WW. Retrograde amnesia after electroconvulsive therapy: a temporary effect? *J Affect Disord*. 2011;132:216–22.
26. Sobin C, Sackeim HA, Prudic J, Devanand DP, Moody BJ, McElhiney MC. Predictors of retrograde amnesia following ECT. *Am J Psychiatry*. 1995;152:995–1001.
27. Peretti CS, Danion JM, Grange D, Mobarek N. Bilateral ECT and autobiographical memory of subjective experiences related to melancholia: a pilot study. *J Affect Disord*. 1996;41:9–15.
28. Squire LR. ECT and memory dysfunction. In Lerer B, Weiner RD, Belmaker RH (Editors), *ECT: Basic Mechanisms*. London: John Libbey: 1984, pp. 156–63.
29. Sackeim HA, Devanand DP, Prudic J. Stimulus intensity, seizure threshold, and seizure duration: impact on the efficacy and safety of electroconvulsive therapy. *Psychiatr Clin North Am*. 1991;14:803–43.
30. Weiner RD, Rogers HJ, Davidson JR, Squire LR. Effects of stimulus parameters on cognitive side effects. *Ann N Y Acad Sci*. 1986;462:315–25.
31. Freeman CP, Kendell RE. Patients' experiences of and attitudes to electroconvulsive therapy. *Ann N Y Acad Sci*. 1986;462:341–52.
32. Squire LR. Memory functions as affected by electroconvulsive therapy. *Ann N Y Acad Sci*. 1986;462:307–14.
33. Calev A. Neuropsychology and ECT: past and future research trends. *Psychopharmacol Bull*. 1994;30:461–9.
34. Squire LR, Shimamura AP, Graf P. Independence of recognition memory and priming effects: a neuropsychological analysis. *J Exp Psychol Learn Mem Cogn*. 1985;11:37–44.
35. Calev A, Cohen R, Tubi N, Nigal D, Shapira B, Kugelmass S, et al. Disorientation and bilateral moderately suprathreshold titrated ECT. *Convuls Ther*. 1991;7:99–110.
36. Stoudemire A, Hill CD, Morris R, Martino-Saltzman D, Markwalter H, Lewison B. Cognitive outcome following tricyclic and electroconvulsive treatment of major depression in the elderly. *Am J Psychiatry*. 1991;148:1336–40.
37. Johnstone EC, Deakin JF, Lawler P, Frith CD, Stevens M, McPherson K, et al. The Northwick Park electroconvulsive therapy trial. *Lancet*. 1980;2:1317–20.
38. McDonald IM, Perkins M, Marjerrison G, Podilsky M. A controlled comparison of amitriptyline and electroconvulsive therapy in the treatment of depression. *Am J Psychiatry*. 1966;122:1427–31.
39. Gangadhar BN, Kapur RL, Kalyanasundaram S. Comparison of electroconvulsive therapy with imipramine in endogenous depression: a double blind study. *Br J Psychiatry*. 1982;141:367–71.
40. Bidder TG, Strain JJ, Brunschwig L. Bilateral and unilateral ECT: follow-up study and critique. *Am J Psychiatry*. 1970;127:737–45.
41. Rami-Gonzalez L, Salamero M, Boget T, Catalan R, Ferrer J, Bernardo M. Pattern of cognitive dysfunction in depressive patients during maintenance electroconvulsive therapy. *Psychol Med*. 2003;33:345–50.
42. Tsourtos G, Spong J, Stough C. The effects of electro-convulsive therapy on the speed of information processing in major depression. *J Affect Disord*. 2007;103:263–6.
43. MacQueen G, Parkin C, Marriott M, Begin H, Hasey G. The long-term impact of treatment with electroconvulsive therapy on discrete memory systems in patients with bipolar disorder. *J Psychiatry Neurosci*. 2007;32:241–9.

44. Russell JC, Rasmussen KG, O'Connor MK, Copeman CA, Ryan DA, Rummans TA. Long-term maintenance ECT: a retrospective review of efficacy and cognitive outcome. *J ECT*. 2003;19:4–9.
45. Krueger RB, Sackeim HA, Gamzu ER. Pharmacological treatment of the cognitive side effects of ECT: a review. *Psychopharmacol Bull*. 1992;28:409–24.
46. Lerer B, Shapira B. Optimum Frequency of Electroconvulsive Therapy: Implications for Practice and Research. *Convuls Ther*. 1986;2:141–4.
47. Lerer B, Shapira B, Calev A, Tubi N, Drexler H, Kindler S, et al. Antidepressant and cognitive effects of twice- versus three-times-weekly ECT. *Am J Psychiatry*. 1995;152:564–70.
48. Rao KM, Gangadhar BN, Janakiramaiah N. Nonconvulsive status epilepticus after the ninth electroconvulsive therapy. *Convuls Ther*. 1993;9:128–9.
49. Devanand DP, Decina P, Sackeim HA, Prudic J. Status epilepticus following ECT in a patient receiving theophylline. *J Clin Psychopharmacol*. 1988;8:153.
50. Glenisson L, Auriacombe M, Fernandez T, Auriacombe S, Gomez F, Uzandisaga D, et al. [Adverse seizure reactions after electroconvulsive therapy. Study of personal cases and review of the literature]. *Encephale*. 1998;24:1–8.
51. Weiner RD. Convulsive therapy: 50 years later. *Am J Psychiatry*. 1984;141:1078–9.
52. Devanand DP, Dwork AJ, Hutchinson ER, Bolwig TG, Sackeim HA. Does ECT alter brain structure? *Am J Psychiatry*. 1994;151:957–70.
53. Hickie I, Scott E, Mitchell P, Wilhelm K, Austin MP, Bennett B. Subcortical hyperintensities on magnetic resonance imaging: clinical correlates and prognostic significance in patients with severe depression. *Biol Psychiatry*. 1995;37:151–60.
54. Devanand DP, Prudic J, Sackeim HA. Electroconvulsive Therapy-Induced Hypomania is Uncommon. *Convuls Ther*. 1992;8:296–8.
55. Devanand DP, Fitzsimons L, Prudic J, Sackeim HA. Subjective side effects during electroconvulsive therapy. *Convuls Ther*. 1995;11:232–40.
56. DeBattista C, Mueller K. Sumatriptan prophylaxis for postelectroconvulsive therapy headaches. *Headache*. 1995;35:502–3.
57. Dinwiddie SH, Huo D, Gottlieb O. The course of myalgia and headache after electroconvulsive therapy. *J ECT*. 2010;26:116–20.
58. Sackeim HA. Comments on the "half-age" method of stimulus dosing. *Convuls Ther*. 1997;13:37–43.
59. Gomez J. Subjective side-effects of ECT. *Br J Psychiatry*. 1975;127:609–11.
60. Sackeim HA, Ross FR, Hopkins N, Calev L, Devanand DP. Subjective side effects acutely following ECT: associations with treatment modality and clinical response. *Convuls Ther*. 1987;3:100–10.
61. Shapira B, Calev A, Lerer B. Optimal use of electroconvulsive therapy: choosing a treatment schedule. *Psychiatr Clin North Am*. 1991;14:935–46.
62. Crider BA, Hansen-Grant S. Nonconvulsive status epilepticus as a cause for delayed emergence after electroconvulsive therapy. *Anesthesiology*. 1995;82:591–3.
63. Fink M. Optimizing ECT. Encephale. 1994;20:297–302.
64. Ghaziuddin N, Kutcher SP, Knapp P, Bernet W, Arnold V, Beitchman J, et al. Practice parameter for use of electroconvulsive therapy with adolescents. *J Am Acad Child Adolesc Psychiatry*. 2004;43:1521–39.
65. Cohen D, Paillere-Martinot ML, Basquin M. Use of electroconvulsive therapy in adolescents. *Convuls Ther*. 1997;13:25–31.
66. Ghaziuddin N, Laughrin D, Giordani B. Cognitive side effects of electroconvulsive therapy in adolescents. *J Child Adolesc Psychopharmacol*. 2000;10:269–76.
67. Walter G, Rey JM. An epidemiological study of the use of ECT in adolescents. *J Am Acad Child Adolesc Psychiatry*. 1997;36:809–15.

68. Bloch Y, Sobol D, Levkovitz Y, Kron S, Ratzoni G. Reasons for referral for electroconvulsive therapy: a comparison between adolescents and adults. *Australas Psychiatry*. 2008;16:191–4.
69. de la Serna E, Flamarique I, Castro-Fornieles J, Pons A, Puig O, Andres-Perpina S, et al. Two-year follow-up of cognitive functions in schizophrenia spectrum disorders of adolescent patients treated with electroconvulsive therapy. *J Child Adolesc Psychopharmacol*. 2011;21:611–9.
70. Rey JM, Walter G. Half a century of ECT use in young people. *Am J Psychiatry*. 1997;154:595–602.
71. Cohen D, Taieb O, Flament M, Benoit N, Chevret S, Corcos M, et al. Absence of cognitive impairment at long-term follow-up in adolescents treated with ECT for severe mood disorder. *Am J Psychiatry*. 2000;157:460–2.
72. Ghaziuddin N, Dumas S, Hodges E. Use of continuation or maintenance electroconvulsive therapy in adolescents with severe treatment-resistant depression. *J ECT*. 2011;27:168–74.
73. Ghaziuddin N, King CA, Naylor MW, Ghaziuddin M, Chaudhary N, Giordani B, et al. Electroconvulsive treatment in adolescents with pharmacotherapy-refractory depression. *J Child Adolesc Psychopharmacol*. 1996;6:259–71.
74. Taieb O, Flament MF, Chevret S, Jeammet P, Allilaire JF, Mazet P, et al. Clinical relevance of electroconvulsive therapy (ECT) in adolescents with severe mood disorder: evidence from a follow-up study. *Eur Psychiatry*. 2002;17(4):206–12.
75. Kutcher SP, Robertson HA. Electroconvulsive therapy in treatment-resistant bipolar youth. *J Child Adolesc Psychopharmacol*. 1995;5:167–75.
76. Moise FN, Petrides G. Case study: electroconvulsive therapy in adolescents. *J Am Acad Child Adolesc Psychiatry*. 1996;35:312–8.
77. Guttmacher LB, Cretella H. Electroconvulsive therapy in one child and three adolescents. *J Clin Psychiatry*. 1988;49:20–3.
78. Schneekloth MD, Rummans T, Logan KM. Electroconvulsive therapy in adolescents. *Convuls Ther*. 1993;9:158–66.
79. Baeza I, Flamarique I, Garrido JM, Horga G, Pons A, Bernardo M, et al. Clinical experience using electroconvulsive therapy in adolescents with schizophrenia spectrum disorders. *J Child Adolesc Psychopharmacol*. 2010;20:205–9.
80. Walter G, Rey JM. Has the practice and outcome of ECT in adolescents changed? findings from a whole-population study. *J ECT*. 2003;19:84–7.
81. Sackeim HA, Prudic J, Devanand DP, Kiersky JE, Fitzsimons L, Moody BJ, et al. Effects of stimulus intensity and electrode placement on the efficacy and cognitive effects of electroconvulsive therapy. *N Engl J Med*. 1993;328:839–46.
82. Sackeim HA, Prudic J, Devanand DP, Nobler MS, Lisanby SH, Peyser S, et al. A prospective, randomized, double-blind comparison of bilateral and right unilateral electroconvulsive therapy at different stimulus intensities. *Arch Gen Psychiatry*. 2000;57:425–34.
83. McCall WV, Dunn AG, Kellner CH. Recent advances in the science of ECT: can the findings be generalized? *J ECT*. 2000;16:323–6.
84. Zervas IM, Calev A, Jandorf L, Fink M. Blood pressure, memory, and electroconvulsive therapy. *Convuls Ther*. 1993;9:14–22.
85. Petrides G, Maneksha F, Zervas I, Carasiti I, Francis A. Trimethaphan (Arfonad) control of hypertension and tachycardia during electroconvulsive therapy: a double-blind study. *J Clin Anesth*. 1996;8:104–9.
86. Devanand DP, Briscoe KM, Sackeim HA. Clinical Features and Predictors of Postictal Excitement. *Convuls Ther*. 1989;5:140–6.

87. Ottosson JO. Use and misuse of electroconvulsive treatment. *Biol Psychiatry*. 1985;20:933–46.
88. Phutane VH, Thirthalli J, Muralidharan K, Naveen Kumar C, Keshav Kumar J, Gangadhar BN. Double-blind randomized controlled study showing symptomatic and cognitive superiority of bifrontal over bitemporal electrode placement during electroconvulsive therapy for schizophrenia. *Brain Stimul*. 2012;6:210–17.
89. Sienaert P, Vansteelandt K, Demyttenaere K, Peuskens J. Randomized comparison of ultra-brief bifrontal and unilateral electroconvulsive therapy for major depression: cognitive side-effects. *J Affect Disord*. 2010;122:60–7.
90. Dunne RA, McLoughlin DM. Systematic review and meta-analysis of bifrontal electroconvulsive therapy versus bilateral and unilateral electroconvulsive therapy in depression. *World J Biol Psychiatry*. 2012;13:248–58.
91. Viswanath B, Narayanaswamy JC, Thirthalli J, Gangadhar BN. Effectiveness of bifrontal ECT in practice: a comparison with bitemporal ECT. *Indian J Psychol Med*. 2011;33:66–70.
92. Kellner CH, Knapp R, Husain MM, Rasmussen K, Sampson S, Cullum M, et al. Bifrontal, bitemporal and right unilateral electrode placement in ECT: randomised trial. *Br J Psychiatry*. 2010;196:226–34.
93. Calev A, Gaudino EA, Squires NK, Zervas IM, Fink M. ECT and non-memory cognition: a review. *Br J Clin Psychol*. 1995;34:505–15.
94. Sackeim HA, Prudic J, Nobler MS, Fitzsimons L, Lisanby SH, Payne N, et al. Effects of pulse width and electrode placement on the efficacy and cognitive effects of electroconvulsive therapy. *Brain Stimul*. 2008;1:71–83.
95. Prudic J, Sackeim HA, Devanand DP, Krueger RB, Settembrino JM. Acute cognitive effects of subconvulsive electrical stimulation. *Convuls Ther*. 1994;10:4–24.
96. Gangadhar BN, Janakiramaiah N, Subbakrishna DK, Praveen J, Reddy AK. Twice versus thrice weekly ECT in melancholia: a double-blind prospective comparison. *J Affect Disord*. 1993;27:273–8.
97. Calev A, Fink M, Petrides G, Francis A, Fochtmann L. Caffeine pretreatment enhances clinical efficacy and reduces cognitive effects of electroconvulsive therapy. *Convuls Ther*. 1993;9:95–100.
98. Stern RA, Nevels CT, Shelhorse ME, Prohaska ML, Mason GA, Prange AJ, Jr. Antidepressant and memory effects of combined thyroid hormone treatment and electroconvulsive therapy: preliminary findings. *Biol Psychiatry*. 1991;30:623–7.
99. Tremont G, Stern RA. Use of thyroid hormone to diminish the cognitive side effects of psychiatric treatment. *Psychopharmacol Bull*. 1997;33(2):273–80.
100. Nobler MS, Sackeim H.. *Electroconvulsive Therapy: Clinical and Biological Aspects*. In Goodnick, PJ (ed.). Predictors of response in mood disorders. Washington, DC: *American Psychiatric Press*; 1996, pp. 177–98.
101. Zervas IM, Calev A, Jandorf L, Schwartz J, Gaudino E, Tubi N, et al. Age-Dependent Effects of Electroconvulsive Therapy on Memory. *Convuls Ther*. 1993;9:39–42.
102. Angst J, Angst K, Baruffol I, Meinherz-Surbeck R. ECT-induced and drug-induced hypomania. *Convuls Ther*. 1992;8:179–85.
103. Walter G, Koster K, Rey JM. Views about treatment among parents of adolescents who received electroconvulsive therapy. *Psychiatr Serv*. 1999;50:701–2.
104. Taieb O, Cohen D, Mazet P, Flament M. Adolescents' experiences with ECT. *J Am Acad Child Adolesc Psychiatry*. 2000;39:943–4.

CHAPTER 9
ECT for Mood Disorders

NEERA GHAZIUDDIN

KEY POINTS

- ECT may be used for the treatment of unipolar and bipolar disorders in children and adolescents.
- Consideration for ECT in the treatment of mood disorders should be based on illness-severity and treatment resistance; severe illness that is likely to jeopardize safety, may take precedence over treatment resistance in some cases.
- Treatment resistance is defined as the failure to respond to two or three adequate medication trials, usually in combination with psychotherapy, if appropriate.
- ECT should not be considered a treatment of last resort for mood disorders in this age group.
- There are no controlled trials of ECT for the treatment of mood disorders in patients <18 years.
- Improved remission rate and lower relapse in mood disorders are more likely with an individualized continuation ECT schedule, following an index course.
- Although ECT is rarely used in prepubertal children, there appear to be no differences in indication or practice.

OVERVIEW

In this chapter, we define treatment resistant mood disorders (TRM) in youth, the factors associated with treatment resistance (TR), the complications of TRM (academic and psychosocial failure, association with substance abuse, illness-continuation into adulthood, recurrence and relapse, and the risk of suicide) and the role of electroconvulsive therapy (ECT). Historical and epidemiological perspectives are presented to underscore the existence of TRM and to compare the criteria used for different age groups when using ECT. Since there are no controlled trials of ECT for the treatment of mood disorders in youth, we stress the need for systematic, multicenter studies to identify best practice and ensure optimum practice. Case vignettes are used where necessary, using fictitious identifiers. [It should be noted that terms such as "children," "youth," and "minors" are used interchangeably and refer to patients younger than 18 years. "Adolescents" refers to individuals who range in age from 12 to 18 years, whereas pre-pubertal children are those below age 12. Due to paucity of data in pre-pubertal children, the majority of the information presented in this chapter is based on experience with adolescents.

The reader is referred to Chapter 5 ("A Practical Guide to Using ECT in Youth") for identifying patients who may benefit from ECT and necessary steps for managing a case.

HISTORICAL PERSPECTIVE

About 5% of adolescents suffer from major depressive disorder (MDD), with some variability in rates, depending on the subject group under study. For instance, higher rates have been identified in association with comorbid psychiatric or medical disorders. The frequency of treatment resistance (TR) or treatment resistant mood disorders (TRM), however, during adolescence remains unknown. Adult studies report considerable variability, depending on how treatment resistance is defined. In one adult study, for instance, TR was defined by the failure to respond to a single antidepressant trial (1). However, the rate was elevated to about 15–20% when the definition included the failure to respond to two adequate antidepressant trials (2).

The lifetime prevalence of bipolar disorder (BP) in adolescents is believed to range from 1% to 3%. There are several diagnostic difficulties in identifying the frequency of BP during adolescence because of considerable skepticism about this disorder, especially outside the United States, and due to important and frequently overlooked differences in the definition of BP between the *International Classification of Disease* (ICD-10) and the *Diagnostic and Statistical Manual* (DSM-IV). As a result, it is more complicated identifying the proportion of BP adolescents who may also meet the criteria for TR.

In the absence of specific data about treatment resistant mood disorders in adolescence, its frequency may be indirectly based on the number of youth who are treated with ECT. However, these figures can be misleading because of considerable national and regional differences in ECT practice. Furthermore, adolescents treated with ECT are a heterogeneous diagnostic group who suffer from a variety of Axis I disorders. Nevertheless, available data about the frequency of ECT use in this group suggest that a small number of adolescents are treated with ECT—about 1% or less of all patients are adolescents. Thompson and Blaine (1987), for instance, found that about 1.5% (n = 500) of all patients treated with ECT (n = 33,384) during 1980 were below the age of 20 years (3). Similarly, Walter and Rey (1997) identified that only 0.93% (n = 42) of all patients treated with ECT during 1990 and 1996 were below 19 years of age (4).

A historic perspective on depression or bipolar disorder in youth suggests that until the late 1980s, these diagnoses were rarely applied to children or adolescents. Unlike DSM-II (American Psychiatric Association, 1968) which did not include mood disorder in youth, DSM-III did include these disorders in its classification system (American Psychiatric Association, 1980, 1987); however, many clinicians continued to instead diagnose adjustment disorders with depressed mood. This was one important reason that may have resulted in the lack of recognition that these disorders during adolescence can be resistant to treatment, often have a recurrent course, and are potentially life-threatening. It is also likely that this diagnostic tradition may have resulted in an overall lag in treatment studies in youth, with none or little research conducted about ECT—probably the most effective treatment for TR mood disorders in any age group.

DEFINITION OF TRM

There is no universally accepted definition of treatment resistant depression or bipolar disorder in adolescents—collectively referred to in this chapter as treatment resistant mood disorders (TRM). Current understanding of TRM is based on case reports and case series, retrospective data, anecdotal experience, and the adult literature. Commonly used definitions include patients (youth or adult) who have failed to respond to several psychotropic agents (at least 2 or 3) administered in adequate dosage and for an adequate duration, usually in combination with psychotherapy. Although this definition is widely applied to adults (5), it is rarely, if ever, applied to adolescents. For instance, Bloch et al. (2008) compared adolescents and adults who had been referred for ECT during a 5-year period. They found that while most adults were referred for treatment resistance, as defined by failure to respond to 2 or 3 agents, adolescents were primarily referred for catatonia or suicidal behaviors and rarely for treatment resistance (6). Similarly, in another study, adolescents with MDD who were treated with ECT (n = 33) had failed to respond to multiple past trials (mean number of psychotropic trials = 8.2 ± 4.2), before they were considered resistant enough for ECT (7).

Due to the absence of clear definitions and treatment guidelines, TRM is often overlooked, thereby missing the opportunity for timely treatment to prevent prolonged morbidity or mortality.

WHEN ECT SHOULD BE CONSIDERED FOR ADOLESCENTS WITH TRM

The reader is referred to Chapter 5 ("A Practical Guide to Using ECT in Minors") for details about patient selection and management. Current literature (summarized in a later section of this chapter) supports the use of ECT in a subgroup of youth with TRM. Severity of illness and associated imminent risk should be the main criteria to consider ECT. ECT should be considered when there is the failure to respond to at least two adequate trials of psychotropic agents, combined with psychotherapy where appropriate. It is important to underscore that ECT should not be considered the treatment of last resort. There is little justification to manage TRM with multiple agents, often lacking in empirical data and associated with unacceptable side effects. In addition, ECT may be used relatively early during the treatment course, even as a first-line treatment, when there is imminent risk of self-harm because of suicidality, when there are concerns about inadequate food or fluid intake, or when there is risk for further deterioration.

RISK FACTORS ASSOCIATED WITH TREATMENT RESISTANCE (UNIPOLAR OR BP ILLNESS)

Relatively little is known about the risk factors for the development of treatment resistant depression in adolescents. A lack of systematic data specific to this age group and difficulty in interpreting publications which have variably defined treatment resistance are the main barriers. Nevertheless, based on a combination of adult and adolescent data and anecdotal reports, factors associated with TR may include chronicity of illness, a failure to achieve symptom remission (remission defined as either the lack of symptoms or the presence of minimal symptoms), symptom severity, comorbid psychiatric conditions, history of trauma or abuse, and certain demographic, clinical, and chronic Axis III medical conditions. Specific diagnoses such as post-traumatic stress disorder (PTSD) or autism spectrum disorder (ASD) may be additional risk factors.

The risk factors for the development of TR mood disorders in adolescents may be best understood in the context of what is known about treatment response. The most systematic examination of predictors of antidepressant response to date are the TADS (Treatment of Adolescent Depression) (8) and the TORDIA studies. The TADs is a multi-site study involving 327 adolescents, 12–17 years old, with a primary diagnosis of MDD. This study identified treatment response to fluoxetine alone, CBT alone, fluoxetine combined with CBT, or pill-placebo alone. It found that response rates were 71% for combined treatment (fluoxetine + CBT), 60.6% for fluoxetine alone, 43.2% for CBT alone, and 34.8% for pill-placebo (8). The subsequent naturalistic phase of the study found that longer treatment over 9 months was superior to shorter-term treatment given over 12 weeks and that combined treatment (fluoxetine + CBT) resulted in earlier improvement, when compared with fluoxetine alone or CBT alone (9). Thus, inadequate treatment duration appears to be a risk factor for early decline. However, it would be premature to conclude that inadequate treatment duration would also result in treatment resistance.

The TORDIA (Treatment of Resistant Adolescent Depression) involved 334 adolescents who had failed to respond to a prior trial of an SSRI (serotonin reuptake inhibitor) and were randomly assigned to either a different medication alone (SSRI or venlafaxine) or a medication switch combined with CBT. Assessment at 12 weeks revealed that combined treatment was superior to medication alone, while response to treatment was more likely in adolescents with less severe depression and lower depression severity, less family conflict, and absence of non-suicidal self-injury (10). After 6 months, the rate of remission was a mere 38.9% and was more likely to occur in adolescents who had lower depression severity, hopelessness, or anxiety (11). Therefore, the findings from TORDIA suggest that adolescents who have failed even a single trial of an SSRI have a relatively low likelihood of achieving remission, despite intensive treatment with an antidepressant combined with CBT over a substantial duration of 6 months. It is worth noting that the illness severity of adolescents who generally receive ECT far exceeds that of patients in the TORDIA study. For instance, a recent retrospective study of TR adolescents (n = 33) treated with ECT found that patients were severely depressed, had attempted suicide on multiple occasions, and had been hospitalized several times (12).

Findings from these adolescent studies suggest that inadequate treatment duration and past history of failure to respond, even to a single antidepressant agent, appear to be associated with poor response to treatment. While variables associated with TR depression in adults include inadequate dosing of antidepressant, poor adherence, and comorbidity with Axis I, II, or III disorders (13); symptoms of melancholia (14); female gender and longer duration of the index episode (15); and psychiatric or medical comorbidity (5).

ECT LITERATURE: TREATMENT OF SEVERE AND/OR TREATMENT RESISTANT MOOD DISORDERS

This section summarizes the ECT literature in adolescents, where ECT was used for the treatment of severe and/or treatment resistant mood disorders. ECT studies in other disorders (psychosis, self-injury, and catatonia) are described in other chapters of this volume. It should be acknowledged that controlled trials of ECT in children or adolescents are lacking and the extant literature is limited to case reports, case series, and studies that are largely retrospective. Nevertheless, the findings indicate that adolescents who are treated with ECT improve significantly following treatment. The reader is referred to Chapter 1 ("The History of Pediatric ECT") to understand the historical and diagnostic traditions that have resulted in the lack of interest in ECT during the past several decades and the paucity of research in this age group.

Bender's (1947) publication about the use of ECT in a mixed diagnostic group of 98 children who were diagnosed with schizophrenia is now considered primarily of historical importance (16) (see additional details in Chapter 1, "The History of Pediatric ECT"). Patients in this group were diagnosed with schizophrenia, using criteria known at the time, and were treated with ECT using more frequent treatment schedules, compared to schedules used at the present time. The majority of patients in this group were improved at follow-up, their cognitive functions remained unchanged (in the subgroup that was retested), and no deaths were reported. However, this work received mixed reviews and, in part, resulted in a ban on ECT in California (17). However, it also stimulated research in the field and set the stage for later studies.

This initial study was followed mostly by single case reports that found ECT to be helpful in the treatment of severe mood and other disorders in adolescents. The only publication that reported a relatively poor outcome to ECT in youths involved four cases, where only one out of the four cases had responded favorably. The three remaining cases did not respond and also suffered from prolonged seizures lasting up to four minutes (18).

A renewed interest in ECT has been apparent, starting in the late 1980s to early 1990s. Using key words "ECT" and "adolescents," a Medline search identified a fivefold increase in the number of publications, with 357 during 1986 to 2012, compared with only 73 during 1960 to 1985. While the earlier publications during 1960 to 1985 had included only a few cases, more recent studies have included a larger number of cases and improved information about the diagnoses and ECT.

The sections that follow describe key publications about ECT in adolescents with mood disorders. Studies described here had included four or more cases and contained systematic information about the diagnoses and the treatment. This information is additionally summarized in Tables 9.1 and 9.2. Table 9.1 includes studies that did not have a comparison group (7, 19–25), while Table 9.2 summarizes studies that included a comparison group (6, 26–29).

ECT in Mood Disordered Adolescents: Studies Without a Comparison Group

1. Guttmacher and Cretella (1988) in a retrospective study, reported four adolescents, ranging in age from 12 to 15 years, who had been treated with ECT during the previous 10 years (19). They reported that only one patient out of four was improved. Two of the four patients were treated, primarily

Table 9.1. ECT IN ADOLESCENTS WITH MOOD DISORDERS: STUDIES WITHOUT A COMPARISON GROUP

Study	n; age in years	Affective disorder/ other diagnoses	Electrode placement	Response/Remission	Side effects	Observations/comments
Guttmacher & Cretella, 1988	4; range = 12 to 15	Depression= 2 Schizophrenia = 1	UL	1 out of 4	Seizures >4 minutes	Prolonged seizures may be due to antipsychotic and/or tricyclic agents given around ECT
Paillere-Martinot et al., 1990	9; range = 15 to 19	Depression = 4 Bipolar = 3 Psychosis = 2	BL	7 out of 9	Minor	
Ghaziuddin et al., 1996	11; mean = 16.3 ± 1.7	11/11	BL = 2 UL = 4 Mixed = 5	Response = all Remission = 7	Minor, Tardive seizure = 1	
Moise & Petrides, 1996	13; range = 16 to 18	8/13	BL = 8 UL = 4 Mixed = 1	10 out of 13	Prolonged Seizures = 3 cases	1 non-responder received a single treatment
Cohen & Paillere-Martinot, 1997	21; range = 13 to 19	MDD = 10 Mania = 4 Schizophrenia = 7	BL = 21	Depression = all Mania = 3 of 4 Schizophrenia = 3 of 7	Minor	Effective for manic and depressive episodes 40% relapse at 1 year
Walter & Rey, 1997	42; <19 years		UL = 30 BL = 5 Mixed = 12		Minor; 2 courses ended prematurely due to SE	Depressive symptoms improved irrespective of diagnosis Improvement apparent around treatment 3
Strober et al., 1998	10; range = 13 to 17	MDD = 10	UL = 2 BL = 1 Mixed = 7	Response = all Remission = 6	Minor	6 out of 9 followed up were in remission at one year
Ghaziuddin 2011	33	33/0	BL	Response = 97% Remission = 60%	Minor	
Ghaziuddin & Dumas, 2011	6	MDD = 6	BL	Response = 5 out of 6 Remission = 4 out of 6	Minor	Longer treatment possibly associated with remission No adverse effects on cognition

*Studies with 4 or more cases are included; UL = unilateral; BL = bilateral.

with unilateral ECT (including the one who improved), one with bilateral (BL) ECT, while electrode placement was not reported in one case. Other findings included unusually prolonged seizures lasting up to four minutes. A possible cause of these prolonged seizures may have been the medications received prior to, or during, ECT. For instance, all the patients had received tricyclic antidepressants and/or antipsychotic agents just prior to ECT and, except for one case, these medications had been continued during ECT.

2. Palliere-Martinot et al. 1990, in a retrospective examination, identified 9 adolescents, aged 15 to 19 years (depression = 4, bipolar disorder = 3, acute psychosis = 2), who were treated with BL ECT during a 3-year period (20). Eight out of nine patients had a positive response; however, one adolescent relapsed one month after treatment. Side effects included mild confusion lasting less than 4 hours in three cases, headache in two cases, asthenia and sedation in two cases, and subjective amnesia in three cases.
3. Ghaziuddin et al. (1996), in a retrospective study, reported 11 adolescents (females = 10, male = 1) with a mean age = 16.3 ± 1.7 years who were treated with ECT (number of treatments = 8 to 15) for severe mood disorders (MDD = 9, BP = 1, organic mood disorder = 1) (21). ECT was administered after the failure to respond to at least three trials with psychotropic medications. Comorbid psychiatric disorders were common (present in 8 out of 11 cases; dysthymia = 4, anxiety disorders = 5, anorexia nervosa = 2, personality disorder = 1). In addition, one youth suffered from insulin-dependent diabetes mellitus (IDDM). Treatment was initiated using BL electrode placement in two cases, while electrode placement was switched to BL position in 5 out of 9 who were started with UL (unilateral electrode) placement. Prolonged seizures, greater than 2.5 minutes, were observed in 13 out of a total of 135 treatments. All patients were improved following ECT on a standardized depression rating scale and global assessment of functioning scale. Neuropsychological testing was completed 1–5 days prior to starting and was repeated 1–5 days after the completion of ECT. Areas that declined statistically included attention, delayed passage recall, and verbal fluency. Motor speed, on the other hand, was statistically improved, while no changes were observed in areas of memory quotient, orientation, passage learning, visual or associative learning, or visual delayed recall. One youth suffered from a single seizure, 6 hours after an ECT treatment; however, no additional seizures were noted during a 6-month follow up, during which he was weaned off prophylactic phenytoin (started after the seizure). Remaining side effects were minor and were limited to the day of treatment.
4. Moise and Petrides (1996), in a retrospective study, reported 13 adolescents, who ranged in age from 16 to 18 years and had been treated with ECT, using their institutional adult protocol during 1983 to 1993 (22).

The adolescents had failed to respond to at least two psychotropic agents. Diagnoses were depression = 1, bipolar disorder = 4, catatonia with affective symptoms = 2, psychotic disorder = 2, schizophreniform disorder = 3, schizophrenia = 1. Prior psychopathology was present in 70%, while history of substance abuse was reported in 9 out of 13 cases. One patient had a concurrent diagnosis of Klien Levin syndrome (morbid episodes of sleep, hypersexuality, irritability, agitation, and auditory hallucinations), while another patient suffered from psoriasis. BL electrode placement was used in eight, UL in four, and one patient was treated with mixed electrode placement (UL followed by BL). Ten patients were deemed responders, with maximum benefit in cases with an affective disorder or non-specific psychosis. At 3-year follow-up, 5 out of 8 patients were asymptomatic, while relapse was noted in 2 cases within a year, despite ongoing maintenance pharmacotherapy. There were no adverse side effects, including problems with cognition, although standardized cognitive testing was not performed.

5. Cohen et al. (1997) conducted a retrospective examination of 21 adolescents (age range = 13–19) who had received ECT during 1984 through 1995 (23). Diagnoses were 10 youth diagnosed with depression, 4 with mania, and 7 with schizophrenia. Five cases were diagnosed with comorbid medical conditions (osteoid osteoma of iliac bone = 1, IDDM and hypothyroidism = 1, Downs syndrome = 1, mental retardation due to neonatal hypoxia = 1, Factor VII deficiency = 1). The mean number of treatments was = 9.5 (range = 3–15). In comparison with boys, girls needed a lower electrical charge to elicit seizures lasting 30 seconds (121 mC in females vs. 310 mC in males, $p \leq 0.05$). All 10 youths with depression improved upon completion of ECT; 3 out of 4 with mania improved, and 3 out of 7 youth with schizophrenia also improved. ECT was more effective in the treatment of both unipolar and bipolar disorders, but less effective for schizophrenia. Memory deficits were apparent by treatment 7; however, none was reported at the time of discharge. A high relapse rate of 40% was found at one-year follow-up.
6. Walter and Rey (1997) identified 42 youth, 18 years old or younger, who had received 49 treatment courses during 1990 to 1996, at any hospital in the state of New South Wales, Australia (24). There was a high rate of comorbid Axis I disorders among a third of this group, and Axis I with a co-occurring Axis II disorder were found in one-quarter of the courses. However, there was little physical illness in this group. In all 49 courses, the treatment was discussed with the patient and the family by more than one psychiatrist, although patients in 14 courses were incapable of giving consent; a child psychiatrist was involved in 30 of 49 courses. Unilateral electrode placement was used in the majority, the mean number of treatments was = 9.5 ± 3.5, mean EEG seizure duration in seconds = 55.7, and

the majority were receiving one or more psyschotropic medications during treatment. Good response was defined as GAF = 70 or higher. Findings from this study included that gender, diagnostic uncertainty, or substance abuse did not predict response. Although depressive symptoms improved irrespective of the diagnosis, a diagnosis of a mood disorder and involuntary status were associated with good response, while a personality disorder diagnosis was negatively associated with good response. Improvement was noted early during the treatment course—as early as after an average of 2.8 treatments. Minor side effects were reported in the majority, although two courses ended prematurely: one due to memory difficulty and a second due to nausea, vomiting, and aches and pains. No persistent cognitive difficulties were reported; memory difficulties were reported in 22%, but were not verified by standardized testing. In summary, ECT was rapidly effective with response noted within the first few treatments, side effects were minor, and depressive symptoms responded to ECT, irrespective of the diagnosis.

7. Strober et al. (1998) conducted an open prospective study in 10 adolescents (females = 7) with treatment resistant psychotic depression who were treated during 1978 to 1996 (30). Adolescents were assessed at baseline by two child and adolescent psychiatrists, and were diagnosed with MDD with psychotic features. Six youth had experienced a prior affective episode (mania or hypomania = 3; minor or major depression = 3). Persistent suicidal ideation was reported by all cases and was present up to the time prior to starting ECT; this included four cases who had engaged in serious, deliberate self-harm while being hospitalized (three had refused to eat, requiring nasal-gastric tube feeding). As part of the hospital-mandated pre-ECT evaluation, three child psychiatrists agreed with the recommendation to treat with ECT. Mixed electrode placement (UL and BL placement) was used in the majority (n = 7), while two cases were exclusively treated with UL and one case with BL. Statistically significant improvement was seen in the entire group, using the Hamilton Depression Rating scale (31), which was noted by the third week of treatment. Nine out of 10 were considered as responders at the 3-week time-point, while 6 out of the 10 youths were in remission at the end of the treatment course. Antidepressant treatment was started at the end of ECT in all 10 cases. Follow-up was conducted at one year in 9 patients who were available. Two cases had relapsed despite pharmacotherapy, at 9 and 11 months respectively, while one patient had experienced an exacerbation in symptoms at month 4. Six of 9 patients remained free of significant affective morbidity at one year. Only minor side effects were reported.
8. Ghaziuddin (2011) described retrospective data involving adolescents who were all treated at the same institution, from 1989 to 2008, and who were diagnosed with MDD (n = 33; females = 19, males = 14; mean age at

treatment = 15.8 ± 1.5; mean age at first psychiatric contact = 12.7 ± 7; mean duration of depressive episode in months = 20.3 ± 22; number of previous episodes = 0.5 ± 1.8; mean number of psychotropic medication trials = 8.2 ± 4.2; mean number of past suicide attempts = 1.9 ± 2.1; history of completed suicide in a relative was reported in one-third of the group; psychotherapy received by 91%) (7). This was a severely depressed group with a mean CDRS score = 67 ± 17 (the Children's Depression Rating Scale; 32) and mean HRSD score = 21.3 ± 5.5 (Hamilton Rating Scale for Depression; 31). Psychotic symptoms were identified only in 27%, while comorbidity with additional Axis I disorders was present in all but 4 cases. Comorbid anxiety disorders were most common and were identified in 13 cases (39%), followed by disruptive behavior disorders in 8 cases (24%) and pervasive developmental disorders in 7 cases (21%). More than one-half of this group resided with both biological parents (17/33) and one in 5 was in special education. A variety of psychosocial impairments were reported prior to ECT; however, the commonest impairment, endorsed by 29 cases (80%), was in the area of school functioning, followed by self-injury reported by 17 cases (48%). Also common was conflict with parents and siblings. Interestingly, relatively low rates of alcohol or drug use were observed—69% and 74% respectively denied ever having used alcohol or street drugs. Decision to proceed with ECT was made after consensus was reached by three child and adolescent psychiatrists (required by state law). Brief pulse ECT was administered using the MECTA or Thymatron (when MECTA was not available); electrode placement was BL in the majority. Thirty-two cases had a positive response (97%), while remission assessed using Clinical Global Index (CGI = 1 or 2) (33) was noted in 20 cases (60%). Side effects were minor and cognitive side effects compared in a subgroup (pre- and post-ECT testing was compared) of 6 subjects found no change in intellectual functioning, while delayed story recall was found to be improved in 3 cases who completed testing at both time points (12). The author concluded that ECT was effective in the treatment of severe treatment refractory depression in adolescents and that neuropsychological data, although only available for a subgroup, did not suggest cognitive decline.

9. Ghaziuddin, et al. (2011) described six adolescents with MDD who were treated with an index course of ECT (three cases had received two index courses), followed by continuation ECT (treatment given within 6 months of the index course) and/or maintenance ECT (treatment given beyond 6 months of the index course) (12). Patients were two females and four males, who ranged in age from 14 to 17 years (mean ± SD = 15.3 ± 1.2) and were treated with BL treatment (mean number of treatment ± SD = 37 ± 4.7). Psychotropic medications were discontinued during treatment, and five out of the six patients were hospitalized during the index course. One youth had refused to be hospitalized; however, a risk-benefit assessment favored

treatment on an out-patient basis, versus involuntary hospitalization; this patient was closely supervised at home and was not considered at high risk for suicide. Continuation/ maintenance course was administered during out-patient visits with closely monitored evaluations every one to two weeks. Four of six cases achieved remission (minimal or no symptoms) while one case was considered a responder (50% improvement). Neuropsychological testing was completed prior to and following ECT (4 to 81 weeks after the completion of ECT). Comparison of results at two time-points revealed that there was no decline in intellectual function, short term memory or verbal memory; in fact, long-term delayed recall was significantly improved. The authors concluded that longer treatment courses may achieve remission, without resulting in adverse cognitive effects.

ECT in Mood Disordered Adolescents: Studies with a Comparison Group

1. Kutcher and Robertson (1995) compared treatment outcome in a group of hospitalized adolescents (n = 22) who were diagnosed with BP disorder (acute mania or depression) and were either treated with ECT (n = 16) or received standard care (n = 6). All 22 adolescents were initially offered ECT; however, 6 declined and thus received pharmacotherapy while remaining hospitalized (26). Cases that were treated with ECT had a positive response, and their length of hospitalization was one-half that of the group that had received standard care (73.8 vs. 176 days). The shorter hospital stay could be translated to a considerable cost saving expressed in Canadian dollars; $58,608 spent for the ECT group, compared with $143,264.00 spent on group that received standard care. The authors concluded that ECT was both effective and a less expensive treatment option.
2. Stein et al. (2004) compared retrospective data for two groups who had been treated with ECT; 36 adolescents were compared with randomly selected adults, also treated with ECT (27). Findings included that the majority of adolescents were treated for affective disorders, including life-threatening symptoms such as catatonia or suicidality (adults, on the other hand, were more likely to be treated for schizophrenic disorders); 61% of adolescents had improved in response to ECT, and 58% did not need hospitalization during the following year, whereas rates for adults were 83% and 49% respectively; both groups did not suffer significant side effects; adolescents were more likely to be hospitalized for a longer period prior to being treated with ECT and were less likely than adults to complete treatment (80% adults vs. 60% adolescents had completed treatment). Findings of this study indicated that clinician are more cautious about using ECT in adolescents (based on longer hospitalization prior to ECT) and the side effects experienced in both age groups are broadly similar. However, for reasons

Table 9.2. ECT STUDIES IN ADOLESCENTS WITH MOOD DISORDERS: STUDIES WITH A COMPARISON GROUP

Authors	n/ age in years	Affective disorder/ other diagnoses	Electrode placement	Response or Remission	Side effects	Observations/Comments
Kutcher & Robertson, 1995	16/ mean = 19.2	16/16	Predominantly BL (87%)	Yes	28% reported side effects; Headache was commonest side effect	Adolescents treated with ECT were compared with those who refused ECT. Greater improvement in youth who accepted ECT
Stein et al., 2004	36/mean ± SD = 17.5 ± 1.9	17/16	Mixed	Yes	Manic switch = 3 Prolonged seizures = 2	Adolescents compared with adults treated with ECT
Bloch et al., 2001	24/ range = 13 to 19	5/ mixed	BL	Remission = 58%	No serious SEs	Compared with adults started on ECT on the same day
Bloch et al., 2008	13/range = 13 to 20	33%/ 67%	BL	Yes	Not reported	Adolescents compared with adults treated with ECT
Taieb et al., 2002	11/< 19	11/0	Not reported	Yes	Not reported	Retrospective study, comparing educational and social outcome with matched psychiatric controls

*Studies with >4 cases are included.
BL = bilateral.

that are unclear, lower response rate was seen in adolescents. Adolescents were also more likely than adults to end treatment prematurely.

3. Bloch et al. (2001) compared records of 24 consecutively treated adolescents, from 1991 to 1995, with a group of 33 adults who had started ECT on the same day (28). Findings included that the technique used in adolescents was essentially the same as in adults and that ECT was equally effective in both age groups. However, adolescents were more likely to belong to the "psychotic spectrum," while adults were more commonly in the "affective spectrum." There was no difference in serious side effects.
4. Taieb et al. (2002) compared 11 adolescents treated with BL ECT (depression = 6, mania = 5) with matched psychiatric controls (matched on age, gender, school level, and diagnosis) (34). Both groups were followed for a mean duration 5.2 years after ECT. Findings included (1) all adolescents at follow-up, with exception of 2 in the control group, had developed BP disorder; (2) 15/22 had experienced an additional episode of mood disorder; (3) the groups did not differ on social or school functioning; and (4) the impact on school functioning was related to the severity of mood disorder rather than to ECT. In addition to demonstrating the deleterious effect of the severity of the mood disorder on functioning, the study findings also underscored the high rates of switch from unipolar to BP mood disorder in this age group.
5. Bloch et al. (2008) examined records of 13 adolescents (age range = 13 to 20 years) with 56 adults (age range = 22 to 80 years) who were treated with bilateral ECT during 1996 to 2002; clinical evaluation was used to determine the total number of treatments (6). Group differences included a higher number of affective disorders in adults (approximately 60%), compared with a lower number of adolescents with affective illness (33%); lack of response to pharmacotherapy was more common among adults (85.5%) in comparison to adolescents (46.2%); adolescents compared with adults were more likely to receive ECT for catatonia (23.3% vs. 7.1%) or suicidal behavior (23.3% vs. 5.4%); adolescents were likely to have received a fewer number of antidepressant trials compared to adults (0.7 ± 0.8 vs. 2.1 ± 1.8); and ECT was similarly effective in the two age groups. In summary, this study found that despite being equally effective in the two age groups, there were important differences in referral-reasons for ECT at the center where this study was conducted. It is unclear if the age-related differences are specific to certain centers or whether similar differences exist across centers.

A Review Study of ECT in Adolescents

Rey and Walter (1997) published probably the most comprehensive review so far of the ECT literature in adolescents; their paper included all studies in this age group that were published in the English language and studies in other languages that were translated (35). Sixty studies involving youth, which included 396 patients, had been published by 1997. The authors rated the studies, using an overall quality score, based on information included in various domains of each study. Among these publications, the majority were single case reports (60%) and the overall quality of information was poor, but better quality was noted in more recent studies. The improvement rates in response to ECT were 63% for depression, 80% for mania and catatonia respectively, and 43% for schizophrenia. The authors concluded that ECT in adolescents seems to be as effective as in adults and side effects in this age group are also not substantially different from those in adults. They did not find any deaths directly related to ECT. However, a 16-year-old girl died 10 days after the cessation of ECT. This patient had continued to receive an antipsychotic agent despite the diagnosis of neuroleptic malignant syndrome (NMS), which was likely the main cause of her death.

Summary of ECT Studies in Mood Disordered Adolescents

The published literature indicates that the majority of youth treated with ECT for the treatment of severe and/or treatment resistant mood disorders are females who suffer from severe depressive symptoms and who are impaired in multiple areas of functioning. They have a history of failure to respond to several psychotropic agents, usually combined with psychotherapy, and commonly suffer from a range of comorbid psychiatric disorders; however, medical comorbidity is infrequent. As far as the administration of ECT is concerned, ideal electrode placement seems to vary by study, although there appears to be a preference for BL placement over UL placement in more recent studies. Clinically meaningful response tends to occur early and may be as early as after the first few treatments. Many adolescents achieve full remission, and the remission rates may be enhanced by using individualized continuation ECT with pharmacotherapy and psychotherapy, if appropriate. Prolonged seizures may be more likely when psychotropic medications are continued during ECT, especially those with known seizure-lowering effects. On the whole, though, side effects are minor and infrequent.

These data indicate that despite considerable evidence of efficacy, there are considerable shortcomings, which include a relatively small number of cases in each study, lack of controlled or prospective data, absence of comparison groups in the majority of the studies, and lack of systematic follow-up information. The ECT technique currently used in adolescents is derived from experience in adults. Therefore, systematic examination of treatment variables specific to adolescents, is essential to identify the safest and the most effective parameters.

TREATMENT RESISTANCE AND THE ROLE OF ECT

Unipolar Depression

A selective serotonin reuptake inhibitor (SSRI) combined with evidence-based psychotherapy (CBT or IPT) is regarded as the first-line treatment of moderate to severe adolescent depression. Failure to respond to one or two SSRIs is often followed by treatment with a noradrenergic antidepressant. Other agents may be added to the regimen of adolescents who do not respond to monotherapy, such as, antipsychotics, anticonvulsants, lithium, stimulants, and so on. The choice of the augmentation agent is not backed by empirical data and is often based upon the symptoms, the side effect profile, and the preference of the clinician. Information about depressed adolescents who do not respond to standard treatments is limited and, given the lack of data, may only be derived from trials that report response (50% improvement) or remission rates (minimal or no symptoms).

Approximately 71% of adolescents may respond to an initial combination treatment (fluoxetine and CBT) by the end of a 12-week period (8), although remission rates may be higher when treatment is administered over a longer duration (9). In one study, adolescents who had not responded to an initial SSRI were randomized to either a different SSRI with and without CBT or to venlafaxine with and without CBT. Treatments were administered over a 6-month period and the resultant remission rate was 38.9% (11). Based on these figures, it can be hypothesized that 18 adolescents with MDD, out of every 100 diagnosed and treated, may not achieve remission (defined as none or few symptoms), despite receiving evidence-based interventions. The rates may be even higher when severely ill adolescents are exclusively studied, because the above rates involved less severe forms of depression. In addition, data suggest that many depressed adolescents who are non-responders and/or fail to achieve remission to antidepressant treatment, also experience a personal burden of illness, and pose a significant public health problem. It is, therefore, surprising that the treatment of the most severe forms of depression with ECT is either omitted from treatment algorithms for depression, or given only a cursory mention. For instance, nationally recognized guidelines, such as those of the Amercian Academy of Child and Adolescent Psychiatry Practice Parameters for the assessment and treatment of children and adolescents with depression do not include ECT as a treatment option (36).

The practice of prescribing alternative antidepressants or augmenting agents, when adolescents do not respond to two or more antidepressants, is confusing for treating clinicians due to the lack of controlled studies in this age group and the possibility that similar to young adults (18–24-year-olds), adolescents may be less responsive than adults to noradrenergic antidepressants (37). Similarly, other commonly used agents such as antipsychotic agents, antiepileptic medications, stimulants, or lithium have also not been systematically studied in adolescents who suffer from TR depression. The frequently reported use of antipsychotic agents in adolescents with TR depression is exclusively based on observation in adults who had received adjunctive treatment with these agents, after failing to respond to antidepressant monotherapy (38, 39). Furthermore, antipsychotic agents are associated with substantial side effects, such as weight gain and obesity, an elevated risk for diabetes mellitus, possible adverse effects on neurocognition and elevated fatality rates shown in post-marketing data (40). Antiepileptic drug (AED) mood stabilizers, which are also used for augmenting antidepressants, are associated with adverse effects on behavior and cognition found in some agents in this class (41). Additionally, an increased risk of suicidality has been associated with AEDs, resulting in a "black box" warning by the US Food and Drug Administration (FDA) (42).

The frequently used practice of changing from one antidepressant to another when there is inadequate response is a widely used practice, although it has its own limitations and needs to be examined further in adolescents. For instance, the STAR-D trial in adults found lower efficacy when patients were switched to a different agent after failing to achieve remission with the initial agent. Furthermore, while one in three adults had achieved remission following the first antidepressant trial, the rates became progressively lower with each successive trial (43). It is possible that even lower remission rates may apply to adolescents, especially because younger patients may be less likely to respond to noradrenergic antidepressants.

In summary, about one in every four or five adolescents diagnosed with MDD may not respond to two sequentially used antidepressant agents administered in adequate dose and duration. The lack of clear guidelines, absence of controlled data, and substantial side effects associated with commonly used augmentation strategies are challenges that need to be addressed in the treatment of severe adolescent depression. Switching treatment from one antidepressant to another when there is inadequate response should be done thoughtfully because of the risk of increasing treatment resistance with a greater number of antidepressants. Some adolescents in this group are likely to benefit from ECT. However, lack of controlled trials of ECT in adolescents and inadequate training of child and adolescent psychiatrists in this area are important barriers that prevent its timely use.

Based on the currently available information, ECT may be a reasonable choice for some patients in this subgroup, when there is failure to respond to two or three antidepressant trials administered in combination with evidence-based psychotherapy. In practice, most child and adolescent psychiatrist do not consider ECT, even for the most severe forms of depression and despite the failure to achieve adequate response to treatment. Possible reasons that ECT is rarely considered are discussed in detail in Chapter 1, "The History of Pediatric ECT," and Chapter 3, "ECT and Stigma."

Bipolar Disorders

There are no studies about treatment resistant BP during adolescence. According to treatment guidelines, the pharmacotherapy of BP disorder of adolescents during manic, depressive, or mixed states is essentially similar to that of adults and should be based on the illness phase, symptom profile, past history of response, and patient/parental preference. Commonly recommended medications include lithium, valproate, lamotrigine, or risperidone (44, 45). A major drawback of these recommendations is that medications are relatively less well studied in adolescents than in adults and may be associated with significant side effects.

Although as many as one in five adults with BP report onset of symptoms before the age of 18 years, the diagnosis and treatment is often delayed by several years (46). A prolonged prodromal phase, sometimes lasting up to a decade, during which non-specific symptoms (irritability, sleep problems, depression, anxiety) may be present, is partly responsible for this problem (47). Additionally, unipolar depression is often the first sign of BP disorder in adolescents, especially in those with an elevated familial risk (48), which may result in many unsuccessful antidepressant trials. Furthermore, variants of BP illness, when incorrectly treated as unipolar depression, have been recognized as a factor leading to the development of treatment resistance (49). Another likely factor is the diagnostic confusion with schizophrenia, due to frequently present psychotic symptoms in adolescents with BP disorder (50). Earlier reports had cited that up to 50% of adolescents with BP may be misdiagnosed with schizophrenia. Therefore, both delayed and inaccurate diagnosis of BP during adolescence appears to hamper the recognition of treatment resistance and its effective management.

Based on the extant literature, BP disorder may be effectively treated with ECT (see Tables 9.1 and 9.2). Furthermore, due to an elevated rate of conversion to BP disorder, found during follow-up of adolescents who had presented with TR depression (34), it is suggested that a high index of suspicion for BP is warranted in this group. It is noteworthy that ECT is rarely included as a treatment option for BP adolescents, including in the American Academy of Child and Adolescent Psychiatry Practice Parameters for the Assessment and Treatment of Children and Adolescents with BP (51).

Based on the existing literature, it is reasonable to expect that adolescents with TR BP would likely present with either a history of failure to respond to multiple antidepressants, or with worsening symptoms, when treated as unipolar depression (see Case Vignette I). However, systematic examination of this group is necessary before any generalizations can be made.

CASE VIGNETTE 1: ADOLESCENT MALE WITH TREATMENT RESISTANT DEPRESSION WHO DEVELOPED HYPOMANIA TWO YEARS FOLLOWING ECT

KM (12) is a 15-year-old who presented with a diagnosis of MDD and a one-year history of worsening depression, failure to respond to two SSRI and two noradrenergic antidepressants combined with psychotherapy. At the time of assessment for ECT, he had deteriorated from being a highly functional adolescent, who had excelled academically and socially, to become severely withdrawn from school, friends, and family, and he was unable to attend school. His family history was positive for bipolar disorder in a second-degree relative. He was diagnosed with severe MDD with catatonic features and was treated with an index course of 11 bilateral treatments, followed by 25 treatments during a continuation course. He had an excellent response and was treated with duloxetine, methylphenidate, and selegiline during follow-up over 1.5 years. At that point, he developed irritability, difficulty in concentration, reduced sleep, and decline in functioning, resulting in a revised diagnosis of bipolar disorder not otherwise specified. He was treated with a low dose antipsychotic agent with positive outcome and returned to premorbid levels of functioning. He remained highly functional and excelled in multiple areas during follow-up over 22 months, when he dropped out of treatment.

COMPLICATIONS OF TRM DISCUSSED USING CASE VIGNETTES

School-Related Problems

Academic failure and refusal or the inability to attend school is frequently seen in patients who are treated with ECT for TRM. The problems may include poor school attendance, varying from weeks, months, to even years, lack of motivation and interest, and difficulty with social functioning. Comorbid anxiety in many instances may predate the mood disorder and is a likely pathway to developing school-related problems. Additionally, a close association has been shown between anxiety and depression in adults (52) and in youth, including those who are at familial risk for later development of major mood disorders (53).

In a case-series of six adolescents with MDD who had received continuation or maintenance ECT following an index course, severe difficulty in attending school was noted prior to treatment (12). Four of the six cases suffered from anxiety disorders that had resulted in school avoidance, dating back 2–3 years prior to treatment with ECT. In these cases, intermittent school avoidance was evident as early as in grade school (4th or 5th grade) and had become persistent by middle school, resulting in a complete inability to attend school. In the remaining two cases, their poor school attendance was more likely associated with repeated or prolonged hospitalizations. One case (out of the six cases) was lost to follow-up: therefore, his pre-treatment school related problems could not be compared to his post-ECT functioning. However, as a group, improvement in depressive symptoms was associated with improved overall functioning and a greater ability to tolerate behavior modification for the treatment of anxiety. This overall improvement also resulted in successful school attendance, using a combined approach with pharmacotherapy and rigorous behavior modification (exposure and response prevention) following ECT. The authors concluded that behavior modification was impossible prior to ECT, due to the severity of mood symptoms. This case series underscored the importance of treating underlying mood symptoms before school-related problems may be treated. Clearly, only a few cases of school non-attendance would meet the illness-severity criteria to receive ECT and in no way should ECT be regarded as a treatment for school-related problems, unless accompanied by severe TRM.

Both long-standing school problems (case vignette 2) and short-standing problems, clearly limited to illness onset, may also be seen (case vignette 3).

CASE VIGNETTE 2: LONG-STANDING SCHOOL REFUSAL IN A PATIENT WITH MDD AND COMORBID SOCIAL PHOBIA

A 14-year-old female with MDD and social phobia was reported in the above publication as case #3, or BG (12). BG was noted to be anxious about school starting at age 11 years. Additional symptoms included worsening depression, self-injurious behaviors (SIB), and suicide attempts. ECT was recommended based on the severity of her symptoms, lack of response to multiple antidepressant trials in combination with CBT, and high risk for suicide based on positive family history of completed suicides in a first-degree and two second-degree relatives. The patient's depressive and anxiety symptoms improved with ECT, which was followed by pharmacotherapy (lithium, selegiline patch, and quetiapine) combined with CBT and behavior modification (exposure and response prevention). As her ECT frequency was slowly tapered down, her therapist worked closely with the patient's school counselor, using a graded approach and helping her return to school, starting with 1-hour attendance that was progressively increased over months. In addition, the patient was permitted to take brief breaks when feeling overwhelmed, and the family was instructed that the patient should remain in school even if she reported "feeling ill." During follow-up over 2 years, the patient continued to receive pharmacotherapy and CBT, she was functioning with minimal symptoms of depression or anxiety, and was able to tolerate a shortened school day with excellent academic performance.

CASE VIGNETTE 3: SCHOOL-RELATED PROBLEMS CLEARLY LIMITED TO DEPRESSION ONSET ONE YEAR EARLIER

KG is a 15-year-old male who had developed depression and anxiety one year prior to his presentation. He had become progressively depressed after learning that his sister had been molested and experiencing family conflict that followed when these facts were revealed. At presentation, his symptoms included increased withdrawal from family, peers, and previously enjoyed activities, sad mood, guilt, anhedonia, increased crying, lack of interest in academic work, and suicidal ideation. Additionally, he had declined from being an A student to where he was failing several classes and was no longer attending school. Treatment with ECT (recommended based on illness severity and risk of suicide) resulted in resolution of depressive symptoms and improved functioning that included return to his previous academic level. At one year follow-up, he continued to receive outpatient treatment that included an antidepressant and psychotherapy and was reported to excel in multiple areas.

Suicidal Behaviors

Suicidal ideation, suicidal behaviors, and death by suicide are relatively common among adolescents diagnosed with unipolar or bipolar mood disorders. Adolescents as a group display one of the highest rates of completed suicide, with suicide as the third leading cause of death (CDC, 2009). Data suggest that suicide intent (SI) and depressed mood may be the two most ECT-responsive symptoms (54). Ninety percent of individuals who die by suicide suffer from depression, which is identified as a leading associated cause. Although strategies for the prevention of suicide must remain multifactorial, effective treatment of the mood disorder is essential. Furthermore, data suggest that adolescents who kill themselves while receiving an SSRI may not have received these agents long enough to derive adequate benefit. Therefore, the rapid speed of response associated with ECT is an important factor worth consideration when selecting a treatment for an adolescent who is imminently suicidal and at elevated risk due to additional vulnerability factors (family history of completed suicide, repeated attempts with a realistic likelihood of death, medical and/or psychiatric comorbid conditions). Whereas, the relatively slow speed of treatment response associated with most pharmacological agents is a factor that argues against conventional treatment in these instances.

ECT may be considered relatively early during a treatment course for some adolescents with unipolar or bipolar illness who are at imminent risk for suicide. Although the term "imminent risk" is poorly defined, published data support that factors such as recurrent SI, repeated suicide attempts, severe depression (characterized by guilt, hopelessness, irritability, or sleep disturbance), comorbid diagnoses (substance abuse, anxiety, and conduct disorders) and positive family history of death by suicide may be used in estimating the degree of risk for suicide.

The following cases involve suicidal adolescents, who had different outcomes following ECT; case "LI" (vignette 4) had an excellent response, while case "IW" (vignette 5) did not benefit from ECT.

CASE VIGNETTE 4: ECT IN AN IMMINENTLY SUICIDAL ADOLESCENT WITH TREATMENT RESISTANT DEPRESSION AND EXTENSIVE FAMILY HISTORY OF SUICIDE

LI is a 12-year-old female with normal intellectual functioning, with no history of abuse or trauma and a history of migraine headaches. She was hospitalized with the diagnoses of MDD, dysthymia, and social phobia, and with a 3-year history of depression with suicidal thoughts. Her family history was highly significant for mood disorders and suicide in three maternal generations; maternal grandmother and maternal great grandparents had committed suicide while maternal great grandfather had committed murder-suicide. LI's mother suffered from severe depression and had been in treatment since she was an infant. The patient had not responded to treatment with venlafaxine, bupropion, sertraline, and lithium combined with weekly psychotherapy. Approximately 3 months after her initial presentation, she was treated with 16 bilateral treatments due to lack of response, repeated hospitalization with symptom-worsening, and escalating suicidality evidenced by an antidepressant overdose and a second overdose with an OTC agent. LI improved following ECT; however, she took one more drug overdose within the first 4 weeks of ECT. She was followed closely while receiving pharmacotherapy and psychotherapy. Her diagnosis was changed subsequently, around age 18 years, from MDD to BP II, due to hypomania, mood swings, and uncharacteristic risk-taking behaviors and reduced sleep. At this point mood stabilizers (lamotrigine and aripiprazole) were initiated, resulting in a positive response. During the total follow-up period spanning 9 years following ECT received at age 12 years, there were no further hospitalizations or suicide attempts. At the time of writing this report, LI had self-discontinued all psychotropic medications over the previous 2 years and, although she continued to function well in multiple areas, she was advised that close follow-up was highly recommended.

CASE VIGNETTE 5: ECT IN AN IMMINENTLY SUICIDAL ADOLESCENT WITH MDD, EATING DISORDER, PTSD, AND HISTORY OF SEXUAL ABUSE

MW is a 16-year-old female with symptoms of MDD with psychotic features, dysthymia, PTSD related to past history of sexual abuse, eating disorder NOS (restricting and purging behaviors), and alcohol abuse (drank periodically, until intoxicated). Multiple and severe symptoms had failed to respond to citalopram with risperidone, bupropion, venlafaxine, aripiprazole, clonazepam, and carbamazepine, all of which had been administered in adequate dose and adequate duration, in conjunction with weekly psychotherapy during the previous one year. She had made four suicide attempts at the time of her initial presentation, was reporting constant suicidal thoughts, and was no longer able to attend school despite being an above average student in the past. Based on the severity of her symptoms and the lack of response to combined treatment with pharmacotherapy and psychotherapy, she was treated with 18 bilateral ECT. This was followed by pharmacotherapy with fluoxetine and aripiprazole and ongoing psychotherapy. The patient was advised continuation ECT with a slow taper-down regimen; however, she declined this option. She was subsequently placed in a residential facility because of residual symptoms. Although she did well on completion of the residential program, the depressive symptoms recurred within a few weeks, despite ongoing treatment. The patient continued to refuse an additional course of ECT. At the time of her last follow-up at our clinic, MW had made 3–4 additional suicide attempts.

Substance Abuse

A positive association is known between depression and substance abuse, with peer delinquency as one of the strongest predictors. However, it is unclear whether substance abuse including alcohol is more common across all types and severity of mood disorders, or whether these behaviors are limited to certain illness subtype and/or illness severity. Large scale studies have found that the likelihood of substance abuse may increase, particularly in the presence of anxiety and with a higher number of comorbid psychiatric conditions (55).

In adolescents with severe mood disorders who were treated with ECT, one study found that 37% met criteria for substance abuse (24). However, another study found, where all patients had been treated at the same institution, that alcohol and substance abuse were relatively less frequent at the time of evaluation for ECT (31% endorsed ever having used alcohol and 26% admitted using illicit drugs). Some adolescents may become dependent on prescription medications when there are coexisting prominent somatic symptoms associated with mood disorders, which offers additional challenges to treatment.

Treatment with ECT in adolescents who have comorbid alcohol or substance use can be complicated for a variety of reasons. First, there is a known association between alcohol abuse and lowered seizure threshold, although an association between lower seizure threshold and marijuana is less well established. Second, substance abuse involving many illicit or prescription drugs may result in prolonged seizures. Because younger age is associated with a lower seizure threshold, youth with substance abuse disorders may be at additional risk for excessively long seizures, resulting in post-treatment confusion. Third, comorbid substance abuse may be associated with poor treatment compliance, resulting in an inadequate ECT course. Therefore, it is important that any adolescent with a substance abuse problem is identified prior to starting ECT, an adequate wash-out is completed prior to initiating ECT, and treatment targeting the substance abuse problem be included during follow-up.

The following case describes some of the practical difficulties that may be encountered in youth with a comorbid substance abuse disorder.

CASE VIGNETTE 6: ECT IN AN ADOLESCENT WITH INSULIN DEPENDENT DIABETES MELLITUS (IDDM) AND TR DEPRESSION, GENERALIZED ANXIETY DISORDER (GAD), AND SUBSTANCE ABUSE

This case illustrates psychiatric and medical comorbidity and the challenges due to substance abuse encountered during treatment.

SX is a 16-year-old male who presented with a 2-year history of depression and anxiety that had developed a few months following his diagnosis of IDDM. His parents denied any behavior or emotional problems prior to his medical diagnosis. At presentation, his IDDM was moderately well controlled and SX had not suffered any episodes of hypoglycemia or diabetic ketoacidosis. However, his hemoglobin A1c was elevated.

Psychiatric symptoms included loss of interest, reduced pleasure, initial and middle insomnia, fatigue, reduced appetite, somatic complaints, low self-esteem, increased guilt, several suicide attempts that he refused to discuss, and severe anxiety accompanied by avoidance of school, eating in public places, and other social situations. SX denied any symptoms of hypomania or mania. He admitted to binge drinking and daily use of marijuana, starting several months prior to his evaluation for ECT. Past unsuccessful treatment trials included five different antidepressants, antipsychotic agents, and mood stabilizers in adequate dose and duration. He was diagnosed with treatment resistant MDD, generalized anxiety disorder, and alcohol and marijuana abuse.

His birth and development were unremarkable, and he came from an intact family with no evidence of major psychopathology in any first- or second-degree relative. After the diagnostic evaluation, he was hospitalized for ECT and was treated with 14 BL treatments. ECT resulted in response (improved sleep and irritability). Unfortunately,ECT had to be discontinued on discovery that he was using K2 (a synthetic cannabinoid). The patient was followed up for approximately 6 months during which he continued to be depressed and angry and became more neglectful of his diabetic care. He started to refuse all psychiatric treatment and admitted to not caring about the risks of increasingly poor diabetic care and worsening depression. The patient was lost to follow-up after 6 months of ECT.

Illness Chronicity and Relapse

The majority of depressive and other mood disorders remit with conventional treatment (medications, psychotherapy) within 7–9 months. However, persistent or chronic depression is more likely to result in negative outcomes. Although it is difficult to predict which adolescents are at an elevated risk for chronicity, several baseline clinical variables appear to be associated with this outcome. These include severity of depression, comorbid anxiety, lower perception of self-efficacy, suicidal ideation and behaviors, symptoms of obsessive-compulsive disorder (OCD), and history of childhood abuse (56, 57). In the experience of the author, comorbid anxiety disorders and autism spectrum disorders appear to be relative common diagnoses in adolescents with chronic TRM. Successful outcome with ECT is more likely when comorbid psychiatric diagnoses and problem behaviors are correctly identified and treated appropriately.

CASE VIGNETTE 7: CHRONIC DEPRESSION IN A CASE WITH COMORBID GAD, PDD-NOS, AND SCHOOL REFUSAL

TR is a 16-year-old male with MDD with symptom onset at age 8 years and comorbid diagnoses that included GAD and ASD (12). His ASD diagnosis was missed prior to his presentation for treatment at our center; as a result he had never received any academic support or interventions for his social and language deficits. Symptoms of ASD included lack of age-appropriate reciprocity in social interactions and pragmatic deficits, use of pedantic speech with difficulty in understanding humor or sarcasm. He did not report any restricted interests or behaviors, however. It was noteworthy that because of severe symptoms, patient had not attended school since the 6th grade. The patient was treated with ECT, based on the severity of his depression, multiple unsuccessful antidepressant trials given in combination with supportive psychotherapy over many years, and an elevated risk for completed suicide based on a positive family history in a second-degree relative. This patient received 25 BL ECT during an index course and 7 treatments during a continuation course. Pharmacotherapy was re-initiated as his treatment frequency was reduced to once per week. He received lamotrigine and quetiapine combined with supportive therapy, relaxation and exposure and response prevention. The patient remained free of depression over follow-up at 1.5 years. During this time he was able to graduate from school and participated in some limited social activities (family get-togethers, able to enjoy a TV show with the family), which he had not done in many years. We concluded that effective treatment of depression, anxiety, and providing remedial education were important factors that resulted in successful outcome in an otherwise chronically ill male with treatment resistant depression and ASD. It should be noted that there was no change in his core symptoms of ASD; however, he experienced significant improvement in mood symptoms.

CONCLUSION

Treatment resistant mood disorder in adolescence is a debilitating illness that may be successfully treated with ECT, when treatment resistance is correctly identified. Comorbid psychiatric disorders are common in this subgroup and require appropriate interventions, often following the successful treatment of the mood disorder. Larger scale and prospective studies, including longitudinal follow-up, are essential to identify important illness and treatment variables in this age group.

QUESTIONS AND ANSWERS

1. *When should an adolescent or a pre-adolescent child with a mood disorder be referred for ECT?*

   ECT should not be considered a treatment of last resort. Multiple treatment failures are possibly associated with worsening future outcome. Illness severity and treatment resistance are the two most important referral criteria. Illness severity may take precedence over adequacy of past treatments, especially in patients who appear to be in imminent danger.

2. *Does ECT change the course of a mood disorder?*

   It is generally believed that effective treatment, until remission of symptoms is achieved, may improve the long-term outcome of mood disorders. Lack of complete remission is associated with poor functioning of the adolescent and a greater number of future recurrences, which may also become less responsive to treatments.

3. *Is it essential to differentiate whether the young person has bipolar or unipolar depression prior to starting ECT?*

   No, it is not essential. In many cases, it may be difficult to identify the exact type of mood disorder because full-blown episodes associated with BP may not be evident until the late teens or the twenties. Youth who eventually develop BP may have a greater likelihood of positive family history, may have worsening or lack of response to antidepressants, and may experience either frank hypomania or marked increase in irritability during ECT.

DISCLOSURE

Dr. Neera Ghaziuddin has no conflicts to disclose. She is funded for unrelated studies by the Centers for Disease Control (CDC) and receives institutional funding from the University of Michigan.

REFERENCES

1. Fava M, Davidson KG. Definition and epidemiology of treatment-resistant depression. *Psychiat Clin NA*. [Review]. 1996 Jun;19(2):179–200.
2. Burrows GD, Norman TR, Judd FK. Definition and differential diagnosis of treatment-resistant depression. *Int Clin Psychop*. [Review]. 1994 Jun;9 Suppl 2:5–10.
3. Thompson JW, Blaine JD. Use of ECT in the United States in 1975 and 1980. *Am J Psychiatry*. May 1987;144(5):557–62.

4. Walter G, Rey JM. An epidemiological study of the use of ECT in adolescents. *J Am Acad Child Adoles Psychiat*. 1997 Jun;36(6):809.
5. Fava M. Diagnosis and definition of treatment-resistant depression. *Biol Psychiat*.[Research Support, Non-U.S. Gov't Review]. Apr 15, 2003;53(8):649–59.
6. Bloch Y, Sobol D, Levkovitz Y, Kron S, Ratzoni G. Reasons for referral for electroconvulsive therapy: a comparison between adolescents and adults. *Australas Psychiatry*.[Comparative Study Research Support, Non-U.S. Gov't]. 2008 Jun;16(3):191–4.
7. Ghaziuddin N, ed. Treatment Resistant Depression in Adolescents in Symposium, Treatment Resistant Depression: a roadmap for effective care (Chair: Greden JF). Honolulu, Hawaii: American Psychiatric Association; 2011.
8. March J, Silva S, Petrycki S, Curry J, Wells K, Fairbank J, et al. Fluoxetine, cognitive-behavioral therapy, and their combination for adolescents with depression: Treatment for Adolescents With Depression Study (TADS) randomized controlled trial. [see comment]. *JAMA*. 2004 Aug 18;292(7):807–20.
9. March J, Silva S, Curry J, Wells K, Fairbank J, Burns B, et al. The Treatment for Adolescents With Depression Study (TADS): outcomes over 1 year of naturalistic follow-up. *Am J Psychiatry*. [Multicenter Study Randomized Controlled Trial Research Support, N.I.H., Extramural]. Oct 2009;166(10):1141–9.
10. Asarnow JR, Emslie G, Clarke G, Wagner KD, Spirito A, Vitiello B, et al. Treatment of selective serotonin reuptake inhibitor-resistant depression in adolescents: predictors and moderators of treatment response. *J Am Acad Child Adoles Psychiat*. [Comparative Study Multicenter Study Randomized Controlled Trial Research Support, N.I.H., Extramural]. 2009 Mar;48(3):330–9.
11. Emslie GJ, Mayes T, Porta G, Vitiello B, Clarke G, Wagner KD, et al. Treatment of Resistant Depression in Adolescents (TORDIA): week 24 outcomes. *Am J Psychiatry*. [Randomized Controlled Trial Research Support, N.I.H., Extramural]. 2010 Jul;167(7):782–91.
12. Ghaziuddin N, Dumas S, Hodges E. Use of continuation or maintenance electroconvulsive therapy in adolescents with severe treatment-resistant depression. *J ECT*. 2011 Jun;27(2):168–74.
13. Rush AJ, Thase ME, Dube S. Research issues in the study of difficult-to-treat depression. *Biol Psychiat*. [Research Support, Non-U.S. Gov't Review]. Apr 15, 2003;53(8):743–53.
14. Malhi GS, Parker GB, Crawford J, Wilhelm K, Mitchell PB. Treatment-resistant depression: resistant to definition? *Acta Psychiatrica Scandinavica*. [Research Support, Non-U.S. Gov't]. Oct 2005;112(4):302–9.
15. Kennedy N, Paykel ES. Treatment and response in refractory depression: results from a specialist affective disorders service. *J Affect Disorders*. 2004 Jul;81(1):49–53.
16. Bender L. One hundred cases of childhood schizophrenia treated with electric shock. *Trans American Neurol Assoc*. 1947;72:169.
17. Rice J. Berkeley to vote on banning electroshock therapy. Associated Press. August 24, 1982.
18. Guttmacher LB, Cretella H. Electroconvulsive therapy in one child and three adolescents. *J Clin Psychiat*. [Case Reports]. Jan 1988;49(1):20–3.
19. Guttmacher LB, Cretella H. Electroconvulsive therapy in one child and three adolescents. *J Clin Psychiat*. Jan 1988;49(1):20.
20. Paillere-Martinot ML, Zivi A, Basquin M. Use of electroconvulsive therapy in adolescence. *Encephale*. Sep-Oct 1990;16(5):399.

21. Ghaziuddin N, King CA, Naylor MW, Ghaziuddin M, Chaudhary N, Giordani B, et al. Electroconvulsive treatment in adolescents with pharmacotherapy-refractory depression. *J Child Adoles Psychop*. 1996;6(4):259.
22. Moise FN, Petrides G. Case study: electroconvulsive therapy in adolescents.see comment. *J Am Acad Child Adoles Psychiat*. 1996 Mar;35(3):312.
23. Cohen D, Paillere-Martinot ML, Basquin M. Use of electroconvulsive therapy in adolescents. *Convulsive Therapy*. 1997 Mar;13(1):25.
24. Walter G, Rey JM. An epidemiological study of the use of ECT in adolescents. *J Am Acad Child Adoles Psychiat*. [Research Support, Non-U.S. Gov't]. 1997 Jun;36(6):809–15.
25. Strober M, Rao U, Pataki C, DeAntonio M. Complete remission of "treatment resistant" severe melancholia in adolescents with phenelzine: two case reports. *J Affect Disorders*. Jul 1998;50(1):55.
26. Kutcher S, Robertson H. Electroconvulsive therapy in treatment-resistant bipolar youth. *J Child Adoles Psychop*. 1995;5(3):167–75.
27. Stein D, Kurtsman L, Stier S, Remnik Y, Meged S, Weizman A. Electroconvulsive therapy in adolescent and adult psychiatric inpatients—a retrospective chart design. *J Affect Disorders*. Nov 1, 2004;82(3):335–42.
28. Bloch Y, Levcovitch Y, Bloch AM, Mendlovic S, Ratzoni G. Electroconvulsive therapy in adolescents: similarities to and differences from adults. *J Am Acad Child Adoles Psychiat*. [Comparative Study Evaluation Studies]. Nov 2001; 40(11):1332–6.
29. Taieb O, Flament MF, Chevret S, Jeammet P, Allilaire JF, Mazet P, et al. Clinical relevance of electroconvulsive therapy (ECT) in adolescents with severe mood disorder: evidence from a follow-up study. *Eur Psychiatry*. Jul 2002;17(4):206.
30. Strober M, Rao U, DeAntonio M, Liston E, State M, Amaya-Jackson L, et al. Effects of electroconvulsive therapy in adolescents with severe endogenous depression resistant to pharmacotherapy. *Biol Psychiat*. Mar 1, 1998;43(5):335.
31. Hamilton M. A rating scale for depression. *J Neurol Neurosur Ps*. 1960;23:56–62.
32. Poznanski EO, Grossman JA, Buchsbaum Y, Banegas M, Freeman L, Gibbons R. Preliminary studies of the reliability and validity of the children's depression rating scale. *J Am Acad Child Psychiat*. [Research Support, U.S. Gov't, P.H.S.]. Mar 1984;23(2):191–7.
33. Guy W. ECDEU Assessment Manual for Psychopharmacology-Revised (DHEW Publ No ADM 76-338). In: Department of Health, Education, and Welfare, Public Health Service, Alcohol, Drug Abuse and Mental Health Administration, NIMG Psychopharmacology Research Branch, Division of Extramural Research Program. Rockville, MD; 1976, pp. 218–22.
34. Taieb O, Flament MF, Chevret S, Jeammet P, Allilaire JF, Mazet P, et al. Clinical relevance of electroconvulsive therapy (ECT) in adolescents with severe mood disorder: evidence from a follow-up study. *Eur Psychiatry*. [Research Support, Non-U.S. Gov't Validation Studies]. Jul 2002;17(4):206–12.
35. Rey JM, Walter G. Half a century of ECT use in young people. *Am J Psychiatry*. [Review]. May 1997;154(5):595–602.
36. Birmaher B, Brent DA, Benson RS. Summary of the practice parameters for the assessment and treatment of children and adolescents with depressive disorders. American Academy of Child and Adolescent Psychiatry. *J Am Acad Child Adoles Psychiat*. [Guideline Practice Guideline]. Nov 1998;37(11):1234–8.
37. Mulder RT, Watkins WGA, Joyce PR, Luty SE. Age may affect response to antidepressants with serotonergic and noradrenergic actions. *J Affect Disorders*.

[Clinical Trial Multicenter Study Randomized Controlled Trial Research Support, Non-U.S. Gov't]. Sep 2003;76(1–3):143–9.

38. Berman RM, Fava M, Thase ME, Trivedi MH, Swanink R, McQuade RD, et al. Aripiprazole augmentation in major depressive disorder: a double-blind, placebo-controlled study in patients with inadequate response to antidepressants. *CNS Spectrums*. [Comparative Study Randomized Controlled Trial Research Support, Non-U.S. Gov't]. Apr 2009;14(4):197–206.
39. El-Khalili N, Joyce M, Atkinson S, Buynak RJ, Datto C, Lindgren P, et al. Extended-release quetiapine fumarate (quetiapine XR) as adjunctive therapy in major depressive disorder (MDD) in patients with an inadequate response to ongoing antidepressant treatment: a multicentre, randomized, double-blind, placebo-controlled study. *Int J Neuropsychop*. [Clinical Trial, Phase III Multicenter Study Randomized Controlled Trial Research Support, Non-U.S. Gov't]. 2010 Aug;13(7):917–32.
40. Nuevo R, Chatterji S, Fraguas D, Verdes E, Naidoo N, Arango C, et al. Increased risk of diabetes mellitus among persons with psychotic symptoms: results from the WHO World Health Survey. *J Clin Psychiat*. [Interactive Tutorial Multicenter Study Randomized Controlled Trial Research Support, Non-U.S. Gov't]. Dec 2011;72(12):1592–9.
41. Coppola G, Verrotti A, Resicato G, Ferrarelli S, Auricchio G, Operto FF, et al. Topiramate in children and adolescents with epilepsy and mental retardation: a prospective study on behavior and cognitive effects. *Epilepsy Behav*. [Clinical Trial]. Feb 2008;12(2):253–6.
42. Bagary M. Epilepsy, antiepileptic drugs and suicidality. *Curr Opin Neurol*. [Review]. Apr 2011;24(2):177–82.
43. Rush AJ. Limitations in efficacy of antidepressant monotherapy. *J Clin Psychiat*. 2007;68 Suppl 10:8–10.
44. Bramness JG, Groholt B, Engeland A, Furu K. The use of lithium, valproate or lamotrigine for psychiatric conditions in children and adolescents in Norway 2004-2007: a prescription database study. *J Affect Disorders*. [Research Support, Non-U.S. Gov't]. Oct 2009;117(3):208–11.
45. Geller B, Luby JL, Joshi P, Wagner KD, Emslie G, Walkup JT, et al. A randomized controlled trial of risperidone, lithium, or divalproex sodium for initial treatment of bipolar I disorder, manic or mixed phase, in children and adolescents. *Arch Gen Psychiat*. [Randomized Controlled Trial Research Support, N.I.H., Extramural]. May 2012;69(5):515–28.
46. Berk M, Dodd S, Callaly P, Berk L, Fitzgerald P, de Castella AR, et al. History of illness prior to a diagnosis of bipolar disorder or schizoaffective disorder. *J Affect Disorders*. [Multicenter Study Research Support, Non-U.S. Gov't]. Nov 2007;103(1–3):181–6.
47. McNamara RK, Nandagopal JJ, Strakowski SM, DelBello MP. Preventative strategies for early-onset bipolar disorder: towards a clinical staging model. *CNS Drugs*. [Research Support, N.I.H., Extramural Review]. Dec 2010 1;24(12):983–96.
48. Hillegers MH, Reichart CG, Wals M, Verhulst FC, Ormel J, Nolen WA. Five-year prospective outcome of psychopathology in the adolescent offspring of bipolar parents. *Bipolar Disorders*. [Research Support, Non-U.S. Gov't]. 2005 Aug;7(4):344–50.
49. Amsterdam JD, Hornig-Rohan M. Treatment algorithms in treatment-resistant depression. *Psychiat Clin NA*. [Review]. 1996 Jun;19(2):371–86.

50. Carlson GA, Fennig S, Bromet EJ. The confusion between bipolar disorder and schizophrenia in youth: where does it stand in the 1990s? *J Am Acad Child Adoles Psychiat.* [Research Support, U.S. Gov't, P.H.S.]. May 1994;33(4):453–60.
51. McClellan J, Werry J. Practice parameters for the assessment and treatment of children and adolescents with bipolar disorder. American Academy of Child and Adolescent Psychiatry. *J Am Acad Child Adoles Psychiat.* [Guideline Practice Guideline]. Oct 1997;36(10 Suppl):157S–76S.
52. Aina Y, Susman JL. Understanding comorbidity with depression and anxiety disorders. *J Am Osteopath Assoc.* May 2006;106(5 Suppl 2):S9–14.
53. DelBello MP, Geller B. Review of studies of child and adolescent offspring of bipolar parents. *Bipolar Disorders.* [Review]. Dec 2001;3(6):325–34.
54. Patel M, Patel S, Hardy DW, Benzies BJ, Tare V. Should electroconvulsive therapy be an early consideration for suicidal patients? *J ECT.* 2006 Jun;22(2):113–5.
55. Kessler RC, Walters EE. Epidemiology of DSM-III-R major depression and minor depression among adolescents and young adults in the National Comorbidity Survey. *Depress Anxiety.* [Research Support, Non-U.S. Gov't Research Support, U.S. Gov't, P.H.S.]. 1998;7(1):3–14.
56. Gordon MS, Tonge B, Melvin GA. Outcome of adolescent depression: 6 months after treatment. *Aust NZ J Psychiat.* [Randomized Controlled Trial Research Support, Non-U.S. Gov't]. Mar 2011;45(3):232–9.
57. Uher R, Caspi A, Houts R, Sugden K, Williams B, Poulton R, et al. Serotonin transporter gene moderates childhood maltreatment's effects on persistent but not single-episode depression: replications and implications for resolving inconsistent results. *J Affect Disorders.* [Research Support, N.I.H., Extramural Research Support, Non-U.S. Gov't]. Dec 2011;135(1–3):56–65.

CHAPTER 10

ECT for Schizophrenia Spectrum Disorders

YUVAL BLOCH, DANIEL STEIN, AND GARRY WALTER

KEY POINTS

- When acute psychotic symptoms are part of a young person's presentation early in an illness course, distinguishing between schizophrenia spectrum disorders (SSD) and affective spectrum disorders can be difficult.
- ECT is used more commonly in affective disorders than in SSDs, both in adults and in adolescents.
- Antipsychotic medications are more effective than ECT in treating SSDs, both in adults and in adolescents.
- Clozapine is more effective than ECT in treating resistant schizophrenia.
- ECT is beneficial and probably accelerates the treatment response when used as an "add-on" to medications in adults suffering from treatment resistant schizophrenia, and the available evidence also supports these findings in adolescents.
- The predominance of catatonic, positive, and affective symptoms is a predictor of a more favorable response to treatment compared to the predominance of negative symptoms and low premorbid functioning. Nevertheless, using ECT as an add-on to atypical antipsychotics may be a valuable therapeutic alternative for SSDs resistant to pharmacotherapy, especially in cases where there is a predominance of "non-negative" symptoms.
- ECT is a relatively safe procedure, not only for adults but also for adolescents suffering from SSD.
- In (preadolescent) children with SSD, there is sparse information about ECT.
- While the clinical use of ECT in adolescents with SSDs is broadly similar to its use in adults for the same indication, higher acuity and life-threatening situations (specifically high risk of suicide or catatonia) may be more common indications for ECT in adolescents.

OVERVIEW

In this chapter, we will briefly mention pharmacotherapy for SSDs, then summarize the data on ECT in the treatment of adults with SSD. This is followed by consideration of available knowledge, experience, and recommendations in relation to SSD in children and adolescents. Two concluding vignettes focus on some of the issues covered in the chapter.

INTRODUCTION

Schizophrenia spectrum disorders (SSDs) are conditions in which psychotic symptoms, which may include delusions, hallucinations, and disorganized thought process, speech, and behavior, are the central feature of the disturbance. In SSDs, the psychosis cannot be explained by a mood disorder (such as psychotic depression or a manic episode with psychotic features), and it is not related to the effect of a substance (as in substance-induced psychosis) or to a known medical condition (as in psychosis secondary to a thyroid disorder, for example). The differentiation within SSDs—between schizophrenia, schizophreniform disorder, and brief psychotic episode—is based on the pervasiveness and duration of the psychotic symptoms. Schizoaffective disorder is part of the SSD and is typified by the combination of full-blown schizophrenic and affective symptoms. Psychotic disorder not otherwise specified (psychotic disorder NOS) is the SSD default category. There are conflicting data about the prevalence of SSD in adolescents; the estimated prevalence of schizophrenia is 0.1–0.2% (1).

Schizophrenia is a severe mental disorder, with a prolonged and often taxing course, that significantly affects the lives of patients and their families. The type and clustering of the symptoms from which the patient suffers influences the prognosis and therapeutic decisions. Early age of onset (such as childhood or adolescence), low overall baseline functioning, and an insidious course are considered poor prognostic signs. Although affective symptoms are considered a good prognostic sign, these symptoms are associated with a high risk of suicidal behavior. When severe, this affective cluster is a suitable target for ECT in both adult and adolescent SSD patients.

From the classic subtypes of schizophrenia, catatonic type schizophrenia, typified by either a paralysis-like state, or a hyperactive, hypervigilant motor state, is usually associated with a good response to ECT. The distinction between "positive" symptoms (such as auditory hallucinations and persecutory delusions) and "negative" (or deficit) symptoms (including social withdrawal, reduced motivation, loss of energy [anergia], inability to feel pleasure [anhedonia], and difficulties in expressing emotions and in taking care of oneself) is very relevant when making therapeutic decisions. Positive schizophrenic symptoms are associated with a much better response to ECT.

SSD, sometimes referred to as "non-affective psychosis," is considered a "weaker" indication for ECT than "affective psychosis." At the same time, it is important to remember that there is a relative lack of diagnostic stability regarding psychotic disorders in adolescents (2–7). In a 10-year follow-up study of 470 patients hospitalized with a first psychotic episode (7), of whom approximately half were adolescents, about half (50.7%) of the patients had a diagnostic shift during follow-up. Whereas a diagnosis of schizophrenia and bipolar disorder was relatively stable—respectively, 89.2% and 77.8% of those patients maintained their initial diagnosis—less than 50% of patients diagnosed with psychotic depression at baseline maintained this diagnosis at follow-up. Most shifts in the psychotic depression category were to schizophrenia and schizoaffective disorder (23 of 77 patients). This diagnostic change highlights the need to take into account the presence and combination of affective and psychotic symptoms in adolescents, beyond the immediate diagnostic label, if considering ECT.

The severity and deteriorating course of schizophrenia and schizoaffective disorder have encouraged the search for effective early intervention strategies; this is particularly relevant in children and adolescents, in order to prevent future deterioration.

PHARMACOTHERAPY

Treatment of SSDs always demands an integrated therapeutic approach. The timing and use of biological treatments must never ignore psychosocial interventions. We will focus in this brief discussion on currently relevant pharmacological alternatives to the use of ECT. At the time of writing, a total of 21 studies support the role of antipsychotic medications in treating SSD in minors. Of these, eight are double blind placebo (or sub-therapeutic dose) controlled studies encompassing more than 800 young persons suffering from SSDs and using a variety of second generation antipsychotics (SGAs) (8–22).

The conclusions drawn from these studies are:

1. SGAs are superior to placebo in the short term (9, 11, 12, 14–17). A beneficial effect of first generation antipsychotics (FGAs) is also largely supported.
2. There is a growing awareness of the severity of adverse effects of these medications, including extrapyramidal side effects and tardive dyskinesia, metabolic syndrome (including hyperglycemia and hyperlipidemia), weight gain, hyperprolactinemia, hepatotoxicity, seizures, and adverse cardiovascular and hematological effects.
3. A sizable minority of patients (20–30%) do not achieve symptomatic remission with SGAs and FGAs, that is, positive symptoms persist despite two adequate trials of antipsychotic medications.

4. Clozapine has an advantage (8, 10, 13, 18, 19, 23) in treatment-refractory schizophrenia. A larger percentage of adolescents than adults develop adverse effects with clozapine, particularly neutropenia (23). In addition, there is growing awareness of clozapine resistant schizophrenia in younger patients (8, 10, 18, 23).

In summary, antipsychotic medications are only partially effective in treating SSDs in children and adolescents, and have troubling side effects. Accordingly, it is important to assess the efficacy and adverse effect profile of other forms of treatment, such as ECT, in these patients.

THE USE OF ECT IN ADULT PATIENTS DIAGNOSED WITH SCHIZOPHRENIA

For over 60 years, there have been small- to medium-scale controlled studies of the use of ECT in adults suffering from SSD. Well-conducted meta-analyses (24–26) summarize evidence from randomized controlled trials (RCTs) about ECT in adult patients with schizophrenia.

1. Meta-analyses combining results from sham controlled studies suggest that ECT is effective in the treatment of adult patients with schizophrenia:
   a. When ECT is compared with placebo or sham ECT, more people improve with actual ECT by the end of the treatment course (n = 392, 10 RCTs, risk ratio (RR) 0.76 random 95% confidence interval [CI] 0.59 to 0.98, numbers needed to treat [NNT] 6 CI 4 to 12). The short-term superiority of ECT is demonstrated mainly with clinical global impression assessments and, to a lesser extent, with the brief psychiatric rating scale (BPRS).
   b. The use of ECT may result in a significantly shorter time to improvement than sham ECT, as assessed by reduction in BPRS scores midway through the course of treatment. This early advantage of ECT may be maintained at short-term follow-up (6 weeks post treatment).
   c. There is limited evidence that ECT may result in fewer relapses in the short run than sham ECT (n = 47, 2 RCTs, RR fixed 0.26 CI 0.03 to 2.2), and a greater likelihood of discharge from inpatient treatment (n = 98, 1 RCT, RR fixed 0.59, CI 0.34 to 1.01).
2. When ECT is directly compared with antipsychotic medications (total n = 443, 10 RCTs), results favor pharmacotherapy (n = 175, 3 RCTs, RR fixed "not improved at the end of ECT course" 2.18 CI 1.31 to 3.63).
3. The combination of ECT and neuroleptic mediations results in an increase in the number of patients who had improved at the end of treatment

compared to patients treated with ECT alone (n = 183, 6 RCT, RR 0.81 fixed CI 0.66 to 1.00, I-squared 44.6%) (27–31). Recent open studies (32–38) and reviews that summarize the results of both open and controlled studies (39–41) also emphasize that combining ECT with antipsychotic medications appears to be effective and preferable over either treatment alone in patients with medication-resistant chronic schizophrenia. This is particularly the case when adding ECT to second generation neuroleptics (35) such as clozapine (33, 41), olanzapine, and risperidone (37). Some studies (42) have shown that in patients with schizophrenia who are unresponsive to clozapine, ECT may be preferred to other neuroleptics.

4. ECT as an add-on to pharmacotherapy has been shown to accelerate the speed of remission (36, 43–45), although the early advantage of ECT is likely not maintained at medium- (6 months) and long-term (1 year) post-treatment follow-up.
5. The most frequent indication to augment pharmacotherapy with ECT is in patients with medication-refractory schizophrenia (26, 46, 47). While several recent open studies (48–50) report beneficial effects of this combination only for "positive" symptoms of schizophrenia, a few studies have shown that adding ECT to antipsychotic medications, particularly to second generation neuroleptics, may also improve negative symptoms (37, 51).
6. Most studies suggest that shorter duration of the psychotic episode, better premorbid function, and fewer negative symptoms are predictors of a better response to ECT in patients with treatment resistant schizophrenia (47, 49, 50). A recent review (41) suggests that catatonic symptoms are the most responsive to ECT, followed by positive symptoms such as paranoid delusions and affective symptoms.
7. In relation to long-term effects and maintenance ECT, only one RCT (52) has found that continuation ECT (in combination with pharmacotherapy) may be beneficial in the long-term course of patients with schizophrenia who had improved with treatment of the acute phase. By contrast, Matheson et al. (46) have noted in their review that although there is good evidence supporting a significant, although small, improvement in global symptoms in patients with schizophrenia treated with ECT, with or without concurrent antipsychotics (RR = 0.76) in the short term (up to 3 months post-treatment), there is no evidence for long-term (usually 12 months) therapeutic effects. In the same vein, other open studies (34, 53) and meta-analyses (43) have indicated that ECT-antipsychotic combinations might be better than antipsychotics alone in the first few weeks of treatment, but not at long-term follow-up.
8. In terms of predictors of long-term improvement, Chanpattana and Andrade (54), in their meta-analysis of ECT in patients with schizophrenia (not confined only to RCTs), suggest that a 3-week post-ECT

stabilization period identifies patients who will maintain improvement at later periods. Several open studies in treatment-resistant patients with schizophrenia receiving maintenance ECT combined with neuroleptics have shown that early improvement in psychopathology, quality of life and functioning with acute treatment may predict the maintenance of these changes at long-term (mostly one year) follow-up (32, 37, 41, 48, 55–57).

9. The relapse rate of patients treated with maintenance ECT-neuroleptics has been found to be significantly lower in comparison to patients treated only with medications (56). This finding is of considerable clinical relevance when bearing in mind that long-term adverse effects with the ECT-neuroleptic combination, including cognitive adverse effects, are generally infrequent and mild (36, 39, 46, 56), and no greater than for ECT alone (35, 40).
10. Unilateral and bilateral ECT have been found to be equally effective in terms of global improvement (n = 78, 2 RCTs, RR fixed "not improved at end of course of ECT" 0.79 CI 0.45 to 1.39). Nevertheless, as there is only limited research on unilateral ECT in schizophrenia with most RCTs using bilateral rather than unilateral placement, bilateral ECT remains at present the most frequently used method in treating schizophrenia (47).
11. The data with respect to the number of ECT treatments required for improvement are equivocal. Three trials (28, 29, 58) suggest that ECT courses of up to 12 treatments, given in combination with antipsychotics, may be sufficient for a significant clinical improvement in patients showing limited improvement with medications, when compared with antipsychotics and sham ECT (n = 67, RR fixed 0.30 CI 0.16 to 0.55, I-squared 11%). One trial has shown a significantly greater effect with 20 versus 12 treatments (59) (n = 43, RR 2. fixed 53 CI 1.13 to 5.66).
12. With respect to adverse effects, 8 of the 26 RCTs in Tharyan and Adams's meta-analyses (26) assessed memory functions after ECT, using validated neuropsychological test batteries. The results of these studies are equivocal. No differences in cognitive impairment were found in patients treated with ECT versus medication or placebo, although patients receiving ECT had more complaints of forgetfulness (60). More recent studies comparing patients with schizophrenia treated with maintenance ECT and patients who have never been treated with ECT have also shown no between-group differences in levels of memory, attention, or frontal function impairment (61). Overall, most of the existing literature suggests no significant measurable adverse effects with long-term use of ECT, with or without concomitant psychotropic medications, in adult patients with schizophrenia (39, 46, 62). This is likely the result of the low numbers of ECT administered during continuation treatment (46).

To summarize the adult literature, there is reasonable evidence to support the use of ECT as an add-on treatment for patients suffering from schizophrenia that is resistant to neuroleptic medications. ECT is highly effective for catatonic features and is beneficial also for other positive schizophrenic symptoms, whereas its efficacy for negative schizophrenic symptoms is questionable. Evidence supports a course of 12–20 bilateral treatments being effective in the short term and safe; unilateral treatment might be effective but has not been adequately studied. Data are insufficient to draw definite conclusions about the long-term efficacy of combined ECT-neuroleptic treatment and of maintenance ECT in adult patients. Despite this limitation, there is presently no clear evidence to dismiss the use of ECT for adult patients with schizophrenia (26).

ECT IN ADOLESCENT PATIENTS SUFFERING FROM SSDs

Although the adult ECT literature may serve as a guide, development—from both neurobiological and socio-psychological perspectives—requires that treatment provided for adolescents is based on studies conducted in adolescents. With respect to (pre-adolescent) children, it is noteworthy that SSDs, and specifically schizophrenia, are very rare and there is reluctance to administer ECT, even if withholding ECT may endanger lives. Unsurprisingly, there is almost no valid evidence for the use of ECT in children suffering from schizophrenia, as defined according to modern nosology. Data about ECT in young people are scarce. There are no RCTs comparing ECT in children and adolescents with SSDs to sham ECT and/or neuroleptic medications. Most of the publications are case reports or case series. Some studies have attempted to use adult patients treated with ECT in the same center as a comparison group (63–65) or a matched group of adolescents who have not been treated with ECT (66). Other studies either include adolescents diagnosed with SSD among adolescents with other psychiatric diagnoses) (67–71), or combine adolescent and young adult patients suffering from schizophrenia (42, 57).

More recent studies have included objective measures and follow-up data (66, 72). One recent prospective study focused on newly diagnosed psychosis and raised questions about the therapeutic validity of discriminating between affective psychosis and SSD early in the disease course (73).

Box 10.1 summarizes the findings of some of the more important reports about ECT in adolescents diagnosed with SSDs; in each study, we convey the main "take home message," allowing for the various methodological limitations.

INDICATIONS AND EFFICACY

In 1997, Rey and Walter (68) conducted a meticulous systematic review of all reported cases (396 patients in 60 studies) of ECT in patients under the age

Box 10.1: STUDIES ON ECT IN SCHIZOPHRENIA SPECTRUM DISORDERS IN CHILDREN AND ADOLESCENTS

Rey and Walter 1997 (68)

Design Extensive systematic review of all published cases of ECT in patients under age 18.[a] Safety procedures and adverse effects similar to adults.

Participants 396 patients, data on diagnosis and outcome present in 205 patients

Diagnosis 36 schizophrenia, 2 schizoaffective, 24 catatonia,[b] 4 NMS[c]

Outcome Rates of improvement: 42%—schizophrenia; 63%—depression; 80%—mania; 80%—catatonia

Take home messages

ECT is used less often for SSD and is less effective for SSD than for affective diagnoses and catatonia.

ECT is effective in catatonia and NMS beyond the psychiatric diagnosis.

Walter and Rey 1997 (67)

Design Epidemiological survey of a 5-year experience in a region with approximately 6 million inhabitants[a]

In all patients, ECT was given as a "last resort" after failure of pharmacotherapy; most patients treated with medications in addition to the ECT.

Participants 42 patients received 47 ECT courses.

Diagnosis 18 SSD

Outcome Rates of improvement: 28%—SSD; 66%—affective disorder. Improvement in affective symptoms: 70% of SSD patients.

Take home messages

ECT is less effective for SSD than for affective diagnoses.

However, it is effective in the treatment of mood symptoms as part of SSD.

Bloch et al. 2001 (63)

Design Comparative chart review.[a] All adolescents received bilateral ECT. All patients received ECT as an add-on to medications.

Participants 25 adolescents and 33 adults

Diagnosis Adolescents: 4 catatonic schizophrenia; 4 schizoaffective; 11 non-catatonic schizophrenia

Outcome 58% improvement in the adolescent group (most diagnosed with SSDs); in 67%, no re-hospitalization in the following year.

Take home messages

ECT is effective in adolescents suffering from SSDs.

(*continued*)

Box 10.1: (CONTINUED)

Stein et al. 2004 (64)
Design Comparative chart review[a]
Participants 36 adolescents and 57 adults
Diagnosis Adolescents: 7 catatonic schizophrenia and 12 non-catatonic schizophrenia
Course of ECT 33/37 adolescents were treated with bilateral ECT in comparison to 17/57 adults (because of severe deterioration in the first 4 adolescents treated with unilateral ECT).
Outcome 58% of adolescents with schizophrenia improved (with better results on the CGI[e] for adolescents with affective disorders). In 68% of the improved adolescents with SSD, no re-hospitalization at 1 year.
Side effects ECT was discontinued in 20% of the adolescents (manic switch, prolonged seizures, and headaches) but in only one adult patient.

Take home messages
In adolescents ECT is effective in treating SSDs, although less effective than for affective disorders.

ECT is generally safe in adolescents, although there were more discontinuations due to adverse effects, compared with adults.

Baeza et al. 2010 (72)
Design Retrospective chart review
Participants 13 adolescents diagnosed with SSDs
Diagnosis 5 paranoid schizophrenia, 2 disorganized schizophrenia, 2 catatonic schizophrenia, 2 undifferentiated schizophrenia, 2 schizoaffective disorder
Reason[d] 8-severity and lack of response to past treatment with 2 to 3 medications over 10 to 34 weeks; 4 catatonia; 1 NMS[c]
ECT Informed consent of legal guardian for ECT
Propofol for anesthesia
Bilateral at threshold, number of sessions 13. 9 ±4.3 (M>F)[f]
Mean duration of seizures 43.9s.d.16.9 seconds (F>M)[g]
Outcome Most patients (53.8%) had a 20% reduction in PANSS,[h] but not on the negative subscale. Significant improvement also on CGI[e].
No deterioration at 6 months follow-up in comparison to the end of the ECT course.
At 6 months, 12 patients treated with antipsychotics, 7 with maintenance ECT.

(*continued*)

Box 10.1: (CONTINUED)

Side effects Generally mild: headache (12.9%), myalgia (0.5%), disorientation (0.5%), agitation (0.5%).

On continuous ECT, there were unexpected convulsions with changes in the EEG in one patient treated successfully with valproate.

Take home messages

ECT is effective, but not for negative symptoms.

Data on maintenance ECT are inconclusive.

de la Serna 2011 (66)

Design Longitudinal follow-up

Participants 9 SSD adolescents treated with ECT and neuroleptics; 9 patients treated with neuroleptics alone.

Diagnosis Schizophrenia (7 patients) and schizoaffective disorder (2 patients) in both groups

Outcome Benefit was maintained after 2 years; both groups improved from baseline; no between-group difference in improvement.

Side effects No significant between-group differences in mental state.

Take home messages

ECT is safe in adolescents suffering from SSDs.

No long-term cognitive impairment.

Zhang et al. 2012 (73)

Design Case control prospective study

Participants 112 patients between the ages of 13 and 20

Diagnosis Acute psychosis—hallucinations, delusions or severe thought disorder: Symptoms for less than 1 year; Pharmacotherapy for less than 1 month.

Protocol: Patients were matched for age and sex. Randomization was 2:1. (Antipsychotics and ECT, n = 78; Antipsychotics alone, n = 34) Medications—mainly second generation antipsychotics.

ECT Informed consent from adolescent and guardian.

Propofol for anesthesia. Unilateral at threshold.

Three times a week for up to 14 sessions.

Outcome ECT treated group:

Shorter hospital stay. Discharge based on predetermined PANSS[h] evaluation of positive symptoms, insight, and judgment.

Improved condition at 2 and 7 weeks from baseline, based on PANSS.

Improved sleep quality, correlated with total and positive PANSS scores.

Negative symptoms did not improve.

Side effects Most patients in both conditions had side effects.

The ECT treated group suffered from more transient headaches and dizziness.

(continued)

Box 10.1: (CONTINUED)

Take home messages

ECT is a safe and tolerable intervention in adolescents with first-episode psychosis, and shows greater efficacy when combined with antipsychotic pharmacotherapy vs. pharmacotherapy alone.

[a] *Outcomes were based on diagnosis; the more general findings on ECT in adolescents are also described in this review.*

[b] *Patients suffering from catatonia were grouped together irrespective of diagnosis; diagnosis included schizophrenia, affective disorders, and medical conditions.*

[c] *Neuroleptic malignant syndrome.*

[d] *Reason relates to defining the reason for referral to ECT and treatment course before referral.*

[e] *CGI-clinical global improvement scale.*

[f] *M>F: males had significantly more sessions than females.*

[g] *Significantly longer EEG seizure duration in female than male patients.*

[h] *Positive and Negative Syndrome Scale*

of 18. A clear diagnosis and outcome could be found for only 154 patients (and for an additional group of 51 bipolar patients with mixed presentations). Thirty-six (less than a quarter) of these 154 patients were diagnosed with schizophrenia, and another 2 with a schizoaffective disorder. In that review, ECT was generally found to be effective and well tolerated, but the diagnosis for which ECT was least effective was schizophrenia: significant improvement or remission occurred in only 42% of the adolescents with schizophrenia, as opposed to 63% of the patients diagnosed with depression and 80% of the patients diagnosed with mania or catatonia. The comparatively less frequent use and more limited efficacy of ECT in adolescents with schizophrenia is in accordance with most of the subsequent studies.

In another study, Walter and Rey (67) used an epidemiological survey of hospital charts in New South Wales (NSW), Australia, to identify patients under the age of 18 treated with ECT. Forty-two patients were treated in NSW in the period 1990–1995, and had a total of 49 courses (7 patients had 2 courses). Only 5 out of 18 (28%) ECT courses for patients with SSD resulted in a remission or a significant improvement, in comparison to 19 of the 29 courses in patients with affective spectrum disorders (66%). In the analysis of their data, Walter and Rey (67) evaluated efficacy according to both diagnosis and symptoms, and differentiated between affective and psychotic symptoms. ECT was effective in 7 of 10 (70%) courses for affective symptoms in patients with SSDs (6 patients with depression in schizophrenia, 4 with schizoaffective disorder). In 5 out of 18 treatment courses in which ECT was considered effective for psychotic symptoms in patients suffering from SSD, two patients were diagnosed with catatonic schizophrenia and one with depression in schizophrenia.

This differentiation underscores the importance of the type of symptoms for which ECT is given, beyond the psychiatric diagnosis per se. Bloch et al. (63) studied 24 consecutive adolescent patients treated with ECT over the years 1991–1995. While 19 of these adolescents were diagnosed with SSDs, 4 of the 19 were diagnosed with catatonic schizophrenia, and another 4 with a schizoaffective disorder, supporting the notion that ECT is mainly used to treat affective and catatonic symptoms. In a later study, this group (65) followed 13 adolescents over six years who had been treated with ECT. Nine patients were diagnosed with SSDs (5 with schizophrenia and 4 with schizoaffective disorder). However, when looking beyond diagnosis to the reason for referral (excluding resistance to pharmacotherapy), catatonia (3 patients) and severe suicidal risk (3 patients) were much more common in this adolescent group than in a comparison group of adult patients hospitalized in the same facility. In keeping with these findings, Stein et al. (64) compared 36 adolescent patients treated by ECT over a 6-year period with 57 adult ECT recipients. Nineteen patients (53%) were diagnosed with SSDs. In relation to the reason for ECT referral, the prevalence of acute life-threatening conditions was far more common in adolescents than in the adult group: catatonia in 9 patients, severe suicidal risk in 12, resistant psychotic depression in 9, and agitation in another 6 (the respective numbers in the 57 adult patients were 6, 13, 13, and 25). Later case reports have supported the use of ECT for treating schizophrenia with catatonic features (57, 74–76). Other case reports relate to the effect of ECT in cycloid or acute confusion psychosis, and assert that both include many catatonic features (77, 78).

Recent studies (72, 73), using evaluations with the potential to distinguish among the different symptom clusters of schizophrenia (e.g. the Positive and Negative Syndrome Scale; PANSS), support the impression of earlier research that improvement in SSD is mainly for positive symptoms. Baeza et al. (79) studied 13 adolescents with SSDs before and 6 months after ECT. Clinical response (20% or greater reduction in PANSS total scores at 6-month end point) was achieved in just over half (54%) of the patients. However, only scores on the positive rather than negative symptom PANSS subscale improved significantly following ECT. Zhang et al. (73) conducted a prospective case control study of the first episode period of one month or less. Patients were matched in groups of three for age and gender, and then randomized by 2:1 to receive a course of ECT in addition to pharmacotherapy (78 patients) or to continue only with pharmacotherapy with no sham ECT. The combined ECT-medication group had a significantly shorter duration of inpatient treatment compared to the controls (mean ± SD of 23.2 ± 8.2 days vs. 27.3 ± 9.3 days, $p = 0.018$). The response rate over 7 weeks was significantly greater in the ECT-treated group than in the controls, with a cumulative response rate of 74.3% versus 50.0%. Improvement was significantly greater in the add-on ECT group on objective sleep measures; these correlated with a significant improvement on total PANSS, positive symptoms, and general psychopathology scores, but not with the negative symptom score.

The lack of response of negative symptoms to ECT helps to explain the treatment's lack of long-term impact in the majority of cases of SSD. When long-term outcome (6 months to 2 years) is measured by indicators of the overall condition, such as general function (67, 68), the results of ECT are disappointing—patients remain ill. However, improvement in positive symptoms will often be maintained with continued pharmacotherapy after the ECT course (63, 64, 79).

To summarize the data for young persons, ECT is used more effectively for affective disorders than for SSDs. In the treatment of SSDs, ECT is likely to be beneficial for catatonic, affective, and positive symptomatology, but not for negative symptoms.

ADVERSE EFFECTS

In relation to the adverse effects of ECT in the treatment of adolescents with SSDs, it should be noted that most study samples do not distinguish between SSDs and other indications for ECT. Most studies suggest that the side effects of ECT in adolescents and adults are similar. In the study by Baeza et al. (79), only mild and transient side effects were documented; these included headache (12.9% of the 13 SSD patients), myalgia (0.5%), disorientation (0.5%), and agitation (0.5%). Zhang et al. (73), in a study of 112 adolescents with a first episode of psychosis, found ECT to be generally well tolerated; adverse effects were more prevalent in recipients of an add-on, unilateral ECT protocol compared to control patients treated with neuroleptics (transient headache 29% vs. 2%, and dizziness, 19% vs 3%, respectively).

Two issues require specific mention regarding adolescents with SSD who are treated with ECT. First, ECT in these patients is usually given as an add-on to antipsychotic pharmacotherapy. Antipsychotics, depending on the specific medication used, may lower the seizure threshold. Although most antipsychotic medications will be used in adolescents with psychotic symptoms (when those symptoms are, for example, a component of psychotic depression or a manic episode), clozapine (with a dose dependent effect on convulsive threshold) is more commonly used in SSDs than in other disorders with psychotic symptoms. Perhaps the lower convulsive threshold in ECT (related to age) and co-administration of pharmacotherapy, with a similar effect, explain the higher prevalence of prolonged seizures (seizures lasting more than 180 seconds) and tardive seizures (seizures arising in the first 24–48 hours after ECT) in adolescents (80) with SSD treated with the combination of ECT and clozapine. Baeza et al. (72) describe a case of delayed convulsions with changes in the EEG following combined ECT-clozapine treatment that normalized and stabilized with valproate. Similar reports are found in case reports and case series (63, 64, 81, 82).

The second issue pertains to the fact that a cluster of cognitive symptoms makes up part of the diagnosis of schizophrenia, and cognitive decline is a frequent outcome of the disorder. The possible effects of ECT on the cognition of young SSD patients need to be interpreted in this light (61, 62, 83–86). De la Serna (66) presented a 2-year follow-up of nine adolescents with SSD treated with ECT and neuroleptics, matched to nine adolescents with SSD treated only with neuropleptics. In follow-up cognitive assessment, both groups had improved significantly in the semantic category of the verbal fluency task and digits forward. Moreover, at follow-up no significant differences were found between the two groups in any clinical or cognitive variable assessed.

In summary, ECT is generally a safe treatment for adolescent patients diagnosed with SSDs. The likelihood of the combination of ECT and antipsychotic medications to potentially lower the convulsive threshold requires close attention.

ETHICS AND CONSENT

Ethics and consent warrant careful consideration in any discussion on ECT in young persons and are discussed in detail in Chapter 4 of this volume. In most respects, the issues in the young patient with SSD are no different from young patients with other diagnoses. However, since the use of ECT is not as well established in adolescents suffering from SSDs compared to adolescents with other disorders, prudence in its use and other opinion(s) are particularly relevant (86–89).

TECHNIQUE

Knowledge about optimal technical parameters for the use of ECT in adolescents diagnosed with SSD is very limited. We have a better understanding from the adult literature about the potential advantages of ultra-brief stimulation and unilateral electrode placement at six times the seizure threshold, to enhance efficacy and safety (75, 90–93). With respect to the anesthetic agent employed, early studies of ECT in adolescents with SSD have mainly used methohexital (64), whereas later studies have used propofol (72, 73). Succinylcholine has generally been the muscle relaxant of choice. Electrode placement has been bilateral in most studies (57, 63–66, 72). An exception is the study of Zhang et al. (73), which used unilateral ECT at threshold for early intervention in acute psychosis. The American Academy of Child and Adolescent Psychiatry (AACAP) recommendations (89) state that it is preferable to commence with right unilateral, and switch to bilateral placement if there is no significant response. In cases where the danger to the patient's life or health is severe, it is possible to start with bilateral placement. Since these resistant, acute, and dangerous circumstances are common in patients with SSD referred for ECT, it is not surprising that this technique is used in most naturalistic studies.

The ECT course of adolescent patients generally entails 10–20 treatments, given 2–3 times a week (94). It is our impression that the adolescent patient with SSD may require a longer ECT course than the patient with an affective disorder. Whereas the mean number of ECT sessions in the review by Rey and Walter (68), in which most of the described patients were diagnosed with affective disorder, was 9.6, in studies with a higher proportion of patients with SSD (e.g. 63, 64, 79), the mean number of sessions has been greater (14.5 ± 4.8, 17.03 ± 5.9 and 13.9 ± 4.3 sessions, respectively). Data on maintenance ECT in young patients with SSD are extremely limited (74). However, when longer follow-up has been reported, it has been found that several patients have continued with ECT. For example, in the study by Baeza et al. (79), 7 of the 13 patients treated with ECT at the acute stage (53.8%) received continuation ECT at 6 months after the initial assessment. At 2-year follow-up, none of the 9 patients assessed had continued with ECT, and no patients received more than 20 ECT treatments in total (66).

WHEN IS ECT RELEVANT FOR TREATING ADOLESCENTS WITH SSD? A STEP-BY-STEP "DECISION TREE"

Schizophrenia and schizoaffective disorder generally have a lengthy course, and ECT does not provide a permanent "cure" for these disorders. Further, it is apparent that our knowledge about the use of ECT in treating SSD adolescents is limited. The evidence for antipsychotic medication in adolescents with SSD in adolescents is far more robust than the evidence for ECT. When used to treat SSD in adults, ECT is usually used as an "add-on" to pharmacotherapy in medication-resistant patients.

Thus, the first consideration with an adolescent suffering from SSD who is referred to ECT is: Why use ECT rather than pharmacotherapy?

1. Resistance to Antipsychotic Medications

This is the commonest reason for the use of ECT in an adolescent suffering from SSD (65, 72). Use of ECT in these circumstances is consistent with practice parameters for the assessment and treatment of children and adolescents diagnosed with schizophrenia: ECT should be used as a last resort after pharmacotherapy (including a trial of clozapine) has failed. What is "resistance to pharmacotherapy?" Currently accepted criteria for treatment resistance (based on definitions used for adult patients) require that the adolescent be persistently ill with schizophrenia, with relentless positive symptoms (such as hallucinations or delusions) despite adequate antipsychotic drug treatment (23). Prior to ECT, we will generally have trialed at least 2–3 courses of antipsychotic medication (ensuring adequate trial duration and medication dose), including a trial of clozapine for at least a few months due to the possibility of late response. Indeed, in some of the more recent reports, patients are referred to ECT after showing resistance to clozapine (66, 74).

2. Intolerance of Antipsychotic Medications

Antipsychotic medications may cause significant adverse effects for many young patients. Awareness about weight gain, metabolic side effects, and other adverse events associated with second generation antipsychotics is increasing. A change in medication is often helpful to reduce these effects. Because ECT generally does not replace medications, but is used as an add-on strategy, its advantage in this context is limited.

3. Management of Acute Life- or Health-Threatening Conditions Likely Requiring Immediate Response

Acute, often reversible, life- or health-threatening conditions are perhaps the most relevant scenario for the use of ECT in adolescents with SSDs.

A. *Neuroleptic malignant syndrome (NMS)* is an idiosyncratic, life-threatening complication of treatment with antipsychotic drugs that is characterized by fever, severe muscle rigidity, and autonomic and mental status changes. Since NMS is caused by neuroleptic therapy, its treatment requires that the neuroleptics be ceased (95, 96). Silva et al. (97) reviewed 77 published cases of NMS with first generation antipsychotics and Neuhut et al. (98) examined 20 cases of NMS with atypical antipsychotics in adolescents. The psychiatric diagnoses for which these patients received pharmacotherapy in the review of Silva et al. (97) included schizophrenia (24.3%), schizoaffective disorder (5.4%), bipolar disorder (17.6%), and other psychotic diagnosis (23.0%); in 17.6% of the cases, there was no mention of psychiatric diagnosis. Nine of the 77 patients received ECT for the management of NMS. Comparing the outcome of the different treatments for NMS, the authors note that there were no deaths in the group treated with ECT (7 of the 77 patients with NMS died as a result of the NMS). In some of the patients in this study, ECT was unsuccessful in shortening the course of NMS. Neuhut et al. (98) reviewed patients under the age of 18 who suffered from NMS related to the use of second generation antipsychotic medications (only English-published studies were included in these reviews): 13 of the 20 patients described had been diagnosed with SSDs, and 5 patients treated with ECT for their NMS showed a favorable outcome. We support these reviewers' suggestion that ECT is probably underutilized for the treatment of NMS in adolescents.

B. *Catatonic features*. As discussed in Chapter 11 ("ECT for Catatonia in Autism"), studies on ECT in adolescents not uncommonly include patients with a catatonic syndrome, as a feature of SSD, an affective disorder, or possibly an independent diagnosis (57, 63, 64, 68, 74, 76–79, 87, 99, 100). Catatonic features usually appear abruptly and have an acute, severe, and sometimes life-threatening course, as patients with this condition may stop eating and drinking. In comparison to other psychiatric treatments, ECT has onset of action that may be evident as early as within the first 1–3 weeks of commencement of therapy (i.e., 6–9 sessions). ECT is thus of potential benefit in the management of catatonia. In keeping with accepted practice guidelines (89), ECT should be considered in an adolescent suffering from abrupt, life-threatening catatonic features, even if the "pharmacotherapy resistant" criterion is not established.

C. *Severe suicidality*. ECT may be one of the only psychiatric therapies with an "antisuicidal" (i.e., beyond "antidepressant") effect (101). Its relatively early impact is highly important in the severely suicidal patient. However, in many patients suicidal intent and behavior often follow a chronic course. In a register-based cohort study of a mainly adult population, there were comparatively more completed suicides the week after concluding ECT (102). ECT per se was probably not the culprit; rather, it is likely that ECT increased the energy level of patients who were otherwise still depressed and that energized patients were then able to successfully suicide, as is sometimes the case with completed suicide in patients with severe depression on antidepressant medication (102). Nevertheless, prudence is necessary when planning maintenance therapy after a successful course of ECT for depressed suicidal adolescents.

D. *Florid psychosis*. As discussed earlier, this indication is related to "severe agitation" or "cycloid psychosis." ECT will generally be used for this situation due to poor response to courses of antipsychotic medications, non-compliance with pharmacotherapy, or when agitation becomes life- or health-endangering.

To conclude, in adolescents diagnosed with SSDs, ECT is likely most useful in life- or health-threatening conditions such as NMS, catatonia, severe suicidal risk, and severe agitation. Not only is ECT beneficial in these conditions, but its relatively rapid effects render it as being of particular merit.

NEW DIRECTIONS IN ECT FOR SSD

Most studies on ECT in adolescents with SSD regard its use in this population as a late treatment option. Still, in recent years, efforts have been geared toward preventing or minimizing the deteriorating course of schizophrenia. In this respect, the first psychotic episode is a time when interventions can potentially improve the prognosis for many patients. There is evidence that reduction of time to commence therapy in a psychotic episode may represent an important predictor for better prognosis (103).

In a recent large-scale prospective case-controlled study (73), ECT was used as an early intervention strategy to improve the poor outcome often associated with schizophrenia. The results (see Box 10.1) seem promising, with shorter hospital stay in patients receiving unilateral ECT as an add-on to phamacotherapy, suggesting an accelerated treatment response when compared with patients treated with medication alone.

The evidence for the safety of ECT may encourage extending research from the study of ECT in medication-resistant patients or acute life-endangering conditions to the use of ECT as one of a number of procedures to improve the overall outcome in younger patients with a first psychotic episode. Increasing knowledge about the optimal ECT parameters in the use of this treatment in adolescents still needs be addressed, especially when ECT is employed at an early stage in the management of psychosis. In line with this suggestion, research into newer techniques for brain stimulation, such as transcranial magnetic stimulation and direct current stimulation, for these indications should also be encouraged.

The following case vignettes, drawn from the authors' experience, are examples when ECT was considered the most optimum treatment option and the decision making process was complex.

CASE VIGNETTE

Jason, the first of three children, was 14 years old and a good student in 8th grade. He came from an intact, well-adjusted, upper middle class family. There was no family history of psychiatric disorders, and his development had been normal. He was referred for psychiatric evaluation for the first time in his life at the age of 14 years. In the weeks preceding the evaluation, he became confused, feeling as if planes "use" him and send him special vibrations to be broadcast on TV. At the evaluation, affective symptoms were not prominent. Jason was diagnosed with a schizophreniform disorder, and had a period of home hospitalization, in which he stayed at home under the continuous supervision of a responsible adult, with regular meetings with his psychiatrist and daily phone conversations involving the psychiatrist with his family. He was started on risperidone, which was gradually increased to 3 mg daily. In the first weeks, there was an improvement in his psychosis and he managed to return to school. Later, he developed severe extrapyramidal side effects, with severe prolonged and deforming dystonia. Attempts to lower the dose of risperidone and to add anticholinergic medications were unsuccessful. He was switched to olanzapine, but remained highly psychotic with considerable weight gain, severe sedation, and no improvement in dystonia. The continuation of this condition necessitated hospitalization in a psychiatric day center.

The following treatment options were considered at this point: (1) ECT; (2) Clozapine; (3) change to a first generation antipsychotic medication; (4) change to a different atypical antipsychotic medication; (5) washout of all antipsychotic agents; (6) mood stabilizers; and (7) benzodiazepines. Because Jason was diagnosed with schizophrenia, mood stabilizers were not considered as a suitable option. Medical and neurological consultations were sought and these did not reveal any significant findings. Jason's condition deteriorated in the course of an attempt to taper off medications, and benzodiazepines had no effect. An attempt with a first generation antipsychotic medication was considered inappropriate due to the risk of worsening the extrapyramidal syndrome. Treatment with a different second generation antipsychotic was considered questionable due to the pervasive and ongoing deterioration in condition.

Due to the presence of severe, fulminant psychosis and severe antipsychotic-induced extrapyramidal movements, treatment choices considered were ECT and clozapine. Jason was overwhelmed with fear in relation to ECT, and therefore clozapine was initiated after obtaining informed consent from Jason's family. Treatment with clozapine resulted in remission, which was maintained over the next 3 years, until Jason developed severe neutropenia (less than 400 neutrophils/cm^3 detected in a routine blood count). Jason was then hospitalized to a pediatric ward. Clozapine was tapered down, but hematopoietic growth factors were required to stabilize his hematological condition. Jason was started on quetiapine and the dose was gradually increased to 800 mg/d. However, he continued to deteriorate over the following weeks; he became paranoid and was violent toward family members for the first time. Jason was hospitalized in a closed psychiatric ward and switched to clozapine, but his condition continued to deteriorate. The next change in treatment entailed a combined regimen of olanzapine 25 mg/d and clonazepam. Although he was less agitated, Jason's severe paranoid psychosis persisted.

The hematology consultant considered that re-challenge with clozapine was too risky, as were other antipsychotic agents, such as ziprasidone (noting that aripiprazole was not available at the time). Finally, having exhausted all possible options, ECT was suggested.

Since Jason's therapists wanted to avoid the raised convulsive threshold associated with benzodiazepines, he was tapered off clonazepam. Jason was successfully treated with a course of 11 bilateral ECT sessions combined with olanzapine. He was discharged, and ECT was gradually stopped. On follow-up, he remained in a stable condition for the next 5 years, and had continued treatment with olanzapine 20 mg/d. There were no longer active psychotic symptoms, he worked part-time, and he was taking courses at a nearby college. Jason's affect was blunted, and it was difficult for him to adjust to change. However, he stated that he did not like to remember the past, adding "I feel ECT helped me to push away my disease."

CASE VIGNETTE

Linda was hospitalized at the age of 17 years, due to prolonged and distressing ideas of reference, that caused her to stop eating and drinking. Linda's mother had been diagnosed with schizophrenia. Linda's early development was described as normal. In elementary school, children would tease and mock her because she was "slow, strange and had silly beliefs and fears." At the age of 13, she was seen for the first time by a child and adolescent psychiatrist, and was initially diagnosed with an undifferentiated psychosis, and later with schizophrenia. She received six full trials of antipsychotic medications with partial, transient improvement. Paranoid symptoms were pervasive and persistent.

In the inpatient department, a trial of clozapine was discontinued because of deterioration in Linda's mental state. Her movements became very slow, she would freeze on occasions (these periods lasting several minutes), and she started to refuse food and general assistance.

Linda was diagnosed with catatonia. Her food avoidance had become dangerous and she was deemed to be resistant to psychotropic medication, including clozapine. At this point, ECT was initiated. Immediate improvement commenced after two treatments—improvement was noted in food intake and there was also greater fluidity of movements. After five sessions, Linda refused to continue with ECT, developing overwhelming fear of the procedure. She was stabilized with risperidone, and was returned to a rehabilitation program.

CONCLUSION

ECT in a young person with SSD may not be the first treatment that comes to a clinician's mind. Nevertheless, as outlined in this chapter, in certain situations the treatment may be effective and indeed lifesaving. Furthermore, the treatment is safe. Clinicians need to familiarize themselves with the literature surrounding the use of ECT in this patient group, and some of the specific issues around its use in SSD compared to patients with other psychiatric diagnoses. Further studies will help to inform treatment in this area.

QUESTIONS AND ANSWERS

1. *What are the main indications for ECT in schizophrenia spectrum disorder (SSD)?*

   Indications for the use of ECT in SSD are based on the combination of specific symptoms, severity of symptoms, and dangers from or lack of response to pharmacotherapy. ECT is indicated where catatonic, affective, or positive symptoms predominate, there is severe suicidal danger (or food refusal, severe agitation, etc), and pharmacotherapy (including clozapine) has failed or cannot be used safely (for example, in situations of neuroleptic malignant syndrome).

2. *What is the rationale for using ECT in an effort to accelerate treatment response rate early in the course of a young person with SSD?*

   The rationale is the frequent difficulty in diagnosing SSD from affective psychosis early in the course of the disease, the possible therapeutic opportunities in the first episode of these severe disorders, the effectiveness of ECT in many young patients with SSD, and the high safety of modern ECT.

3. *Is ECT as effective in SSD as in mood disorders?*

   No, ECT is less effective in SSD. Affective or catatonic symptoms in SSD are target symptoms for ECT. Negative symptoms of schizophrenia respond less (if at all) to ECT.

4. *Can ECT worsen the short-term or the long-term outcome in patients with SSD?*

   Cognitive deterioration is one of the dreaded potential trajectories of SSD. Since cognitive side effects of ECT may occur in the short term, and some patients report subjective difficulties with memory in the longer term following ECT, awareness about the potential cognitive effects of ECT when treating adolescents suffering from SSD with ECT is always warranted. When used carefully for the appropriate indications and with modern techniques, ECT improves the short-term outcome of these severe psychiatric disorders.

DISCLOSURES

Dr. Yuval Bloch has no conflicts to disclose. He is funded by Shalvata and TAU. Grant Support: National Alliance for Research on Schizophrenia and Depression (NARSAD), 2003 and 2007.

Dr. Daniel Stein has no conflict of interest to report.

Prof. Garry Walter has received research support from Lundbeck and AstraZeneca for a study titled "Psychiatric Evaluation in Primary Care."

REFERENCES

1. Rajji TK, Ismail Z, and Mulsant BH. Age at onset and cognition in schizophrenia: meta-analysis. *Br J Psychiatry.* 2009;195(4):286–93.
2. Correll CU, et al. Prospective study of adolescents with subsyndromal psychosis: characteristics and outcome. *J Child Adolesc Psychopharmacol.* 2005; 15(3):418–33.

3. Fraguas D, et al. Does diagnostic classification of early-onset psychosis change over follow-up? *Child Psychiatry Hum Dev.* 2008;39(2):137–45.
4. Hollis C. Adult outcomes of child- and adolescent-onset schizophrenia: diagnostic stability and predictive validity. *Am J Psychiatry.* 2000;157(10):1652–9.
5. Olfson M, Marcus SC, Wan GC. Treatment patterns for schizoaffective disorder and schizophrenia among Medicaid patients. *Psychiatr Serv.* 2009;60(2): 210–6.
6. Salvatore P, et al. McLean-Harvard International First-Episode Project: two-year stability of DSM-IV diagnoses in 500 first-episode psychotic disorder patients. *J Clin Psychiatry.* 2009;70(4):458–66.
7. Bromet EJ, et al. Diagnostic shifts during the decade following first admission for psychosis. *Am J Psychiatry.* 2011;168(11):1186–94.
8. Kumra S, et al. Childhood-onset schizophrenia. A double-blind clozapine-haloperidol comparison. *Arch Gen Psychiatry.* 1996;53(12):1090–7.
9. Delbello MP, et al. A double-blind, randomized, placebo-controlled study of quetiapine as adjunctive treatment for adolescent mania. *J Am Acad Child Adolesc Psychiatry.* 2002;41(10):1216–23.
10. Shaw P, et al. Childhood-onset schizophrenia: A double-blind, randomized clozapine-olanzapine comparison. *Arch Gen Psychiatry.* 2006;63(7):721–30.
11. Tohen M, et al. Olanzapine versus placebo in the treatment of adolescents with bipolar mania. *Am J Psychiatry.* 2007;164(10):1547–56.
12. Findling RL, et al., A multiple-center, randomized, double-blind, placebo-controlled study of oral aripiprazole for treatment of adolescents with schizophrenia. *Am J Psychiatry,* 2008;165(11):1432–41.
13. Kumra S, et al. Clozapine and "high-dose" olanzapine in refractory early-onset schizophrenia: a 12-week randomized and double-blind comparison. *Biol Psychiatry.* 2008;63(5):524–9.
14. Findling RL, et al. An open-label study of aripiprazole: pharmacokinetics, tolerability, and effectiveness in children and adolescents with conduct disorder. *J Child Adolesc Psychopharmacol.* 2009;19(4):431–9.
15. Kryzhanovskaya L, et al. Olanzapine versus placebo in adolescents with schizophrenia: a 6-week, randomized, double-blind, placebo-controlled trial. *J Am Acad Child Adolesc Psychiatry.* 2009;48(1):60–70.
16. Haas M, et al. A 6-week, randomized, double-blind, placebo-controlled study of the efficacy and safety of risperidone in adolescents with schizophrenia. *J Child Adolesc Psychopharmacol.* 2009;19(6):611–21.
17. Tramontina S, et al. Aripiprazole in juvenile bipolar disorder comorbid with attention-deficit/hyperactivity disorder: an open clinical trial. *CNS Spectr.* 2007;12(10):758–62.
18. Kumra S, et al. Clozapine versus "high-dose" olanzapine in refractory early-onset schizophrenia: an open-label extension study. *J Child Adolesc Psychopharmacol.* 2008;18(4):307–16.
19. Kumra S, et al. Efficacy and tolerability of second-generation antipsychotics in children and adolescents with schizophrenia. *Schizophr Bull.* 2008;34(1):60–71.
20. Findling RL, et al. A prospective, open-label trial of olanzapine in adolescents with schizophrenia. *J Am Acad Child Adolesc Psychiatry.* 2003;42(2):170–5.
21. Findling RL, et al. Efficacy and safety of quetiapine in adolescents with schizophrenia investigated in a 6-week, double-blind, placebo-controlled trial. *J Child Adolesc Psychopharmacol.* 2012;22(5):327–42.

22. Findling RL, et al. Double-blind maintenance safety and effectiveness findings from the Treatment of Early-Onset Schizophrenia Spectrum (TEOSS) study. *J Am Acad Child Adolesc Psychiatry.* 2010;49(6):583–94; quiz 632.
23. Kranzler HN, et al. Treatment-refractory schizophrenia in children and adolescents: an update on clozapine and other pharmacologic interventions. *Child Adolesc Psychiatr Clin N Am.* 2006;15(1):135–59.
24. Tharyan P. Electroconvulsive therapy for schizophrenia. *Cochrane Database Syst Rev.* 2000(2):CD000076.
25. Tharyan P, Adams CE. Electroconvulsive therapy for schizophrenia. *Cochrane Database Syst Rev.* 2002(2):CD000076.
26. Tharyan P, Adams CE. Electroconvulsive therapy for schizophrenia. *Cochrane Database Syst Rev.* 2005(2):CD000076.
27. Naidoo D. The effect of reserpine (serpasil) on the chronic disturbed schizophrenic: a comparative study of Rauwolfia alkaloids and electroconvulsive therapy. *J Nerv Ment Dis.* 1956;123(1):1–13.
28. Brandon S, et al. Leicester ECT trial: results in schizophrenia. *Br J Psychiatry.* 1985;146:177–83.
29. Abraham KR, Kulhara P. The efficacy of electroconvulsive therapy in the treatment of schizophrenia: a comparative study. *Br J Psychiatry.* 1987; 151:152–5.
30. Sarkar P, et al. An exploratory evaluation of ECT in haloperidol-treated DSM-IIIR schizophreniform disorder. *Convuls Ther.* 1994;10(4):271–8.
31. Goswami U, Kumar U, Singh B. Efficacy of electroconvulsive therapy in treatment resistant schizophreinia: a double-blind study. *Indian J Psychiatry.* 2003;45(1):26–9.
32. Kho KH, et al. Electroconvulsive therapy for the treatment of clozapine nonresponders suffering from schizophrenia: an open label study. *Eur Arch Psychiatry Clin Neurosci.* 2004;254(6):372–9.
33. Gazdag G, Kocsis-Ficzere N, Tolna J. The augmentation of clozapine treatment with electroconvulsive therapy. *Ideggyogy Sz.* 2006;59(7–8):261–7.
34. Havaki-Kontaxaki BJ, et al. Concurrent administration of clozapine and electroconvulsive therapy in clozapine-resistant schizophrenia. *Clin Neuropharmacol.* 2006;29(1):52–6.
35. Nothdurfter C, et al. The influence of concomitant neuroleptic medication on safety, tolerability and clinical effectiveness of electroconvulsive therapy. *World J Biol Psychiatry.* 2006;7(3):162–70.
36. Masoudzadeh A, Khalilian AR. Comparative study of clozapine, electroshock and the combination of ECT with clozapine in treatment-resistant schizophrenic patients. *Pak J Biol Sci.* 2007;10(23):4287–90.
37. Ravanic DB, et al. Long-term efficacy of electroconvulsive therapy combined with different antipsychotic drugs in previously resistant schizophrenia. *Psychiatr Danub.* 2009;21(2):179–86.
38. Kristensen D, et al. Electroconvulsive therapy for treating schizophrenia: a chart review of patients from two catchment areas. *Eur Arch Psychiatry Clin Neurosci.* 2011;261(6):425–32.
39. Braga RJ, Petrides G. The combined use of electroconvulsive therapy and antipsychotics in patients with schizophrenia. *J ECT.* 2005;21(2):75–83.
40. Haskett RF, Loo C. Adjunctive psychotropic medications during electroconvulsive therapy in the treatment of depression, mania, and schizophrenia. *J ECT.* 2010;26(3):196–201.

41. Zervas IM, Theleritis C, Soldatos CR. Using ECT in schizophrenia: a review from a clinical perspective. *World J Biol Psychiatry*. 2012;13(2):96–105.
42. Greenhalgh J, et al. Clinical and cost-effectiveness of electroconvulsive therapy for depressive illness, schizophrenia, catatonia and mania: systematic reviews and economic modelling studies. *Health Technol Assess*. 2005;9(9):1–156, iii–iv.
43. Painuly N, Chakrabarti S. Combined use of electroconvulsive therapy and antipsychotics in schizophrenia: the Indian evidence: a review and a meta-analysis. *J ECT*. 2006;22(1):59–66.
44. Hustig H,Onilov R. ECT rekindles pharmacological response in schizophrenia. *Eur Psychiatry*. 2009;24(8):521–5.
45. Kellner CH, et al. Continuation electroconvulsive therapy vs pharmacotherapy for relapse prevention in major depression: a multisite study from the Consortium for Research in Electroconvulsive Therapy (CORE). *Arch Gen Psychiatry*. 2006;63(12):1337–44.
46. Matheson SL, et al. Quality assessment and comparison of evidence for electroconvulsive therapy and repetitive transcranial magnetic stimulation for schizophrenia: a systematic meta-review. *Schizophr Res*. 2010;118(1–3):201–10.
47. Phutane VH, et al. Why do we prescribe ECT to schizophrenia patients? *Indian J Psychiatry*. 2011;53(2):149–51.
48. Chanpattana W, Kramer BA. Acute and maintenance ECT with flupenthixol in refractory schizophrenia: sustained improvements in psychopathology, quality of life, and social outcomes. *Schizophr Res*. 2003;63(1–2):189–93.
49. Chanpattana W, Sackeim HA. Electroconvulsive therapy in treatment-resistant schizophrenia: prediction of response and the nature of symptomatic improvement. *J ECT*. 2010;26(4):289–98.
50. Chanpattana W, Chakrabhand ML. Combined ECT and neuroleptic therapy in treatment-refractory schizophrenia: prediction of outcome. *Psychiatry Res*. 2001;105(1–2):107–15.
51. Chanpattana W, et al. Short-term effect of combined ECT and neuroleptic therapy in treatment-resistant schizophrenia. *J ECT*.1999;15(2):129–39.
52. Chanpattana W. Maintenance ECT in treatment-resistant schizophrenia. *J Med Assoc Thai*. 2000;83(6):657–62.
53. Ucok A, Cakr S. Electroconvulsive therapy in first-episode schizophrenia. *J ECT*. 2006;22(1):38–42.
54. Chanpattana W, Andrade C. ECT for treatment-resistant schizophrenia: a response from the far East to the UK. NICE report. *J ECT*. 2006;22(1):4–12.
55. Chanpattana W. Maintenance ECT in schizophrenia: a pilot study. *J Med Assoc Thai*. 1998. 81(1): p. 17–24.
56. Suzuki K, et al. Continuation electroconvulsive therapy for relapse prevention in middle-aged and elderly patients with intractable catatonic schizophrenia. *Psychiatry Clin Neurosci*. 2005;59(4):481–9.
57. Suzuki K, et al. Improvement of psychiatric symptoms after electroconvulsive therapy in young adults with intractable first-episode schizophrenia and schizophreniform disorder. *Tohoku J Exp Med*. 2006;210(3):213–20.
58. Taylor P, Fleminger JJ. ECT for schizophrenia. *Lancet*. 1980;1(8183):1380–2.
59. Baker AA, Game JA, Thorpe JG. Some research into the treatment of schizophrenia in the mental hospital. *J Ment Sci*. 1960;106:203–13.
60. Bagadia VN, et al. Evaluation of cognitive effects of ect (preliminary observations). *Indian J Psychiatry*. 1981;23(4):324–9.

61. Rami L, et al. Absence of additional cognitive impairment in schizophrenia patients during maintenance electroconvulsive therapy. *Schizophr Bull.* 2004;30(1):185–9.
62. Sackeim HA, et al. The cognitive effects of electroconvulsive therapy in community settings. *Neuropsychopharmacology*. 2007;32(1):244–54.
63. Bloch Y, et al. Electroconvulsive therapy in adolescents: similarities to and differences from adults. *J Am Acad Child Adolesc Psychiatry*. 2001;40(11):1332–6.
64. Stein D, et al. Electroconvulsive therapy in adolescent and adult psychiatric inpatients: a retrospective chart design. *J Affect Disord.* 2004;82(3):335–42.
65. Bloch Y, et al. Reasons for referral for electroconvulsive therapy: a comparison between adolescents and adults. *Australas Psychiatry*. 2008;16(3):191–4.
66. de la Serna E, et al. Two-year follow-up of cognitive functions in schizophrenia spectrum disorders of adolescent patients treated with electroconvulsive therapy. *J Child Adolesc Psychopharmacol*. 2011;21(6):611–9.
67. Walter G, Rey JM. An epidemiological study of the use of ECT in adolescents. *J Am Acad Child Adolesc Psychiatry,* 1997;36(6):809–15.
68. Rey JM, Walter G. Half a century of ECT use in young people. *Am J Psychiatry.* 1997;154(5):595–602.
69. Hegeman JM, et al. [The efficacy of electroconvulsive therapy in adolescents. A restrospective study]. *Tijdschr Psychiatr*. 2008;50(1):23–31.
70. Walter G, Rey JM. Has the practice and outcome of ECT in adolescents changed? findings from a whole-population study. *J ECT*. 2003;19(2): 84–7.
71. Paillere-Martinot ML, Zivi A, Basquin M. [Use of electroconvulsive therapy in adolescence]. *Encephale*. 1990;16(5):399–404.
72. Baeza I, et al. Clinical experience using electroconvulsive therapy in adolescents with schizophrenia spectrum disorders. *J Child Adolesc Psychopharmacol.* 2010;20(3):205–9.
73. Zhang ZJ, et al. Electroconvulsive therapy improves antipsychotic and somnographic responses in adolescents with first-episode psychosis: a case-control study. *Schizophr Res*. 2012;137(1–3):97–103.
74. Consoli A, et al. Moderate clinical improvement with maintenance ECT in a 17-year-old boy with intractable catatonic schizophrenia. *Eur Child Adolesc Psychiatry.* 2009;18(4):250–4.
75. Rhoads JC, et al. The successful use of right unilateral ultra-brief pulse electroconvulsive therapy in an adolescent with catatonia. *Brain Stimul.* 2010;3(1):51–3.
76. Ghaziuddin N, et al. ECT treatment of malignant catatonia/NMS in an adolescent: a useful lesson in delayed diagnosis and treatment. *J ECT.* 2002;18(2): 95–8.
77. Neuhaus AH, et al. Electroconvulsive monotherapy in the treatment of acute confusion psychosis: a case report. *Pharmacopsychiatry*. 2005;38(6):330–2.
78. Neuhaus AH, et al. Electroconvulsive monotherapy in confusion psychosis: a potential standard regimen? *Pharmacopsychiatry.* 2007;40(4):170–1.
79. Baeza I, et al. Electroconvulsive therapy in early adolescents with schizophrenia spectrum disorders. *J ECT*. 2009;25(4):278–9.
80. Chanpattana W, et al. Effects of stimulus intensity on the efficacy of bilateral ECT in schizophrenia: a preliminary study. *Biol Psychiatry*. 2000;48(3):222–8.
81. Bloch Y, Pollack A, Mor I. Should the administration of ECT during clozapine therapy be contraindicated? *Br J Psychiatry*. 1996;169(2):253–4.
82. Glenisson L, et al. [Adverse seizure reactions after electroconvulsive therapy. Study of personal cases and review of the literature]. *Encephale.* 1998;24(1):1–8.

83. Ghaziuddin N, Laughrin D, Giordani B. Cognitive side effects of electroconvulsive therapy in adolescents. *J Child Adolesc Psychopharmacol.* 2000;10(4):269–76.
84. Schat A, et al. Changes in everyday and semantic memory function after electroconvulsive therapy for unipolar depression. *J ECT.* 2007;23(3):153–7.
85. Smith GE, et al. A randomized controlled trial comparing the memory effects of continuation electroconvulsive therapy versus continuation pharmacotherapy: results from the Consortium for Research in ECT (CORE) study. *J Clin Psychiatry.* 2010;71(2):185–93.
86. Garg R, Chavan BS, Arun P. Quality of life after electroconvulsive therapy in persons with treatment resistant schizophrenia. *Indian J Med Res.* 2011;133:641–4.
87. Zisselman MH, Jaffe RL. ECT in the treatment of a patient with catatonia: consent and complications. *Am J Psychiatry.* 2010;167(2):127–32.
88. Baker T. The minor issue of electroconvulsive therapy. *Nat Med.* 1995;1(3):199–200.
89. Ghaziuddin N, et al. Practice parameter for use of electroconvulsive therapy with adolescents. *J Am Acad Child Adolesc Psychiatry.* 2004;43(12):1521–39.
90. Sackeim HA, et al. Effects of stimulus intensity and electrode placement on the efficacy and cognitive effects of electroconvulsive therapy. *N Engl J Med.* 1993;328(12):839–46.
91. Sackeim HA, et al. Effects of pulse width and electrode placement on the efficacy and cognitive effects of electroconvulsive therapy. *Brain Stimul.* 2008;1(2):71–83.
92. Sienaert P, et al. Randomized comparison of ultra-brief bifrontal and unilateral electroconvulsive therapy for major depression: clinical efficacy. *J Affect Disord.* 2009;116(1–2):106–12.
93. Kellner CH, et al. Bifrontal, bitemporal and right unilateral electrode placement in ECT: randomised trial. *Br J Psychiatry.* 2010;196(3):226–34.
94. Shoirah H, Hamoda HM. Electroconvulsive therapy in children and adolescents. *Expert Rev Neurother.* 2011;11(1):127–37.
95. Strawn JR, Keck PE Jr, Caroff SN. Neuroleptic malignant syndrome. *Am J Psychiatry.* 2007;164(6):870–6.
96. Trollor JN, Sachdev PS. Electroconvulsive treatment of neuroleptic malignant syndrome: a review and report of cases. *Aust N Z J Psychiatry.* 1999;33(5):650–9.
97. Silva RR, et al. Neuroleptic malignant syndrome in children and adolescents. *J Am Acad Child Adolesc Psychiatry.* 1999;38(2):187–94.
98. Neuhut R, Lindenmayer JP, Silva R. Neuroleptic malignant syndrome in children and adolescents on atypical antipsychotic medication: a review. *J Child Adolesc Psychopharmacol.* 2009;19(4):415–22.
99. Bertagnoli MW, Borchardt CM. A review of ECT for children and adolescents. *J Am Acad Child Adolesc Psychiatry.* 1990;29(2):302–7.
100. Cizadlo BC, Wheaton A. Case study: ECT treatment of a young girl with catatonia. *J Am Acad Child Adolesc Psychiatry.* 1995;34(3):332–5.
101. Kellner CH, et al. Relief of expressed suicidal intent by ECT: a consortium for research in ECT study. *Am J Psychiatry.* 2005;162(5):977–82.
102. Munk-Olsen T, et al. All-cause mortality among recipients of electroconvulsive therapy: register-based cohort study. *Br J Psychiatry.* 2007;190:435–9.
103. Perkins DO, et al. Relationship between duration of untreated psychosis and outcome in first-episode schizophrenia: a critical review and meta-analysis. *Am J Psychiatry.* 2005;162(10):1785–804.

CHAPTER 11

ECT for Catatonia in Autism

DIRK M. DHOSSCHE, AND LEE E. WACHTEL

KEY POINTS

- Catatonia is currently viewed as a unique neuropsychiatric syndrome characterized by specific motor signs, which can be life-threatening when aggravated by autonomic dysfunction and fever, yet treatable with (high-dose) benzodiazepines and/or ECT, if recognized early.
- Catatonia has been increasingly recognized as a comorbid syndrome of autism at a rate of 12–17% in adolescents and young adults with autism spectrum disorders.
- Additional symptoms, often seen around adolescence in autism, which should alert a clinician for catatonia, are markedly increased psychomotor slowness, which may alternate with excessive motor activity, apparently purposeless, and not influenced by external stimuli, extreme negativism or muteness, stereotypies, peculiarities of voluntary movement, echolalia, or echopraxia.
- Stressful or new life events, the loss of routine and structure, experiences of loss, conflicts with parents, caregivers, or peers, and discrepancies between the ability in the patient and parental expectations (especially in higher functioning autistic youth) are known to precipitate catatonia, which may present in conjunction with other major psychiatric disorders.
- In autistic patients suspected of catatonia, antipsychotic agents and other medications that can induce catatonia should be discontinued due to the risk of worsening catatonia or precipitating neuroleptic malignant syndrome.
- Lacking controlled trials, successful use of benzodiazepines and ECT for catatonia in autism is supported by case reports and case series.
- A benzodiazepine challenge test of 1 or 2 mg lorazepam, administered *per os*, intramuscularly, or intravenously, may be used to verify the catatonia diagnosis.

- Relatively high dosages of lorazepam, up to 24 mg daily, may be necessary for symptom resolution. A slow dose-titration, which does not induce sedation or other side effects, is recommended.
- Bilateral ECT is indicated for the treatment of catatonia, when lorazepam does not bring about rapid relief. Successful treatment of catatonia with ECT appears to require more frequent seizures than for the relief of major depression. In severe or malignant catatonia, daily ECT for 3 to 5 days may be necessary. The number of sessions necessary before substantial improvement or remission may vary between patients. Maintenance ECT is an integral treatment component for sustained symptom remission.
- Preliminary reports support safety and tolerability of maintenance ECT in autistic patients who show stable neuropsychological testing during treatment.

OVERVIEW

This chapter defines catatonia in autism, describes its historical relevance, symptom overlap between catatonia and autism, and theories underlying the overlap between the two syndromes. Additionally, the evaluation process, diagnosis, and treatment of catatonia in patients with autism is described. The use of ECT is recommended in patients who fail to respond adequately to benzodiazepines as first-line treatment. Case vignettes are presented to illustrate clinical experience. It should be noted that there are no controlled trials of ECT for the treatment of catatonia, irrespective of the underlying etiology of the syndrome. We also note that the terms "youth", "children" and "minors" are used interachangeably and refer to patients younger than 18 years. "Adolescents" refers to individuals who range in age from 12 to 18 years, whereas pre-pubertal children are those below age 12. Due to the paucity of data in pre-pubertal children, the majority of the information presented in this chapter is based on experience with adolescents.

AUTISM AND CATATONIA: A HISTORICAL NOTE

The study of autism historically has not included catatonia, yet catatonia and autism share several symptoms. The overlapping symptoms include mutism, echolalia, stereotypic speech and repetitive behaviors, posturing, grimacing, rigidity, mannerisms, and purposeless agitation (1). This separation between the syndromes can be dated back to the original descriptions of autism by Leo Kanner (1894–1981), who stated in 1943 (2) that the newly coined autism "differed markedly and uniquely from anything reported so far." His lead was widely followed and differences between autism and other neurodevelopmental disorders were emphasized (3). The separation of autism from other disorders became anchored in the *Diagnostic and Statistical Manual* (DSM) and the *International Classification of Disease* (ICD) classification systems, discouraging further inquiries into the commonalities between autism, catatonia, psychosis, mental retardation, and other early-onset neurodevelopmental disorders (4).

A notable exception is the work of Karl Leonhard (1904–1988), who proposed a classification system of endogenous psychoses from toddler-age to adulthood, based on patterns of psychomotor disturbances and catatonic symptoms. Helmut Beckmann (1940–2006) and his group further elaborated on this scheme (5). Among the childhood psychomotor psychoses, Leonhard listed *systematic catatonia* (chronic catatonic schizophrenia with poor prognosis), *motility psychosis* (characterized by frequent hyperkinetic phases with psychosis), and *periodic catatonia* (catatonia with an intermittent course of hyperkinetic and akinetic states) (6). Autism was not specified in his classification, but Leonhard described stereotypies, impulsive aggression, self-injurious and disruptive behaviors, lack of expression, negativism, excitement, ambivalence, counter-grasping, mannerisms, peculiar speech patterns including echolalia, and neologisms in children with developmental delay, which he classified as early childhood catatonia, a form of childhood psychosis (7). The descriptions of pediatric periodic catatonia are similar to those of currently accepted autistic impairments in interaction, communication, and restricted behavioral patterns:

> Good contact is elusive; they remain distant, they may smile, their whole face may laugh, but you cannot tell what it means; childhood catatonics appear like foreign bodies which do not fit into the community; development of speech is held back; a constant turning and twisting; these children keep on repeating certain movements; swinging (a ribbon) to and fro with a turning movement of her head. (7)

Today, these children would likely be diagnosed as suffering solely from an autistic disorder.

MODERN DEFINITION OF CATATONIA

The modern view of catatonia regards it as a unique motor dysregulation syndrome, characterized by identifiable signs such as immobility sometimes alternating with excessive, apparently purposeless motor activity that is not influenced by external stimuli, extreme negativism or muteness, stereotypies, peculiarities of voluntary movement, echolalia, or echopraxia (8). The condition may be associated with a number of medical, neurological, toxic or drug-related conditions, and may have an acute or an insidious onset. In its most severe forms, that is, malignant or lethal catatonia, catatonia is accompanied by autonomic dysfunction and fever, and may become life-threatening with imperative need for immediate treatment.

Catatonia was originally described in 1874 by Kahlbaum as a separate brain disorder with a cyclic, alternating, and ultimately progressive course (9). In 1896 (10), Kraepelin incorporated catatonia as a type of dementia praecox or schizophrenia, leading to decades of subsequent misconception that all catatonia indicates concomitant schizophrenia. In the 1970s, various authors described catatonia as a feature of affective disorders in adults, particularly mania (11–13). Recent samples confirm that more than half of catatonic patients have manic-depressive illness (8, 14), while only 10% and 15% of patients with catatonia meet the criteria for schizophrenia. Catatonia also often occurs in medical patients with drug-related conditions or with seizures (15).

There are no controlled treatment studies in catatonia satisfying current standards for evaluating therapies, yet the literature consistently shows positive effects of anticonvulsant drugs, particularly benzodiazepines and barbiturates, and of ECT, regardless of the severity or etiology of catatonia (16–18) or the age of the patient (19–25).

CATATONIA IN AUTISM

Catatonia has been increasingly recognized as a comorbid syndrome of autism, identified at a rate of 12–17% in adolescents and young adults with autism spectrum disorders (26, 27) and with other intellectual disabilities (28, 29). Catatonic symptoms, such as mutism, stereotypic speech, echolalia, stereotypic or repetitive behaviors, posturing, grimacing, rigidity, mannerisms, and purposeless agitation feature prominently in autism. Therefore, a sharp increase in these symptoms, often in adolescence, qualify for a diagnosis of catatonia (27, 30, 31).

In some cases, catatonia may be a feature of another major psychiatric syndrome such as depression (32), bipolar illness (33), or schizophrenia (34), yet many patients do not qualify for a clear diagnosis of mood or a psychotic disorder, often due to the fact that patients are nonverbal and have severe cognitive impairments. Case reports also describe catatonia in pediatric patients with genetic disorders which are characterized by varying degrees of development impairment but the autistic features often do not amount to a full diagnosis of autism; catatonia has been reported in patients with Prader-Willi syndrome (28) and Down syndrome (35).

It is noteworthy that most cases of catatonia in children and adolescents with autism are not associated with underlying medical or psychiatric conditions. For example, in a sample of 58 children and adolescents with catatonia, 18 (31%) had a history of developmental disorder, that is, autism spectrum disorder, intellectual disability, or neurodevelopmental malformation (36). Only two of those had an identifiable underlying medical or psychiatric condition.

Two systematic studies show that catatonia is found in 12–17% of adolescents and young adults with autism (26, 27). Wing & Shah report that 17% of a large referred sample of adolescents and young adults with autism satisfied modern criteria for catatonia (27). Thirty individuals with autism aged 15 years or older met criteria for catatonia, with classic autistic disorder diagnosed in 11 (37%), atypical autism in 5 (17%), and Asperger disorder in 14 (47%). Under age 15, no child demonstrated the full syndrome, although isolated catatonic symptoms were often observed. In the majority of cases, catatonic symptoms started between 10 and 19 years of age. Five individuals had brief episodes of slowness and freezing during childhood before age 10. Obsessive-compulsive and aggressive behaviors preceded catatonia in some cases. Visual hallucinations or paranoid ideas were occasionally reported, but no diagnosis of schizophrenia could be made. This study also emphasized additional symptoms of catatonia that may be particularly characteristic of catatonia in autism, including amotivation, global slowness, prompt-dependence, and prolonged time to complete previously mastered tasks. It is important to recognize these additional symptoms along the catatonic spectrum, because these behaviors otherwise be erroneously attributed to oppositional or "stubborn" behavior.

In the second study, 13 (12%) of 120 autistic individuals, between ages 17–40 years, had clinically diagnosed catatonia with severe motor initiation problems (26). Another four individuals had several catatonic symptoms, but did not meet criteria for the full syndrome. Eight of the 13 individuals with catatonia suffered from autistic disorder; the remaining five were diagnosed with atypical autism. The proportion of those with autistic disorder that were diagnosed with catatonia was 11% (8/73). Fourteen percent (5/35) of those with atypical autism had catatonia.

A recent hospital-based study (37) of 101 child and adolescent psychiatric inpatients with "at risk" diagnoses including any pervasive developmental disorder, psychotic disorder not otherwise specified, intermittent explosive disorder, mental retardation, neuroleptic malignant syndrome or previously diagnosed catatonia found that 18% of patients met criteria for catatonia, based upon three or more symptoms, including unexplained agitation or excitement, disturbed or unusual movements, reduction in movement, reduction or loss of speech, and repetitive/stereotyped movements. The authors emphasized poor recognition of catatonia in these pediatric conditions, including, but not limited to, pervasive development disorders.

Functional regression in daily self-care and social and educational activities may also be a prominent feature of the catatonic presentation in autism.

	AGE	15	16	17	18	19
BEHAVIORS						
Rocking		x	x	x	x	x
Jumping		x	x	x	x	x
Increased obsessions		x	x	x	x	x
Hand flapping			x	x	x	x
Grunting			x	x	x	x
Echopraxia			x	x	x	x
"Disconnected" behavior					x	x
Echolalia					x	x
Rapid finger flicking						x
Screaming and shouting						x
Finger licking/in nose						x
Abnormal gait						x
Food refusal						x
Loss of continence						x
Loss of self-care skills						x
Freezing "like a statue"						x
Staring, delayed response						x
Unprovoked aggression						x
Self-injury						x

Table 11.1 TIMELINE OF SYMPTOM DEVELOPMENT IN P

In many cases, the ability to self-feed, dress and bathe, or participate in previously mastered leisure and educational activities may be sharply compromised. Additionally, continence may be lost (28).

The following case vignette and work samples are demonstrative of the development of catatonia in an autistic youth. Table 11.1 presents a visual representation of symptom development in this patient, and Boxes 11.1 and 11.2 depict educational decline over a 4-month period.

CASE VIGNETTE

P was the product of a full-term pregnancy with normal spontaneous vaginal delivery. Developmental milestones were within normal limits for the first 15 months of life, when he stopped interacting with others and lost acquired speech. He was diagnosed with a pervasive developmental disorder and began intensive early intervention services at a private clinic. He continued to live at home, and attend a specialized school for the next 15 years. P was estimated to have attained upper elementary school skills; at his best, he was learning European capitals and completing multi-digit multiplication.

At age 15, P demonstrated new-onset grunting and other abrupt vocalizations, progressing to repetitive rocking, lunging, head shaking and finger flapping, multiple stereotypies, and hair-combing echopraxia. The symptoms waxed and waned for the next 3 years, although P continued schooling. Three years and five months after symptom onset, P suddenly stopped eating and required to be fed. He was noted to retain food in his mouth for several minutes and would swallow only after extensive prompting. P lost about 50 pounds in the next few months and demonstrated new-onset rigid posturing, which was intermittent and occurred throughout the day. This behavior was particularly evident at meals when utensils would remain suspended in his hand in the air, or he would clamp down so forcefully that staff members feared breaking his jaw, while attempting to pry utensils out. Periods of stupor, slow gait, and shuffling steps became prominent. Academic progress markedly declined in all subject areas. Aggression and self-injury ensued. Unprovoked physical attacks on family and staff necessitated the use of frequent physical restraint, using canvas belts for limb immobilization. Self-injury included frenetic twisting movements of fingers deep into the nares, self-biting of hands, arms, and tongue resulting in wounds. He was no longer able to attend school or to leave home due to the intensity of the behavior dysregulation. Immediately prior to hospitalization for ECT, P was sleeping from 4 am to 10 am, he would then lie or crouch, remaining unresponsive, and required full care in toileting, bathing, and feeding until early evening when he was noted to be acutely agitated, would engage in self-injury and aggressive episodes that were accompanied by leaping, lunging, jumping, screeching, and nonsensical vocalizations. Self-injury escalated to frank loss of oral tissue and tongue bleeding.

Boxes 11.1 and 11.2 are samples of P's speech and input from his speech and language pathologist, who had worked with him in his educational setting for the previous 16 years. These records show a remarkable decline in skill over a 4-month period.

Box 11.1 DECLINE IN MATH PERFORMANCE AND VERBAL OUTPUT OVER 4-MONTHS

On April 2: 2011 it took: P 52 seconds to independently solve the following math Problem, showing all his scratch work and writing the product solution without any assistance:

3786
x251
950,286 3786

On July 21: 2011 it took: P 11 minutes to name the following number:
"5"

•••

In April 2011 P Provided an average of 60 responses during a 30 minute speech session

In July 2011 P Provided an average of 5 responses during a 30 minute speech session

•••

Box 11.2 DECLINE IN READING OVER 4-MONTHS

On April 27, 2011 P orally read the following snip-it. it took him 23 seconds to read it outloud. He read it fluently, with inflection, and without hesitation:

"A post office is a place that takes care of mail, people go to a post office to mail letters and packages. You can buy stamps there, too. Every letter and package is sorted at the post office. A postal carrier takes your mail to your mailbox. Some mail is sent to far away places by plane, train or truck"

On July 12, 2011 it took P 15 miniutes to orally read the following word:

"butter"

He looked at the word and pointed to it repeatedly, then looking at me. It appeared that his mouth was attempting to form the beginnig of the word, but he could not say it. He finally uttered the word in response to extensive cues.

••

On April 27, 2011 it took P 26 seconds to independently generate and write the folowing answer to a comprehension question:

" People can mail letters and packages at a post office"

On April 27, 2011 it took P 23 seconds to independently write the following entry Into his journal:

" I saw Judy,. I read a paragraph and answered comprehension questions"

On July 12, 2011 it took P 17 minutes to write following word:

" train"

It required over 50 cues plus hand-over-hand assistance and redirection.

••

MECHANISM UNDERLYING CATATONIA IN AUTISM

The precise etiology and pathophysiology of catatonia are unknown, yet the overlap between autistic and catatonic symptoms suggest new models of catatonia in addition to the available paradigms (38, 39). Historically, the study of experimental catatonia started in 1928 by de Jong and Barruk, who had induced catatonia in animals by bulbocapnine (40); however, based on current evidence, catatonia studies should be broadened to include models of developmental impairment.

A first new model suggests a developmental framework where the occurrence of catatonia in young children causes irreversible psychopathology, resulting over time in a clinical presentation similar to autistic impairment (41, 42). Prenatal exposure to valproic acid (VPA) is a promising animal model of early-onset catatonia that has also been studied as a model for autism (43). Offspring of female rats injected with VPA on day 12.5 of gestation show brain abnormalities, including smaller cerebella with fewer Purkinje cells. The rats exhibit catatonic-like behaviors appearing before puberty that include lower sensitivity to pain, diminished acoustic prepulse inhibition, repetitive hyperactivity, unresponsiveness, and withdrawal.

A second new model suggests that catatonia may be induced by intense fear, based on observation of animal reflex of tonic immobility (44). This reaction to fear appears to be similar to catatonia observed in children and adolescents, including those with autism, following severe traumatic events (45–47). Shah and Wing (48) found that ongoing stressful experiences often preceded the development of catatonia in autistic young adults. Life events, loss of routine and structure, experiences of loss, conflicts with parents, caregivers, or peers, and discrepancies between parental expectations and functioning of autistic individuals, especially those who are higher functioning, may precipitate catatonia. Observations which support that catatonia may follow overwhelming anxiety due to trauma, or perception of danger, include positive response of catatonia to anxiolytics such as benzodiazepines or barbiturates. Furthermore, psychogenic theories of catatonia (49) are particularly applicable to people with autism due to their increased vulnerability to social, cognitive, and sensory stressors (50, 51). The following case vignette describes the association between stress and catatonia in an otherwise healthy boy with autism.

CASE VIGNETTE

A 14-year-old autistic boy was at his baseline state of somatic and mental health prior to the sudden 2-month absence followed by precipitious return of his mother. Several hours after being reuinited with his mother, the boy ran into the closet, where he became rigid, immobile, and stuporous, repeating the word "moose." He was hospitalized and initially treated with two antipsychotic trials resulting in clinical worsening. Depakote and lorazepam therapies led to symptom resolution.

BENZODIAZEPINES AND ECT ARE EMPIRICAL TREATMENTS OF CATATONIA IN AUTISM

There are no controlled trials of ECT for the treatment of catatonia in autism. The basis for the management of catatonia in autism consists of case reports accumulated over the past 15 years and reliance on research-supported interventions for catatonia in adults without developmental disorders. Many autistic youth who develop catatonia suffer extreme physical compromise, including inability to move and/or excessive motor activity (the two may coexist), difficulty in eating or voiding, development of dangerous cardiovascular and thermoregulatory instability, as well as onset of repetitive, tic-like, self-injurious behaviors with prominent risk of extreme tissue and organ damage.

In many of the reported cases (48, 52–65), ECT resulted in significant symptom relief without altering the underlying autistic pathology (54, 57, 61, 63–65). Other, usually milder, cases have benefited from the use of lorazepam (62), and social, behavioral, and psychological interventions (48).

Prior to the recently reported cases, the only clinical note about the use of ECT in autism is mentioned in O'Gorman's 1970 book (66), in which a single passage mentions the benefits of prolonged courses of ECT in autistic adolescents: "... avoids the rapid deterioration which tends to occur if such an acutely disturbed episode is prolonged." The text reads: "It appears that, in some hands, ECT is very often helpful, but the course of treatment will often have to be intensive and prolonged. Four or five treatments a week for four or even five weeks may be necessary," and "The present writer's practice is to employ this treatment only during acutely disturbed phases in older (adolescent) patients." This mention of ECT does not define the nature of the disturbance, while catatonia is not mentioned at all. It is noteworthy that this book dates from the 1970s, at the nadir of public acceptance of ECT and peak of antipsychiatric and anti-ECT movements (67). This may explain why his insight into the use of continuation ECT in the medical management of autism was lost (54, 57, 61, 64).

EVALUATION, DIAGNOSIS AND TREATMENT OF CATATONIA

Guidelines for the evaluation, diagnosis, and treatment of catatonia in children, adolescents, and young adults with autism are described and depicted in the algorithm in Figure 11.1.

DIAGNOSIS OF CATATONIA IN AUTISM

Catatonia should be suspected in people with autism whenever there is an obvious and marked deterioration in movement, speech, self-care, and practical skills. The overall motor changes can be variable and may consist of either mostly increased, mostly decreased, or mixed increased and decreased output. Earlier studies in adult psychiatric patients (11) have supported a retarded versus excited type of catatonia; however, similar systematic studies in autistic youth are lacking.

The guidelines presented in Table 11.2 are proposed for diagnosing catatonia in autism (68, 69), using the two criteria suggested by Fink and Taylor (8). However, these criteria are adapted to include a longer time criteria (one day instead of one hour for Criterion A, and one week instead of "on two or more occasions") to allow for baseline abnormalities that are frequently present in autistic individuals, including problems with speech, stereotypy, and other motor problems. Malignant catatonia is diagnosed when these symptoms are accompanied by fever and/or autonomic dysfunction.

Several catatonia rating scales have been developed (70) for the assessment of catatonic symptoms. An overview of often-described catatonic symptoms and suggested assessment procedures during a clinical examination is given in Table 11.3. The most commonly used scale for the assessment of catatonia is the Bush-Francis Catatonia Scale (BFCRS) (71), a 23-item standardized instrument that is designed for diagnosis and for assessment of severity. When using the BFCRS, catatonia may be diagnosed when two or more items on the first 17 items

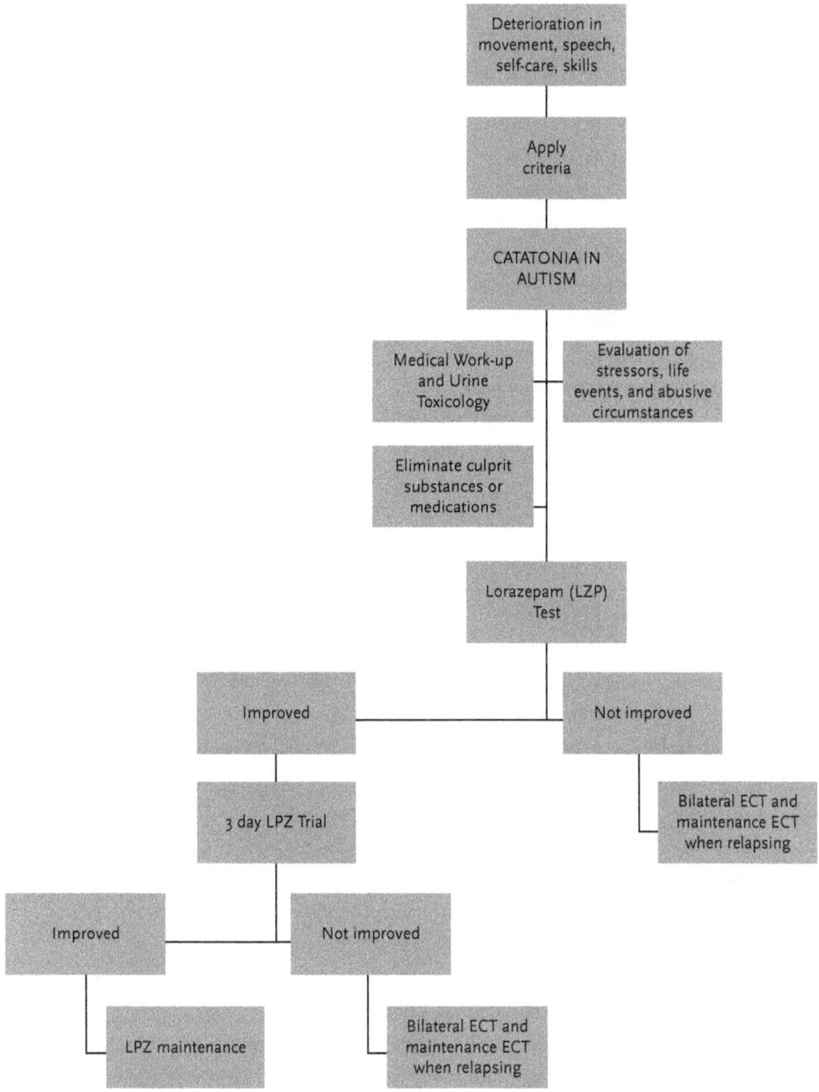

Figure 11.1:
Evaluation, Diagnosis, and Treatment of Catatonia in Autism.

are present. Serial catatonia ratings are useful to detail changes over time and for measuring change during treatment (72) in individual cases and controlled studies. Although the Bush-Francis Catatonia Scale is useful in patients with autism, the scale was developed using a sample of general adult psychiatric patients. There are no catatonia rating scales that have been standardized in patients with autism and in pediatric patients. The KANNER scale, named after Leo Kanner (1894–1981), who described the neuromotor and neurodevelopmental features of autism (2), has been proposed as a unifying instrument for quantifying core

Table 11.2. SUGGESTED DIAGNOSTIC CRITERIA FOR CATATONIA IN AUTISM

Criterion A	Marked change in overall mobility including immobility, increased motor activity (excitement), or a mixed presentation that may include periods of markedly reduced motor activity alternating with excitement, drastically decreased speech, or stupor of at least one day duration, associated with at least one of the following: catalepsy, automatic obedience, posturing, or freezing (abrupt, unexplained cessation of all activity).
Criterion B	In the absence of a change in mobility, drastically decreased speech, or stupor, a marked increase from baseline, for at least one week, of at least two of the following: slowness of movement or speech, difficulty in initiating movements or speech unless prompted, freezing during actions, difficulty crossing lines, inability to cease actions, stereotypy, echo phenomena, catalepsy, automatic obedience, posturing, negativism, or ambitendency.

Table 11.3. DEFINITION OF CATATONIC SYMPTOMS

Excitement	Extreme hyperactivity, apparently non-purposeful
Immobility/stupor	Extreme hypoactivity, immobility and/or minimally responsive
Mutism	Verbally unresponsive or minimally responsive
Staring	Fixed gaze, little or no visual scanning of environment, decreased blinking
Posturing/catalepsy	Maintains posture(s), including mundane (e.g., sitting or standing for hours without reacting)
Grimacing	Maintenance of odd facial expressions
Echopraxia/echolalia	Mimicking of examiner's movements/speech
Stereotypy	Repetitive, non-goal directed motor activity (e.g., finger-play, repeatedly touching, patting or rubbing self)
Mannerisms	Odd, purposeful movements (hopping or walking tiptoe, saluting passers-by, exaggerated caricatures of mundane movements)
Verbigeration	Repetition of phrases or sentences
Rigidity	Maintenance of a rigid position despite efforts to be moved
Negativism	Apparently motiveless resistance to instructions or to attempts to move/examine the patient. Contrary behavior, does the opposite of the instruction.
Waxy flexibility	During reposturing of the patient, patient offers initial resistance before allowing himself to be repositioned (similar to that of bending a warm candle).
Withdrawal	Refusal to eat, drink, and/or make eye contact
Impulsivity	Sudden, inappropriate behavior (e.g., runs down the hallway, starts screaming, or takes off clothes) without provocation. Afterward, cannot explain.
Automatic obedience	Exaggerated cooperation with examiner's request, or repeated movements that are requested once.

(continued)

Table 11.3. (CONTINUED)

Passive obedience (*Mitgehen*)	Raises arm in response to light pressure to finger, despite instruction to the contrary.
Negativism (*Gegenhalten*)	Resistance to passive movement that is proportional to strength of the stimulus; response seems automatic rather than willful.
Ambitendency	The patient appears stuck in indecisive, hesitant motor movements.
Grasp reflex	Strike open palm of patient with two extended fingers of examiner's hand. Automatic closure of patient's hand.
Perseveration	Repeatedly returns to the same topic or persists with same movements.
Combativeness	Usually in an undirected manner, without explanation.
Autonomic abnormality	Abnormality of temperature, blood pressure, pulse rate, respiratory rate, inappropriate sweating.

features of catatonia, across a broad range of neuropsychiatric disorders, including autism and pervasive developmental disorders (73). The scale is comprehensive; however, it is untested and not validated in patients with autism.

Stereotypical movements are common in autistic individuals at their baseline functioning (74, 75); however, a marked increase of stereotypical movements, especially when resulting in self-injury or in conjunction with other catatonic symptoms, should alert the clinician to the possibility of emergent catatonia. Vocal and motor tics are also possible signs of catatonia and, as such, responsive to ECT (76). Tics are defined as sudden and non-rhythmic variants of stereotypic or repetitive movement or vocal abnormalities and are commonly present at a low frequency level in autistic individuals. A stark increase in tics, often accompanied by self-injurious behavior, should prompt an assessment for other symptoms of catatonia. The relations between catatonia, self-injury, and tics and their responsiveness to ECT are discussed in a separate chapter (see Chapter 12, "ECT for Self-injurious Behavior").

DIFFERENTIAL DIAGNOSIS

A detailed history, clinical examination, and application of diagnostic criteria must be used to differentiate catatonia from other well-recognized conditions, syndromes, or disorders featuring psychomotor abnormalities that may overlap with the manifestations of catatonia. Making an adequate differential diagnosis of catatonia is complicated by the fact that there is no biologic marker diagnostic of catatonia. The differential diagnosis of catatonia when motor activity is increased or reduced is shown in Table 11.4. In the next paragraphs, a few annotations on differential diagnosis are made. The reader is referred to an earlier paper for further discussion of the differential diagnosis of catatonia (77).

Table 11.4. DIFFERENTIAL DIAGNOSIS OF PEDIATRIC CATATONIA

Differential diagnosis; when increased motor activity	Acute dystonia Tardive dyskinesia Akathisia Withdrawal-emergent dyskinesias Tics/ Gilles de la Tourette Purposeful, oppositional, or attention-seeking behaviors Conversion disorder Compulsions (in obsessive-compulsive disorder) Epilepsy Delirium
Differential diagnosis; when reduced motor activity	Parkinsonism and morbus Parkinson Malignant hyperthermia Neuroleptic malignant syndrome Serotonergic syndrome Epilepsy Selective mutism Conversion disorder Purposeful, oppositional, or attention-seeking behaviors Status epilepticus Delirium Coma

Some motor manifestations of catatonia such as catatonic excitement, psychomotor retardation, or negativism may be mistaken for purposeful, oppositional, and attention-seeking behaviors that are under full control of the patient and for secondary gain. Decreased speech, muteness, or posturing may be mistaken as indicative of conversion disorder, especially when following stressful events or trauma. It may be difficult in some instances to determine the origin of these behaviors and the degree of control that the patient has over these behaviors, even during longer periods of observation. The catatonia benzodiazepine challenge test, discussed in the treatment section, may be useful in such situations. A profoundly positive response would support a diagnosis of catatonia, although the therapeutic effects of anxiolytics including amytal and benzodiazepines as diagnostic tools and treatment are also known in conversion disorders (78–82). The scope of conversion disorders in patients with autism is largely uncharted territory, and has received even less attention than the issue of catatonia, leading us to favor a diagnosis of catatonia and applying its recommended treatments, which are known to be remarkably effective. A negative challenge test is expected when motor abnormalities represent voluntary behaviors for secondary gain, although there may be mild improvement due to non-specific sedative effects.

Epilepsy and status epilepticus are important differential diagnoses given the symptom overlap between psychomotor seizures and catatonia and the increased prevalence of seizures in catatonic patients (8). In his original description, Kahlbaum reported seizure-like symptoms in catatonia (9). Seizures are also frequent in children and adolescents with autism (83, 84) and catatonia (22, 85); therefore, seizures and catatonia are not mutually exclusive in this population. However, frank epileptic activity is usually absent in electroencephalogram (EEG) recordings in catatonic patients. Typical findings in catatonia include diffuse slowing in patients in catatonic stupor and a dysrythmic EEG in catatonia without stupor. These findings are consistent with non-convulsive status epilepticus that resolves when catatonia remits and support the hypothesis about the underlying cause (39, 86) of this disorder, that there is localized brain excitation in catatonic patients in specific deep brain structures. Furthermore, these abnormalities are not detected by current EEG techniques and improve with anticonvulsant medications, but especially with benzodiazepines and ECT.

PSYCHOLOGICAL AND SOCIAL ASSESSMENT

Children and adolescents with autism who develop catatonia should be assessed for traumatic and abusive events in family and broader environments, in addition to medical causes for catatonia. If traumatic or abusive events are suspected or ascertained, specific preventive actions are indicated, and social or psychotherapeutic interventions may be appropriate when the acute symptoms have abated. Nevertheless, regardless of purported etiology, the presence of catatonia, especially in the more severe forms, is an urgent indication for medical intervention.

CASE VIGNETTE

A 20-year-old autistic man developed multiple symptoms of both catatonia and major depression, after his parents' first extended absence and disruption of his regular routine involving significant daily family interaction. Treatment with antidepressants and lorazepam was immediately beneficial, and extensive preparation with usage of social stories and time lines prevented recurrence of difficulties during a later parental vacation.

LABORATORY AND OTHER INVESTIGATIONS

Various infectious, metabolic, endocrine, neurological, toxic, and autoimmune conditions have been associated with catatonia and must, therefore, be assessed. Proposed basic investigations include a complete blood count and metabolic panel, erythrocyte sedimentation rate, magnetic resonance imaging, electroencephalogram, cerebrospinal fluid analysis, antinuclear antibodies, and urine and organic metabolic testing, with further testing based upon clinical findings (87). Due to the known association between medical-neurological disorders and catatonia, the more invasive tests such as a cerebrospinal fluid analysis should be decided on a case-by-case basis in this subgroup.

A drug screen to detect common illicit and prescribed substances is necessary. Recreational drugs (phencyclidine, mescaline, psilocybin, cocaine, ecstasy, opiates, and opioids), disulfiram, steroids, antibiotic agents (ciprofloxacin), baclofen, and bupropion have been associated with the emergence of catatonia. Withdrawal of benzodiazepines, gabapentin, and dopaminergic drugs, especially if done rapidly, has precipitated catatonia in some patients (8).

MEDICATION MANAGEMENT

All prescribed medications should be evaluated for their potential to induce catatonic symptoms, since many medications can cause catatonia or catatonia-like conditions. Antipsychotic agents should be discontinued because of the reported increased incidence of malignant catatonia or neuroleptic malignant syndrome (NMS) in patients with incipient signs of catatonia (88, 89).

CASE VIGNETTE

A 20-year-old autistic man was hospitalized in catatonic stupor. The patient also demonstrated loud barking and chirping vocal tics. A single dosage of risperidone 1 mg given prior to starting ECT led to marked hypertension. Risperidone was discontinued with prompt return of normotension, and was later successfully re-initiated for both tics and evident psychosis after stabilization with ECT (90).

MEDICAL MANAGEMENT

Simultaneous treatment of catatonia and a drug-induced or medical condition, if any is detected, is generally recommended in addition to supportive measures. For instance, despite the withdrawal of the offending agent, treatment of an underlying infection or metabolic disease, or the removal of a malignancy, as the case may be, catatonia is often noted to persist and requires urgent intervention. Treatment specifically targeting catatonia should not be postponed for elaborate searches for ill-defined or poorly treatable medical conditions. This may be particularly relevant in recent cases of presumed autoimmune entities such as pediatric autoimmune neuropsychiatric disorders associated with streptococcal infections (PANDAS) and anti-NMDA-receptor encephalitis, where catatonic symptoms are evident, yet well-documented anti-catatonic treatments are rejected in favor of novel immunological interventions that are often of little benefit in improving the prominent catatonic presentation (91, 92).

CATATONIA CHALLENGE TEST

As a first step, a benzodiazepine challenge test of 1 or 2 mg of lorazepam may be administered *per os*, intramuscularly, or intravenously, to verify the catatonia diagnosis (8, 18, 72). However, under-utilization of lorazepam in pediatric catatonia has been reported (87). The gamma-aminobutyric acid-A (GABA) receptor modulator zolpidem has also been used as an alternative catatonia challenge test, particularly in Europe (93).

When a single dose of lorazepam is noted to improve catatonia, lorazepam can be prescribed at regular intervals to maintain improvement. Many catatonic patients require relatively high dosages of lorazepam, up to 24 mg daily, for symptom resolution. Our experience shows that in some adolescents with catatonia, doses up to 24 mg daily are tolerated without ensuing sedation, especially when instituted using daily incremental dosages, and result in marked reduction of catatonic symptoms. This suggests that in some cases, catatonia may be associated with high tolerance to benzodiazepines. Careful monitoring in a medical setting for excessive sedation, respiratory compromise, and other side effects is recommended.

USE OF ECT FOR CATATONIA

Three previously published case vignettes are presented regarding the use of ECT for treating catatonia. They also show some of the practical difficulties faced by patients and their families. The first case illustrates difficulties encountered due to the lack of adequate ECT services in some parts of United States. The next two cases highlight the importance of maintenance ECT for achieving sustained remission. Most important, patients with catatonia who are treated with ECT are seriously ill and suffer often from other types of impairment. Therefore, prompt recognition of catatonia and in some cases treatment with ECT are likely to prevent medical complications, such as deep vein thrombosis, pulmonary emboli (96, 97), dehydration, malnutrition, and physical exhaustion.

CASE VIGNETTE (94)

A was a 14-year-old boy with high-functioning autism who presented with a 6-month history of progressive overall slowing of movements, periods of immobility for several minutes, inability to initiate movements without prompting, difficulties ambulating and feeding himself, and occasional encopresis. A would also "get stuck" when going through doorways and stay "frozen" in the car when asked to step outside. A was diagnosed with catatonia by his neurologist. An EEG was completed, which did not show any abnormality.

A was the product of an uneventful pregnancy and met all early developmental milestones. However, he had lost most of his speech at age 13 months and stopped responding to his name. He was diagnosed with autism at age 2 and received early intervention services. A remained nonverbal, but demonstrated above-average intelligence on non-verbal IQ tests (in the range of 140) and excellent school performance.

One month after the onset of symptoms, A was prescribed alprazolam and diazepam for catatonia, without effect. Lorazepam was started subsequently and titrated up to 8 mg thrice daily. A was not sedated on 24 mg of lorazepam, but remained severely impaired and continued to require assistance with ambulation, feeding, and self-care. The parents elected to pursue ECT for their son's condition, as they had heard about other autistic patients who had been diagnosed with catatonia benefiting from ECT. However, they learned that ECT was precluded by law for patients below age 16 in their home state and thus sought ECT out of state.

Examination at the university hospital showed a well-groomed, nonverbal adolescent with increased stereotypies, psychomotor slowing, and episodic immobility. Routine labs were normal, and a CT of the head showed normal brain structures. Catatonia was diagnosed based on published criteria for catatonia and catatonia in autism (68, 69). An independent consulting child psychiatrist and child neurologist concurred with the recommendation for ECT for catatonia after a failed trial of lorazepam. The patient and his parents signed consent for ECT.

An outpatient course of seven bilateral ECT treatments was given with a MECTA 4000 Q device, using methohexital as an anesthetic agent and succinylcholine for muscle relaxation. Seizures were monitored with a single EEG tracing and the cuff method. There were no complications and A improved dramatically, with about 80% reduction of catatonia. After seven ECT, the patient and his parents returned to their home for about one week; however, they returned to the university hospital for an additional four ECT. The acute success of the treatment, along with practical concerns of being away from their home, led the parents to not select M-ECT services.

However, A relapsed quickly, and 6 weeks later the parents returned to the university hospital to resume treatment. A second course of twelve ECT treatments relieved catatonia again and M-ECT was recommended to prevent further relapses. Unfortunately, the practical difficulties of being away from home precluded further treatment at the university hospital. As expected, the patient relapsed within the next few months. The parents have pursued alternative treatments due to lack of local ECT availability, and believe that a number of diverse treatments including high dose folic acid and anti-inflammatory agents have helped A attain a level of functioning that is about 50% of his premorbid, pre-catatonic level. The parents are worried that if catatonia worsens, they will have considerable difficulties accessing ECT treatment in their home state, even when A turns 16, because of limited ECT resources for individuals with developmental disorders.

CASE VIGNETTE (64, 94)

B is an autistic woman adopted from Romania after severe early childhood deprivation who demonstrated intermittent "freezing" episodes and chronic self-injury throughout her childhood before experiencing a profound catatonic deterioration at age 16 involving ongoing posturing, rigidity, mutism, waxy flexibility, negativism, and agitated behaviors including severe self-injury to the point of retinal detachment and traumatic cataract formation, as well as anorexia requiring gastrostomy tube placement for all nutrition and hydration. B was prescribed nearly all US-available psychotropic medications for her presentation before receiving a definitive diagnosis of catatonia. No medication, including benzodiazepines, afforded sustained relief and many trials led to further deterioration.

An acute course of bilateral ECT resolved all symptoms of catatonia as well as nearly completely eradicated dangerous self-injury. B was discharged to an ambulatory ECT setting at a major university medical center free of all catatonic symptoms while receiving ongoing bitemporal ECT at maximal charge, twice weekly, and concomitant citalopram 30 mg daily for intermittent irritability, tearfulness, and decreased interest in activities. The initial treatment plan upon admission to outpatient ECT was to continue bitemporal treatments, decreasing the frequency from the index course and transitioning to once every two weeks for 6 months with a final goal to progressively taper to once monthly maintenance treatments. B was treated with bitemporal ECT twice a week for 6 months at a pulse width of 1, frequency of 60 Hz, duration of 3 seconds, and a current setting of 800 mA for a total charge of 576 mC. During the initial 6 months, decreasing the frequency of ECT was not attempted due to re-emerging symptoms of catatonia, primarily posturing and mutism, as early as the second day after ECT.

After 6 months, ECT frequency was decreased from twice weekly to once weekly. However, after the third week of once weekly ECT, B had a profound deterioration in function, with increased posturing, mutism, and dangerous self-injury, and decreased oral intake. ECT frequency interval was increased to three times a week and olanzapine was added, with little change in catatonic symptoms. Lithium was commenced and titrated up to 450 mg twice daily, at which point B was able to resume twice weekly ECT with sustained resolution of all catatonic symptoms including self-injury. Two further attempts at tapering ECT frequency to once weekly were undertaken but were not successful. During the course of all ECT treatments, anesthesia remained stable. B was pretreated with labetolol 10 mg IV, with induction of anesthesia achieved via methohexital 1.7 mg/kg IV and muscle relaxation with succinylcholine 1.7 mg/kg IV. Once general anesthesia was achieved, she was given flumazenil 0.5 mg IV to reverse the lorazepam in her system and caffeine 250–750 mg IV to potentiate the seizure activity.

In summary, three attempts at decreasing ECT frequency to less than twice weekly during two years of outpatient maintenance ECT resulted in swift return of prominent symptoms of B's catatonia, necessitating return to higher frequency ECT. B has continued ECT on an approximately every-five-day basis for the past six years, with ongoing remission of catatonic symptoms.

CASE VIGNETTE (95)

C is a 14-year-old Caucasian male with prior diagnoses of autism and mild mental retardation whose initial catatonic illness and treatment have been previously described. He premorbidly functioned at a 2nd to 3rd grade academic level, demonstrated near-independence in self-care, actively participated in family and community activities, and was physically healthy. At age 14 years 2 months, however, C began to take increased time to complete academic and routine demands, and required extensive prompting to complete trivial tasks. Intermittently, he would "freeze" and become unresponsive. His movements became progressively slow, and rigidity, posturing, echolalia, and waxy flexibility ensued. Oral intake for both liquids and solids rapidly decreased, and C's body weight decreased from 145 to 110 pounds over 6 months. He was hospitalized several times for IV rehydration.

Prior to the recognition of catatonia, C underwent exhaustive medical and neurological testing, including MRI and CT scans, 24-hour video EEG monitoring, multiple EKGs, echocardiography, Holter monitoring, and extensive laboratory investigations. No etiology was found, although he was documented to have bradycardia with heart rates as low as 40 beats/minute.

Catatonia was ultimately diagnosed after flagrant posturing in a neurologist's office, for which he was prescribed lorazepam. Lorazepam provided immediate relief, but the effects faded despite increased dosage of lorazepam up to 24 mg per day over several weeks. C was admitted to our facility since ECT was not accessible for patients his age in his home state.

On admission, he presented as a cachectic adolescent male with lead-pipe rigidity throughout his body and resistance to movement, requiring 2-person assistance for transitions. Bilateral waxy flexibility was evidenced in the upper extremities. C was mute, and continuously stared downward with frozen facies, unresponsive to verbal or physical prompts or changes in his external surroundings. Posturing in hands and fingers was intermittently observed.

An initial course of 10 right unilateral (RUL) ECT treatments was ineffective; therefore, bilateral ECT was started. The charge dose of 432 mC was eventually increased to 576 mC, which is the maximum deliverable charge using available ECT device. C's motor, verbal, and behavioral symptoms of catatonia improved throughout the 12 bilateral treatments, but his symptoms waxed and waned and concerns remained about nutritional status. After transfer to a pediatrics floor for treatment of dehydration and malnutrition, ECT was suspended as it was inaccessible on the pediatrics service. Within 9 days, C lapsed into a profound catatonic stupor, with rigidity, posturing, staring, mutism, and complete lack of responsiveness, accompanied by hypothermia with core body temperature of 34 °C and profound bradycardia at 24 beats per minute, meeting criteria for malignant catatonia. Bilateral ECT was emergently recommenced using a charge dose of 576 mC. After one treatment, heart rate and temperature normalized. He was also markedly more alert upon waking from his first treatment, and even smiled at the staff. Motor, verbal, and behavioral progress continued with bilateral ECT thrice weekly, although oral intake remained minimal. Olanzapine 1.25 mg BID was initiated to target persistent anorexia, and appetite increased almost immediately.

Treatment was briefly interrupted again when C developed aspiration pneumonia from supplementary nasogastric feedings, resulting in a second transfer to the pediatrics service. C was febrile with maximal temperatures of 40 °C for 48 hours, and amazingly showed a nearly complete remission of all symptoms of catatonia during these two days. The change was remarkable, but short-lived. As C's pneumonia was treated with antibiotics and he returned to an afebrile state after 48 hours, all prior symptoms of catatonia returned.

ECT was resumed within 5 days of pneumonia onset after having a clear chest X-ray, and he showed ongoing improvement. Lithium carbonate was added to his medication regimen and titrated to 450 mg BID, with a resultant serum level of 0.9–1.0 mEq/l. Combined with olanzapine 2.5 mg QAM and 5 mg QHS, ECT frequency was gradually reduced to once weekly with excellent overall sustained symptom remission in terms of systemic, motor, verbal, and behavioral signs of catatonia. C was discharged home, with weekly maintenance ECT for catatonia. Weekly ECT has continued for 3 years since discharge, given the tendency of his catatonic symptoms, including difficulty eating and moving, to remerge approximately on day 5 after each ECT. C actually missed one weekly ECT session during an overseas trip and relapsed into a severe state of delirious mania compounded by significant self-injury, requiring resumption of thrice weekly ECT for two weeks to regain stability.

PRE-ECT LABORATORY AND OTHER INVESTIGATIONS

Routine laboratory tests and an anesthesia consult are required during the pre-ECT workup. Routine imaging studies of the brain are not generally recommended prior to ECT; however, it is acknowledged that, in some hospitals, pre-ECT brain computed tomography (CT) or magnetic resonance imaging (MRI) is mandatory. Additional consultation may be required in selected cases to stabilize general medical issues such as risk of dehydration and hemodynamic abnormalities. Additional details about practical steps prior to, during and following ECT are described in Chapter 5, "A Practical Guide to Using ECT in Minors."

ECT PARAMETERS

General technical issues of ECT and anesthesia parameters in pediatric patients are reviewed in Chapters 5 and 7 (respectively, "A Practical Guide to Using ECT in Minors" and "Anesthesia"). It is imperative to consider two issues, specific to the treatment of catatonia, which extend to pediatric ECT and to autistic youth. First, relief of catatonia often seems to require more frequent seizures than those necessary for the treatment of major depression. The UK standard practice of two seizures a week, although effective for major depression, may not be so for catatonia. In severe or malignant catatonia, daily treatment for 3 to 5 days may be necessary. Second, the efficacy of bilateral (bitemporal or bifrontal) electrode placement is better documented than is unilateral placement. Therefore, based on considerable practical experience, the authors recommend bilateral electrode placement for catatonia in autism. Furthermore, in our experience the number of treatments, before substantial and sustained improvement becomes obvious, cannot be predicted. Therefore, ECT treatment of this patient group must be individually tailored, and the duration and the frequency of treatment should be based on regular assessments, possibly after every 6–12 treatments.

ECT AND CONCURRENT MEDICATIONS

It is recommended that all psychiatric medications should be stopped prior to initiation of ECT, as well as any other non-psychiatric medications, if possible. An exception is when there was a partial response with benzodiazepine treatment, often administered in a high dose; in these instances, ECT and a benzodiazepine may be administered concurrently. Discontinuation or rapid taper of the benzodiazepine may not be advisable at the start of the ECT course, because of a risk of altering the seizure threshold. Concurrent use of lorazepam (or another benzodiazepine) and ECT is then a useful treatment variant. Intravenous administration of flumazenil, a benzodiazepine antagonist, can be used if lorazepam interferes with eliciting seizures during ECT and may be beneficial even if seizures outwardly appear adequate; indeed, use of flumazenil has also been proposed in benzodiazepine-naïve patients for augmentation of ECT effect (98).

MAINTENANCE ECT IN CATATONIA

The case vignettes that are described earlier in this chapter underscore the usefulness of maintenance ECT (M-ECT) for sustained symptom-remission (94). Often the index treatment course is intensive and may last several months. This is usually followed by a maintenance treatment in many cases to avoid relapse. This need for prolonged treatment is reminiscent of the experience of O'Gorman, who reported in the 1970s that intensive and prolonged ECT courses were often necessary to treat acutely disturbed episodes and avoid rapid deterioration in adolescents with autism (66). In cases where catatonia remains undiagnosed or untreated for a prolonged time, the response to ECT is often slow, an expected feature when there are long delays before appropriate treatment is started. The importance of prompt treatment and maintenance ECT also applies to non-autistic populations where ongoing ECT is often imperative to prevent relapse, using various paradigms presented for optimizing M-ECT (99, 100). There are no studies that suggest evidence for structural or histopathological changes during M-ECT (101, 102). Although studies of various cognitive functions demonstrate stability of various longitudinal cognitive measures (103–105), less information is available regarding M-ECT in autism. One case series (94) presents the M-ECT courses of three autistic catatonic patients who received up to 286 maintenance treatments with sustained remission of catatonia and without subjective evidence of decline in cognitive or adaptive skills. One patient was unable to access M-ECT for legal reasons and promptly relapsed into catatonia. While the number of M-ECT delivered to these patients appears high, this finding is considered within the context of a special patient population who are known to have a relatively poor response to psychotropic agents, and possibly a higher overall propensity for treatment resistance.

CASE VIGNETTES

An autistic 21-year-old male, who was severly medically compromised, received 220 M-ECT for catatonia over 2 years, with remarkable recovery and return to baseline psychosocial and educational functioning (106). His global functioning remained stable throughout the entire M-ECT, and comprehensive neuropsychological testing completed at yearly intervals, over 3 years, showed consistent stability without any evidence of cognitive decline. Another report described an 18-year-old male with malignant catatonia in the context of congenital cerebellar dysgenesis in whom neuropsychological testing remained unchanged after2 years following 61 maintenance ECT (107).

CONCLUSION

The use of ECT for catatonia in autism represents a relatively new area of scholarly and clinical focus. Catatonia in autism—a clinical picture that, in itself, has received limited attention—is associated with significant impairment and indeed may be life-threatening. Although not modifying the core symptoms of autism prior to the onset of catatonia, ECT can prove effective for the catatonia if the catatonia fails to respond to first-line treatment with benzodiazepines and there is ongoing significant impairment and/or distress. Some patients may require maintenance ECT to maintain improvement and prevent relapse.

QUESTIONS AND ANSWERS

1. *How common is catatonia in autism?*

   There are a few studies that suggest that catatonia may occur in about one in 7 adolescents and young adults with autism. Although none of these studies has used commonly used catatonia rating scales, catatonia is becoming well documented in a growing number of cases.

2. *How is catatonia diagnosed in people with autism?*

   The diagnosis of catatonia is generally made by applying known clinical signs of catatonia and using standardized catatonia rating scales to assess the scope and the severity of the symptoms. In addition, the diagnosis may be supported by a benzodiazepine challenge test (lorazepam is most commonly used), which is known to result in a marked, albeit temporary, improvement of motor symptoms.

3. *Do all patients with catatonia need treatment with ECT?*

   No. Treatment with ECT may be indicated, however, irrespective of the underlying pathology associated with catatonia, if there is failure to respond to first-line treatment with benzodiazepines and there is ongoing significantly impaired functioning and/or distress.

4. *What medical treatments are used prior to considering ECT?*

   Treatment would depend upon the etiology of catatonia, if an underlying cause is identified. However, medical interventions should include laboratory workup, stopping any psychotropic medication (especially dopaminergic and serotonergic agents) and other medications that are associated with catatonia. Benzodiazepines are the only specific medications used for its treatment.

5. *Does ECT improve the symptoms of autism prior to onset of catatonia?*

   ECT does not resolve or improve core symptoms of autism present prior to onset of catatonia. The expectation is that the child or an adolescent will regain his or her level of functioning prior to the onset of catatonia, if catatonic symptoms resolve completely.

6. *What is the outcome in patients with autism, if catatonia is not treated?*

   The course of untreated catatonia in autism is not well-known, yet the impairment due to catatonia is considerable affecting important areas of self-care and social function. The condition may become life-threatening in cases of malignant catatonia.

7. *How long should the treatment with ECT be continued in patients with catatonia associated with autism?*

   The duration and intensity of ECT varies in each case. There are now a few reported cases who have continued to receive ECT for several years to maintain improvement and to prevent relapse.

8. *Is ECT safe in patients with autism?*

   ECT is considered a safe procedure without any evidence of brain damage, lasting memory loss, or other detrimental effects. Current knowledge may be extended to include the use of ECT in autistic individuals, especially in those who have safely received maintenance ECT for several years.

DISCLOSURES

Dr. Dirk M. Dhossche does not have any conflicts of interest or disclosures to report.

Dr. Lee E. Wachtel does not have any conflicts of interest or disclosures to report.

REFERENCES

1. Kakooza A, Stoppelbein L, Dhossche D. Psychosis in autism. In: Fujii D, Ahmed I, eds. *The Spectrum of Psychotic Disorders: Neurobiology, Etiology and Pathogenesis*. Cambridge: Cambridge University Press; 2006, pp. 233–46.
2. Kanner L. Autistic disturbances of affective contact. *Nervous Child*. 1943;2:217–50.
3. Rutter M. Childhood schizophrenia reconsidered. *J Autism Child Schiz*. 1972; 2:315–37.
4. Turner T. Schizophrenia and mental handicap: a historical review, with implications for further research. *Psychol Med*. 1989;19:301–14.
5. Beckmann H, Franzek E, Stober G. Genetic heterogeneity in catatonic schizophrenia: a family study. *Am J Med Genet B*. 1996;67:289–300.
6. Neumarker K-J. Leonhard and the classification of psychomotor psychoses in childhood and adolescence. *Psychopathology*. 1990;23:243–52.
7. Leonhard K. Early childhood catatonia. In: Beckmann H, ed. *Classification of Endogenous Psychoses and Their Differentiated Etiology*. Vienna: Springer-Verlag; 1999, pp. 330–86.
8. Fink M, Taylor M. *Catatonia: A Clinician's Guide to Diagnosis and Treatment*. Cambridge: Cambridge University Press; 2003.
9. Kahlbaum K. *Die Katatonie oder das Spannungsirresein*. Berlin: Verlag August Hirshwald; 1874.
10. Kraepelin E. *Psychiatrie: Ein Lehrbuch fur Studirende und Aerzte*. 5th ed. Leipzig: Barth; 1896.
11. Morrison J. Catatonia: retarded and excited types. *Arch Gen Psychiat*. 1973;28:39–41.
12. Abrams R, Taylor M. Catatonia: a prospective clinical study. *Arch Gen Psychiat*. 1976;33:579–81.
13. Gelenberg A. The catatonic syndrome. *Lancet*. 1976;1:1339–41.
14. Chalasani P, Healy D, Morriss R. Presentation and frequency of catatonia in new admissions to two acute psychiatric admission units in India and Wales. *Psychol Med*. 2005;35:1667–75.

15. Cottencin O, Warembourg F, de Chouly de Lenclave B, Lucas B, Vaiva G, Goudemand M, et al. Catatonia and consultation-liaison psychiatry study of 12 cases. *Prog Neuro-Psychoph*. 2007;31:1170–6.
16. Fricchione G, Cassem N, Hooberman D, Hobson D. Intravenous lorazepam in neuroleptic-induced catatonia. *J Clin Psychopharm*. 1983;3:338–42.
17. Rohland B, Carroll B, Jacoby R. ECT in the treatment of the catatonic syndrome. *J Affect Disorders*. 1993;29:255–61.
18. Caroff S, Mann S, Francis A, Fricchione G. Catatonia. *From Psychopathology to Neurobiology*. Washington, DC: American Psychiatric Publishing; 2004.
19. Carr V, Dorrington C, Schrader G, Wale J. The use of ECT for mania in childhood bipolar disorder. *Br J Psychiatry*. 1983;143:411–5.
20. Black D, Wilcox J, Stewart M. The use of ECT in children: case-report. *J Clin Psychiat*. 1985;46:98–9.
21. Cizadlo B, Wheaton A. Case study: ECT treatment of a young girl with catatonia. *J Am Acad Child Adoles Psychiat*. 1995;34:332–5.
22. Dhossche D, Bouman N. Catatonia in children and adolescents (letter). *J Am Acad Child Adoles Psychiat*. 1997;36:870–1.
23. Slooter A, Braun K, Balk F, van Nieuwenhuizen O, van der Hoeven J. Electroconvulsive therapy of malignant catatonia in childhood. *Pediat Neurol*. 2005;32:190–2.
24. Lee A, Glick D, Dinwiddie S. Electroconvulsive therapy in a pediatric patient with malignant catatonia and paraneoplastic limbic encephalitis. *J ECT*. 2006;22:267–70.
25. Esmaili T, Malek A. Electroconvulsive therapy (ECT) in a six-year-old girl suffering from major depressive disorder with catatonic features. *Eur Child Adoles Psychiatry*. 2007;16:58–60.
26. Billstedt E, Gilberg C, Gilberg C. Autism after adolescence: population-based 13- to 22-year follow-up study of 120 individuals with autism diagnosed in childhood. *J Autism Dev Disord*. 2005;35:351–60.
27. Wing L, Shah A. Catatonia in autistic spectrum disorders. *Br J Psychiatry*. 2000;176:357–62.
28. Dhossche D, Bouman N. Catatonia in an adolescent with Prader-Willi Syndrome. *Ann Clin Psychiat*. 1997;4:247–53.
29. Verhoeven W, Tuinier S. Prader-Willi syndrome: atypical psychoses and motor dysfunctions. *Int Rev Neurobiol*. 2006;72:119–30.
30. Kakooza-Mwesige A, Wachtel L, Dhossche D. Catatonia in autism: implications across the life span. *Eur Child Adolesc Psychiatry*. 2008;17:327–35.
31. Dhossche D, Reti I, Wachtel L. Catatonia and autism: a historical review, with implications for ECT. *J ECT*. 2009;25:19–22.
32. Wachtel LE, Griffin M, Reti I. Electroconvulsive therapy in a man with autism experiencing severe depression, catatonia, and self-injury. *J ECT*. 2010;96(1):70–3.
33. Wachtel LE, Jaffe R, Kellner CH. Electroconvulsive therapy for psychotropic-refractory bipolar affective disorder and severe self-injury and aggression in an 11-year-old autistic boy. *Eur Child Adolesc Psychiatry*. 2011;20(3):147–52.
34. Volkmar F, Cohen D. Comorbid association of autism and schizophrenia. *Am J Psychiatry*. 1991;148:1705–7.
35. Jap SN, Ghaziuddin N. Catatonia among adolescents with Down syndrome: a review and 2 case reports. *J ECT*. 2011;27(4):334–7.

36. Consoli A, Raffin M, Laurent C, Bodeau N, Campion D, Amoura Z, et al. Medical and developmental risk factors of catatonia in children and adolescents: a prospective case-control study. *Schizophr Res.* 2012;137(1–3):151–8.
37. Ghaziuddin N, Dhossche D, Marcotte K. Retrospective chart review of catatonia in child and adolescent psychiatric patients. *Acta Psychiatr Scand.* 2012;125(1):33–8.
38. Kanes S. Animal models. In: Caroff S, Mann SC, Francis A, Fricchione GL, eds. *Catatonia from Psychopathology to Neurobiology*. Washington, DC: American Psychiatric Publishing; 2004, pp. 189–200.
39. Dhossche DM, Stoppelbein L, Rout UK. Etiopathogenesis of catatonia: generalizations and working hypotheses. *J ECT.* 2010;26(4):253–8.
40. De Jong HH, Barruk H. A clinical and experimental study of the catatonic syndrome (Étude comparative expérimentale et clinique des manifestations du syndrome catatonique). *H Revue neurol.* 1929;21.
41. Dhossche D. Autism as early expression of catatonia. *Med Sci Monitor.* 2004; 10:RA31–9.
42. Dhossche D, Rout U. Are autistic and catatonic regression related? A few working hypotheses involving GABA, Purkinje cell survival, neurogenesis, and ECT. *Int Rev Neurobiol.* 2006;72:55–79.
43. Wagner GC, Reuhl KR, Cheh M, McRae P, Halladay AK. A new neurobehavioral model of autism in mice: pre- and postnatal exposure to sodium valproate. *J Autism Dev Disord.* 2006;36:779–93.
44. Gallup G, Maser J. Tonic immobility: Evolutionary underpinnings of human catalepsy and catatonia. In: Maser J, Seligman M, eds. *Psychopathology: Experimental Models.* San Francisco: Freeman; 1977, pp. 334–57.
45. Dhossche D, Wachtel L. Catatonia in psychiatric illness. In: Fatemi S, Clayton P, eds. *The Medical Basis of Psychiatry.* 3rd ed. Totowa, NJ: Humana Press; 2008, pp. 455–70.
46. Bozkurt H, Mukaddes NM. Catatonia in a child with autistic disorder. *Turk J Pediatr.* 2010;52(4):435–8.
47. Saito S, Yamaga K, Kobayashi T, Kato S. A case of Asperger's disorder with catatonia originally suspected of being catatonic schizophrenia. *Seishin Shinkeigaku Zasshi.* 2011;113:241–7.
48. Shah A, Wing L. Psychological approaches to chronic catatonia-like deterioration in autism spectrum disorders. *Int Rev Neurobiol.* 2006;72:245–64.
49. Moskowitz AK. "Scared stiff": catatonia as an evolutionary-based fear response. *Psychol Rev.* 2004;111(4):984–1002.
50. Dhossche DM, Ross CA, Stoppelbein L. The role of deprivation, abuse, and trauma in pediatric catatonia without a clear medical cause. *Acta Psychiatr Scand.* 2012;125(1):25–32.
51. Dhossche D. Catatonia: the ultimate yet treatable motor reaction to fear in autism *Autism—Open Access.* 2011;1:doi: 10.4172/auo.1000103.
52. Realmuto G, August G. Catatonia in autistic disorder: a sign of comorbidity or variable expression. *J Autism Dev Disord.* 1991;21:517–28.
53. Dhossche D. Catatonia in Autistic Disorders (brief report). *J Autism Dev Disord.* 1998;28:329–31.
54. Zaw F, Bates G, Murali V, Bentham P. Catatonia, autism, and ECT. *Devel Med Child Neurol.* 1999;41:843–5.
55. Brasic J, Zagzag D, Kowalik S, Prichep L, John E, Liang H, et al. Progressive catatonia. *Psychol Rep.* 1999;84:239–46.

56. Hare D, Malone C. Catatonia and autism spectrum disorders. *Autism*. 2004;8:183–95.
57. Ghaziuddin M, Quinlan P, Ghaziuddin N. Catatonia in autism: a distinct subtype? *J Intell Disabil Res*. 2005;49:102–5.
58. Ohta M, Kano Y, Nagai Y. Catatonia in individuals with autism spectrum disorders in adolescence and early adulthood: a long-term prospective study. *Int Rev Neurobiol*. 2006;72:41–54.
59. Cohen D. Towards a valid nosography and psychopathology of catatonia in children and adolescents. *Int Rev Neurobiol.* 2006;72:131–47.
60. Schieveld J. Case reports with a child psychiatric exploration of catatonia, autism, and delirium. *Int Rev Neurobiol.* 2006;72:195–206.
61. Fink M, Taylor M, Ghaziuddin N. Catatonia in autistic spectrum disorders: a medical treatment algorithm. *Int Rev Neurobiol.* 2006;72:233–44.
62. de Winter C, van Dijk F, Verhoeven W, Dhossche D, Stolker J. Autism and catatonia: successful treatment using lorazepam. A case study. *Tijdschrift voor Psychiatrie*. 2007;49:257–61.
63. Bailine S, Petraviciute S. Catatonia in autistic twins: role of electroconvulsive therapy. *J ECT*. 2007;23:21–2.
64. Wachtel L, Kahng S, Dhossche D, Cascella N, Reti I. Electroconvulsive Therapy for catatonia in an autistic girl. *Am J Psychiatry*. 2008;165:329–33.
65. Wachtel LE, Griffin MM, Dhossche DM, Reti IM. Brief report: Electroconvulsive therapy for malignant catatonia in an autistic adolescent. *Autism*. 2010;14(4):349–58.
66. O'Gorman G. *The Nature of Childhood Autism*. 2nd ed. London: Butterworths; 1970.
67. Shorter E, Healy D. Shock therapy: a history of electroconvulsive treatment in mental illness. Piscataway, NJ: Rutgers University Press/University of Toronto Press; 2007.
68. Dhossche D, Shah A, Wing L. Blueprints for the assessment, treatment, and future study of catatonia in autism spectrum disorders. *Int Rev Neurobiol.* 2006;72:267–84.
69. Dhossche D, Wing L, Ohta M, Neumarker K-J, eds. *Catatonia in Autism Spectrum Disorders*. San Diego, CA, and London, UK: Elsevier Academic Pres; 2006.
70. Sienaert P, Rooseleer J, De Fruyt J. Measuring catatonia: a systematic review of rating scales. *J Affect Disord*. 2011;135(1-3):1–9.
71. Bush G, Fink M, Petrides G, Dowling F, Francis A. Catatonia: I: Rating scale and standardized examination. *Acta Psychiatrica Scandinavica*. 1996;93:129–36.
72. Bush G, Fink M, Petrides G, Dowling F, Francis A. Catatonia. II. Treatment with lorazepam and electroconvulsive therapy. *Acta Psychiatrica Scandinavica*. 1996;93:137–43.
73. Carroll B, Kirkhart R, Ahuja N, Soovere I, Lauterbach E, Dhossche D, et al. Katatonia: a new conceptual understanding of catatonia and a new rating scale. *Psychiatry*. 2008;5:42–50.
74. Stoppelbein L, Greening L, Kakooza A. The importance of catatonia and stereotypies in autistic spectrum disorders. *Int Rev Neurobiol.* 2006;72:103–18.
75. Stoppelbein L, Sytsma-Jordan S, Greening L. Correlates of psychomotor symptoms in autism. *Int Rev Neurobiol.* 2005;71:343–57.
76. Dhossche DM, Reti IM, Shettar SM, Wachtel LE. Tics as signs of catatonia: electroconvulsive therapy response in 2 men. *J ECT*. 2010;26(4):266–9.

77. Dhossche DM, Wachtel LE. Catatonia is hidden in plain sight among different pediatric disorders: a review article. *Pediatr Neurol.* 2010;43(5):307–15.
78. McCall WV, Shelp FE, McDonald WM. Controlled investigation of the amobarbital interview for catatonic mutism. *Am J Psychiatry.* 1992;149(2):202–6.
79. Naples M, Hackett T. The amytal interview: history and current uses. *Psychosomatics.* 1978;19(2):98–105.
80. Perry JC, Jacobs D. Overview: clinical applications of the Amytal interview in psychiatric emergency settings. *Am J Psychiatry.* 1982;139(5):552–9.
81. Panzer M, Grunhaus L. The diazepam interview: an underutilized diagnostic procedure? *Ann Clin Psychiat.* 1991;3:73–8.
82. Bleckwenn W. The production of sleep and rest in psychotic cases. *Arch NeuroPsychiatr.* 1930;24:365–72.
83. Bolton PF, Carcani-Rathwell I, Hutton J, Goode S, Howlin P, Rutter M. Epilepsy in autism: features and correlates. *Br J Psychiatry.* 2011;198(4):289–94.
84. Tuchman R, Cuccaro M. Epilepsy and autism: neurodevelopmental perspective. *Current Neurol Neurosci.* 2011;11(4):428–34.
85. Dhossche D, Wilson C, Wachtel L. Catatonia in childhood and adolescence: implications for the DSM-5. *Primary Psychiatry.* 2010;17:35–9.
86. Fink M. The intimate relationship between catatonia and convulsive therapy. *J ECT.* 2010;26(4):243–5.
87. Lahutte B, Cornic F, Bonnot O, Consoli A, An-Gourfinkel I, Amoura Z, et al. Multidisciplinary approach of organic catatonia in children and adolescents may improve treatment decision making. *Prog Neuro-Psychoph.* 2008;32(6):1393–8.
88. Fink M, Taylor M. Neuroleptic malignant syndrome is malignant catatonia, warranting treatments efficacious for catatonia. *Prog Neuro-Psychoph.* 2006;30:1182–3.
89. Seitz DP, Gill SS. Neuroleptic malignant syndrome complicating antipsychotic treatment of delirium or agitation in medical and surgical patients: case reports and a review of the literature. *Psychosomatics.* 2009;50(1):8–15.
90. Consoli A, Benmiloud M, Wachtel L, Dhossche D, Cohen D, Bonnot O. Electroconvulsive therapy in adolescents with the catatonia syndrome: efficacy and ethics. *J ECT.* 2010;26(4):259–65.
91. Dhossche D, Fink M, Shorter E, Wachtel LE. Anti-NMDA receptor encephalitis versus pediatric catatonia. *Am J Psychiatry.* 2011;168(7):749–50; author reply 50.
92. Wachtel LE, Dhossche DM. Challenges of electroconvulsive therapy for catatonia in youth with intellectual disabilities: another tomato effect? *J ECT.* 2012;28(3):151–3.
93. Thomas P, Rascle C, Mastain B, Maron M, Vaiva G. Test for catatonia with zolpidem. *Lancet.* 1997;349:702.
94. Wachtel LE, Hermida A, Dhossche DM. Maintenance electroconvulsive therapy in autistic catatonia: a case series review. *Prog Neuro-Psychoph.* 2010;34(4):581–7.
95. Wachtel L, Griffin M, Dhossche D, Reti I. Electroconvulsive therapy for malignant catatonia in an autistic adolescent. *Autism.* 2010;14(4):349–58.
96. McCall W, Mann S, Shelp F, Caroff S. Fatal pulmonary embolism in the catatonic syndrome: Two case reports and a literature review. *J Clinical Psychiatry.* 1995;56:21–5.
97. Lachner C, Sandson N. A case of catatonia-induced deep venous thrombosis. *Psychosomatics.* 2003;44:512–414.

98. Yi J, Torres J, Azner Y, Vaidya P, Schiavi A, Reti IM. Flumazenil pretreatment in benzodiazepine-free patients: a novel method for managing declining ECT seizure quality. *J ECT*. 2012;28:185–9.
99. Kellner C, Knapp R, Petrides G, Rummans T, Husain M, Rasmussen K, et al. Continuation electroconvulsive therapy vs pharmacotherapy for relapse prevention in major depression: a multisite study from the Consortium for Research in Electroconvulsive Therapy (CORE). *Arch Gen Psychiatry*. 2006;63:1337–44.
100. Petrides G, Dhossche D, Fink M, Francis A. Continuation ECT: relapse prevention in affective disorders. *Convulsive Therapy*. 1994;10:189–94.
101. Lippman S, Manshadi M, Wehry M, Byrd R, Past W, Keller W, et al. 1,250 electroconvulsive treatments without evidence of brain injury. *Br J Psychiatry*. 1985;147:203–4.
102. Scalia J, Lisanby SH, Dwork AJ, Johnson JE, Bernhardt ER, Arango V, et al. Neuropathologic examination after 91 ECT treatments in a 92-year-old woman with late-onset depression. *J ECT*. 2007;23(2):96–8.
103. Devanand DP, Verma AK, Tirumalasetti F, Sackeim HA. Absence of cognitive impairment after more than 100 lifetime ECT treatments. *Am J Psychiatry*. 1991;148(7):929–32.
104. Wijkstra J, Nolen WA. Successful maintenance electroconvulsive therapy for more than seven years. *J ECT*. 2005;21(3):171–3.
105. Zisselman M, Rosenquist P, Curlik S. Long-term weekly continuation electroconvulsive therapy: a case-series. *J ECT*. 2007;23:274–7.
106. Wachtel LE, Reti IM, Dhossche DM, Slomine BS, Sanz J. Stability of neuropsychological testing during two years of maintenance electroconvulsive therapy in an autistic man. *Prog Neuro-Psychoph*. 2011;35(1):301–2.
107. Wachtel D, Dhossche D, Reti IM, Hughes-Wheatland R. Stability of neuropsychological testing during maintenance electroconvulsive therapy. *Pediatr Neurol*. 2012;47(3):219–21.

CHAPTER 12

ECT for Self-injurious Behavior

LEE E. WACHTEL AND DIRK M. DHOSSCHE

KEY POINTS

- Self-injurious behavior (SIB) poses a significant clinical challenge for many patients with autism or other intellectual disabilities.
- SIB may be maintained by operant or environmental factors; in addition, it may be associated with psychiatric, medical, and genetic disorders.
- Some forms of repetitive high-intensity, high-frequency SIB may represent a movement disturbance, best conceptualized as an alternate symptom of catatonia.
- This type of SIB may be exquisitely responsive to ECT with profound patient benefit.
- Multidisciplinary assessment of SIB should be completed before pursuit of ECT.
- Modifications to the ECT protocol may be necessary in pediatric patients with neurodevelopmental disabilities.
- Maintenance ECT is crucial, and poses unique challenges.
- Ethical and legal issues, lack of access to ECT, and stigma are salient obstacles to effective treatment.

"There is no use trying," said Alice; "one can't believe impossible things." "I dare say you haven't had much practice," said the Queen. "When I was your age, I always did it for half an hour a day. Why, sometimes I've believed as many as six impossible things before breakfast."

Lewis Carroll, *Through the Looking Glass*

OVERVIEW

This chapter provides an overview of self-injurious behavior (SIB) in youth with intellectual disability (ID) and other forms of developmental disorders. These behaviors may be maintained by operant reinforcement and by concomitant psychiatric, medical, or genetic conditions. Several recent reports describe the successful use of electroconvulsive therapy (ECT) for the treatment of intractable SIB in children, adolescents, and adults with autism and/or ID (1–6). However, large-scale or controlled studies of such are currently lacking. Self-injury is further explored in relation to stereotypies, tics, and the repetitive movements of catatonia, leading to the proposal that self-injury appears to be an alternate sign of catatonia, with direct implications for effective treatment with ECT. Historical and modern evidence of self-injury as part of the catatonic spectrum is presented, including case presentations of intractable SIB, which was effectively treated with acute and maintenance ECT. Safety and ethical issues, caregiver perceptions, and vistas for future research are reviewed. [We note that the terms, "children" "youth" and "minors" are often used interachangeably to refer to patients younger than 18 years. "Adolescents" refers to individuals who range in age from 12 to 18 years, whereas pre-pubertal children are those below age 12. Due to the paucity of data in pre-pubertal children, the majority of the information presented in this chapter is based on experience with adolescents.]

DEFINITION OF SELF-INJURY

SIB is classically defined as any self-directed action that results in physical harm. In surveys conducted in the United States, it is estimated to occur in 10–50% of individuals with ID (7–9). SIB in ID is demarcated as occurring *without specific suicidal ideation or intent* (10, 11). Common forms of SIB include head-banging, hitting, slapping, punching, biting, kicking, and scratching directed at one or more body surfaces, and often results in frank tissue injury. The frequency and intensity of SIB vary widely; behaviors may occur only a few times per month or year with minimal injury, or may occur several times per day, hour, or even minute, leading to significant bodily harm. Indeed, sequelae of SIB range from mild to profound, and include localized bruising, swelling, bleeding, open wounds with potential for infection, traumatic callous and bony ossification formation, disfigurement, vision impairment resulting from traumatic cataract formation or retinal detachment, hearing loss subsequent to ruptured ear drums, skull fractures, cerebral hemorrhage, development of upper motor neuron sign, and even death

(12, 13). Self-injurious behavior may be particularly dangerous when aimed at the head, given the risk of devastating eye and brain damage. These serious injuries only compound the baseline challenges of the intellectually disabled individual and add significant stress to caregivers, who often resort to heroic measures to prevent ongoing self-injury. Several images of self-injury are shown in Figures 12.1–12.4.

Individuals who engage in one form of self-injury are likely to ultimately engage in additional topographies of SIB. Left untreated, SIB typically becomes more entrenched and treatment-refractory. SIB sharply compromises all aspects of an individual's functioning, and is a major risk factor for placement outside the home and community and in a more restrictive setting. The financial cost of SIB in ID is further estimated in the billions of dollars annually (9, 12, 14, 15). The etiology of this challenging behavior is multifactorial, and multiple traditional models exist. A summary of such is provided below, both for completeness and to alert the reader as to those SIB presentations that are likely responsive to ECT.

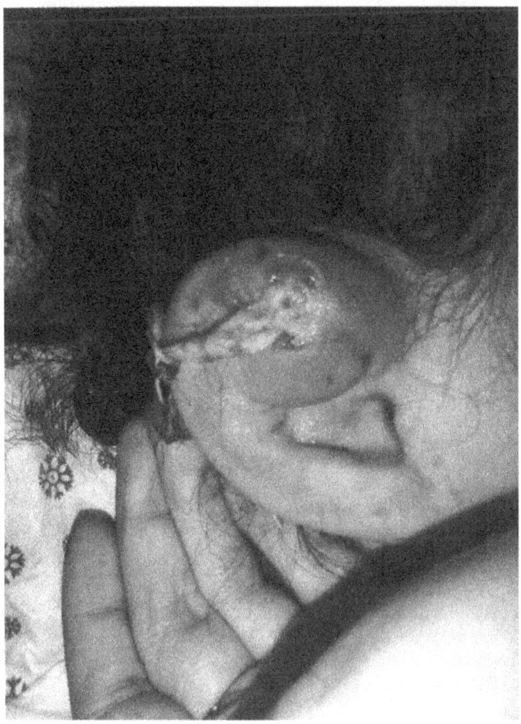

Figure 12.1:
Otic hematoma requiring surgical drainage in an autistic girl.

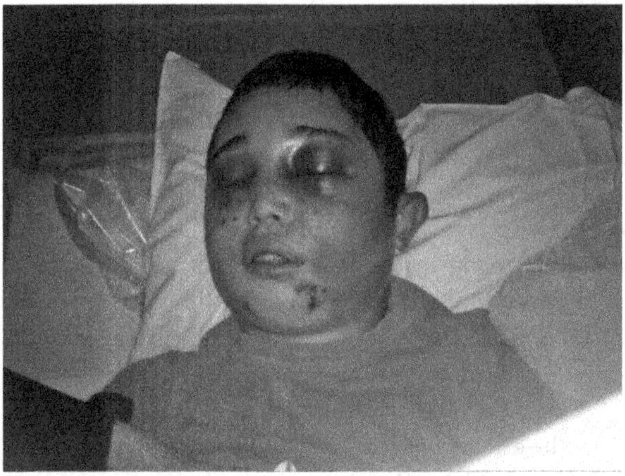

Figure 12.2:
Extreme facial self-injury in an autistic boy.

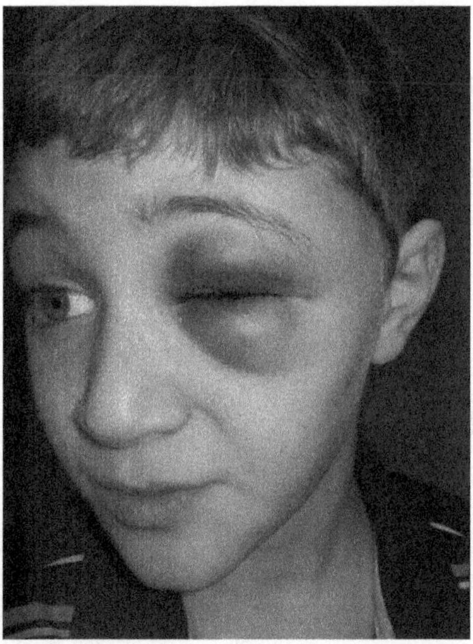

Figure 12.3:
Extreme ocular self-injury in an autistic boy.

CLASSIC THEORIES OF SELF-INJURY

Applied Behavioral Analysis

Over the past half century, the field of applied behavioral analysis has contributed to the assessment and treatment of self-injury, focusing on socially maintained

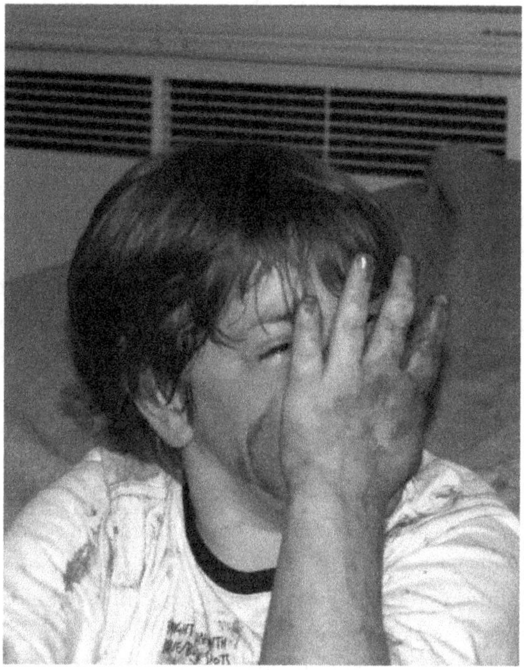

Figure 12.4:
Bloodied face from self-injury in an autistic boy.

SIB (16). Research has shown that there are often discrete operant functions for self-injurious behaviors in individuals with intellectual disabilities, which may typically include access to tangibles and attention, escape from demands, or interruption of preferred activities. Self-injurious behavior may also represent a form of maladaptive communication in individuals with compromised communication skills. A functional behavioral assessment is undertaken to determine the specific operant factors at play, and an individualized treatment protocol developed. Common treatment interventions may include communication training, differential reinforcement for absence of self-injury and/or engagement in desired behaviors, developing appropriate play skills, increasing access to competing items, that is, toys or other implements demonstrated to effectively "compete" with the self-injurious behavior, token economies, level systems, and response reduction procedures. Protective equipment may also be incorporated into a behavioral treatment package on an ongoing or contingent basis (12, 17, 18).

Psychiatry

The presence of self-injury and other challenging behaviors in individuals with intellectual disability has been found predictive of additional psychiatric diagnosis (8, 15), increasing the incidence of discrete psychopathology as much as threefold (19). Conversely, underlying psychiatric disturbance may cause or worsen challenging behaviors in ID (20). Baseline cognitive impairment in itself is regarded as a risk factor for psychopathology (21), and it is recommended that all individuals with ID should be assessed for both problem behaviors and for a full range of *Diasnostic and Statistical Manual* (DSM) psychiatric disorders (22). Specific correlation between self-injurious behaviors and discrete psychiatric diagnoses remains uncertain, with varying results reported in the literature. However, SIB has been associated with depression, hypomania, anxiety, psychosis, and personality disorders. SIB has further been noted with symptoms along the catatonia spectrum, including irritability, odd gestures and mannerisms, stereotypies, pacing, and use of odd/repetitive language. This is of relevance to the later discussion of classification of some self-injury as a sign of catatonia. It is suggested that self-injury may be an "unorthodox" symptom of psychiatric distress, with potential for reduction through diagnosis and treatment of any concomitant psychiatric disorder (23–27).

The comorbidity of self-injury and psychiatric illness invokes the potential utility of targeted psychotropic interventions in the resolution of both entities. Many antidepressants, antipsychotics, and mood stabilizers have been evaluated for effective treatment of corresponding psychiatric disorders, in patients who are intellectually disabled. Furthermore, the best practice recommendations from the American Academy of Mental Retardation (currently the American Association of Intellectual and Developmental Disabilities urge that psychotropic agents be used in a manner that is similar for individuals with ID, for given psychopathology, as in patients without ID (17).

Neurochemical

Further models consider the role of underlying neurochemical disturbance, including dysregulation of dopaminergic, serotonergic and glutamatergic systems, as well as endogenous opioids (28–32). Typical and atypical antipsychotics, including haloperidol, loxapine, thiothixene, thioridazine, and chlorpromazine, have shown benefit in reducing some forms of SIB (33, 34). Risperidone, aripiprazole, zipradisone, and olanzapine have shown efficacy in the reduction of SIB in individuals with autism and other forms of ID (33, 35–38), while clozapine may also help in some cases (39, 40). The tricyclic clomipramine, as well as selective serotonin reuptake inhibitors such as citalopram, fluoxetine, fluvoxamine, paroxetine, and sertraline, have shown benefit in some forms (41, 42). Similarly, opioid antagonist naltrexone has been helpful in some cases (43, 44).

Medical

Medical models of SIB include neuroendocrine dysregulation and altered response to painful stimuli. Support for the neuroendocrine theory is based on rodent, primate, and human data, which have focused upon abnormalities of the hypothalamic-pituitary-adrenal (HPA) axis in subjects with self-injury (45–47). This neuroendocrine model of SIB is particularly attractive because treatment response to ECT is also consistent with the proposed mechanism of action of ECT (48, 49). An alternative medical model of SIB proposes that SIB is a paradoxical pleasurable response to painful stimuli; therefore, this disturbance may be treated using opioid receptor blockade agents, such as naltrexone. This theory proposes that treatment with naltrexone prevents the release of endogenous opioids; therefore, the SIB may not be reinforced as there is no pleasurable sensation. Naltrexone has been shown to be particularly helpful in some cases of severe self-inflicted tissue injury (44, 50).

Additional medical theories of SIB include presence of acute and chronic pain, sensory impairments and epilepsy, which have all been implicated in the pathogenesis of self-injury; however, findings remain equivocal (51–54).

Despite numerous theories regarding the etiology and suggested treatments of self-injury, a significant number of patients display an intractable form of SIB and fail to respond to a myriad of treatments, often across disciplines. Indeed, an expanded understanding of SIB has been urged in the service of these recalcitrant patients who have exhausted conventional models of thinking, reviewed above, and present with ongoing suffering.

SIB as a Sign of Catatonia

The term "catatonia" was first coined by Kahlbaum in 1874 and is currently defined as a neurobiological syndrome. It is characterized by discrete motor, vocal, and behavioral symptoms that may occur in a wide range of psychiatric, neurological, medical, and drug-related conditions. Catatonia can be readily diagnosed and treated, and although it is most frequently associated with mood and psychotic disorders, it is also found in 12–17% of individuals with autism (55, 56). The reader is referred to Chapter 11, "ECT for Catatonia in Autism," for a comprehensive review of the topic.

Recent work has expanded upon the classic theories of self-injury and proposes that in a subgroup of patients who engage in repetitive self-injury, the SIB appears to be a motor disturbance suggestive of catatonia. If the SIB is viewed as a motor sign of catatonia, there are implications for successful treatment with ECT. In a subgroup of patients who typically engage in this form of unstoppable, high-intensity, and high-frequency SIB, the behavior recurs as soon as physical restraint or protective equipment is removed and does not appear to serve any social function. Such patients often engage in self-injury several times per minute in a shockingly staccato-like fashion until physical intervention is used to terminate the behavior. Resultant physical harm may be extreme. Furthermore, this type of SIB may be conceptualized as a stereotypy, which is defined in a medical dictionary as "a persistent, inappropriate mechanical repetition of actions, body postures, or speech patterns, generally occurring without variation in thought processes or ideas." The behavior during a stereotypy is primarily abnormal due to its frequency and/or its intensity, and stereotypy is a recognized symptom of catatonia (57). This form of SIB may be continuous or may occur over a variable duration, interspersed with episodes of relative calmness. In extreme cases, the SIB and associated agitation may be persistent, resulting in exhaustion and medical compromise in addition to devastating physical injury.

It is important to recognize that such involuntary SIB may indeed co-occur with other types of SIB or additional challenging behaviors that are maintained by environmental functions. Indeed, individuals with a given topography of negative behavior are likely to have additional topographies that may complicate the clinical presentation (12).

History

Historical accounts of catatonia in literature over the past two centuries are rich in references to self-injury and are highly instructive for the modern clinician. A comprehensive historical review is provided in Chapter 11, "ECT for Catatonia in Autism." However, the following historical accounts convincingly describe severe SIB in catatonic patients and provide support that these behaviors have been long observed by clinicians. For instance, Bell in 1849 described a patient with delirious mania, providing a vivid description with salient features of self-injury:

> After admission, remained an hour quiet but with an excited, flushed countenance and sparkling eye, as if exerting the utmost self-control; then began to vociferate, howl and stamp, which he continued all night. He bruises and injures himself—beats his head most furiously—scratches open the vein of his arm and bloodies his room extensively—probably loses a quart of blood. (58)

Similarly, Kraepelin in 1896 presented a patient with self-injury in catatonia and included the following description:

> Massive skin abrasions may occur, small and large wounds, because the patient does not abstain from [injuring] his limbs in the slightest, and tries again and again to rip at the exposed patches, tearing off heedlessly the bandages that might hinder him. (59)

Stauder later comments upon concomitant self-injury in malignant catatonia in his 1934 essay "Die Todliche Katatonie" (60), while additional reports of malignant catatonia and self-injury followed over the next two decades (61–63). Interestingly, in his 1950 study of catatonia, Ey discusses "psychomotor discharges" in the form of sudden aggression and self-injurious behaviors, and specifically comments upon stereotypic self-injurious movements including self-scratching, hair-pulling, and self-hitting (64).

A fascinating report from Moscow in 1963 presents seven children from the same extended family who were admitted for psychosis and catatonia compounded by self-injury:

> Their impulsivity grew, often in connection with aggressivity. The patients took on contorted [*verschroben*] poses, froze briefly into fixed positions, and refused food. They became increasingly inaccessible, negativistic. Typical of many of them was their tendency to self-harm: they beat their heads against the wall or the bed-frame, lay in bed so that their necks rested on the bedrail; they pushed on their eyeballs and choked their necks with their hands or a towel, slammed the door on their fingers and so forth. (65)

Leonhard in 1979 used the term "auto-aggressivity," and described self-injury in his classification of childhood catatonia:

> In the beginning of negativistic catatonia in early childhood aggressivity is associated with autoaggressivity. The compulsion may be so strong that the patient must have a nurse close by in order to prevent self-mutilation. The patients hit themselves in the face, knock their heads against hard objects, sometimes bite themselves. Some patients have scars on the face or elsewhere on the body from serious self-inflicted injuries. (66)

These and other historical accounts of SIB in patients with catatonia offer resounding support for self-injury as an alternate symptom of the catatonic presentation, drawing to mind Jorge Santayana's timeless adage, "those who cannot remember the past are condemned to repeat it."

MODERN LITERATURE

Although SIB is not reported as a specific symptom of catatonia, it has been reported to complicate cases of pediatric catatonic, affective, and psychotic illness, with many of these patients experiencing profound global symptom remission with ECT (67–70). In these cases, attention should be paid to eliciting concomitant, classically recognized symptoms of catatonia that further clarify the diagnosis and encourage the clinician to assess for the full range of catatonic symptoms, when presented with intractable repetitive SIB (see Table 12.1 for a summary of this literature).

As previously stated, the early reports did not diagnose self-injury as catatonia; however, later publications have focused specifically on characterization of self-injury in several autistic youth as an alternate sign of catatonia, with profound reduction conferred by ECT (1–4, 71, 72). ECT was first used expressly for self-injury in 1982 in a 25-year-old male with a several-year history of head-directed self-injury who had developed injury-related upper motor neuron signs (5). Similarly, Fink in 1999 reported of a 14-year-old male with intractable head-banging, self-scratching, and mental retardation who experienced a prominent reduction in both forms of self-injury with ECT (48). The children and adolescents described in these reports all demonstrated self-injury of an extreme degree, which had failed to remit over years of myriad behavioral and psychotropic interventions, and had resulted in severe tissue damage, with one patient actually losing an eye as a result of SIB directed to his head. Treatment with ECT resulted in astounding reduction in repetitive self-injury for these patients, allowing them to leave the hospital, abandon restrictive equipment, return to home and school, and resume their developmental trajectories. Two were able to successfully complete retinal re-attachment surgeries without further eye damage or loss of vision (4, 73). One mother shared how ECT allowed her to fulfill one of her simplest dreams of taking all five of her children out for ice cream without her autistic son pounding his face into a bloody pulp, and her husband described ECT as a "game changer" after years of bloody scenes and failed inpatient and outpatient behavioral and psychopharmacological treatment. Another father quipped that his son was finally "released from the shackles of (SIB) hell" (74) via ECT.

The understanding of self-injury as an alternate sign of catatonia has been further clarified through exploration of (1) the relationship between self-injury and stereotypies as catatonic symptoms (75, 76); (2) the concomitance of tics and self-injury in autism and catatonia, with associated reports of profound benefit of ECT in cases of tic disorders accompanied by severe SIB (77–86); and (3) neurochemical theories that suggest that gamma-aminobutyric acid (GABA) dysfunction may be a common biological thread between autism, catatonia, and self-injury, and emphasizing the resounding response of catatonia to treatments that modulate the GABA-A receptor complex, including ECT (55, 87–89). Comprehensive review of such may be found in prior publications (13, 86).

PATIENT SELECTION FOR ECT

Considerable planning and forethought is necessary before a patient with severe, intractable SIB, who is often intellectually disabled, is selected for ECT.

As reviewed at the outset of this chapter, many individuals with ID present with SIB, yet other etiologies may be relevant and must be carefully ruled out. ECT is most certainly not indicated for self-injury maintained by social consequence, although a patient may display SIB as catatonic stereotypy while engaging in occasional SIB that is volitional (the two may coexist and are not mutually exclusive). Concomitant psychiatric and neurochemical disturbance may also be present and should be effectively addressed with psychotropic medications. An interdisciplinary model is considered the golden standard for assessment and treatment and should include comprehensive review of all factors causing and maintaining self-injurious behavior (43, 90). Indeed, it is imperative that any individual presenting with self-injury receives a comprehensive multidisciplinary assessment to fully evaluate the nature of his or her SIB and appropriateness for ECT.

Psychiatric Workup

The patient should be assessed by a psychiatrist familiar with individuals with intellectual disabilities and concomitant behavioral and psychiatric pathology. The goal of psychiatric evaluation is to carefully explore not only the nature of the self-injurious behavior itself, but also additional medical, neurological, psychiatric, and behavioral symptoms that provide further insight into the underlying nature of the patient's presentation and could potentially be addressed through other interventions.

Attention should also be given to assessment of other concomitant ECT-responsive psychiatric conditions, including classic catatonic, affective, and psychotic symptoms. In cases where intractable, repetitive SIB without operant cause is considered an alternate sign of catatonia, it is important to fully assess the patient for additional symptoms of catatonia. Currently, six different catatonia rating scales exist that should be incorporated during a comprehensive assessment. The Bush-Francis Catatonia Rating Scale (BFCRS) is a 23-item scale, which requires the presence of at least 2 items to be present, for at least 24 hours, for the diagnosis to be made (91). The BFCRS is considered valid and reliable, it is the most widely used scale in both research and clinical practice, and it has been modified for usage in pediatric populations (92–94). The KANNER (Katatonia, autism, neuropsychiatric, and neuromovement examination rating) scale was developed expressly for the assessment of catatonia in autism spectrum disorders and is an additional assessment tool, although not yet validated (95). In general, one should diligently assess common symptoms of catatonia such as changes in speech (reduced meaningful speech or echolalia), reduced food or fluid intake, decline in skills including loss of continence (catatonic regression), senseless refusal to participate in previously enjoyed activities (negativism), and other motor disturbances (slowness, posturing, freezing, tics, changes in gait, repetitive or Parkinsonian movements). There is a realistic risk that these less dramatic catatonic symptoms, in patients who engage in extreme SIB, may be overlooked by caregivers and clinicians alike.

The detection of these additional symptoms of catatonia, assist in diagnostic clarification and lend support when a trial of ECT is indicated. The following case vignettes describe clinical scenarios that may be encountered in clinical practice.

CASE VIGNETTE

Q is a 12-year-old boy with autism referred for evaluation for appropriateness of ECT based on an 11-year history of hand-head and hand-eye self-injury occurring at greater than 100 times/minute without physical restraint. Q had exhausted multiple psychotropic and behavioral interventions, and had already suffered a cerebral hemorrhage from self-induced head trauma. Assessment for other symptoms of catatonia revealed intermittent stupor and unresponsiveness, classic steppage gait, and prominent negativism in the form of food refusal, requiring gastrostomy tube placement.

The following case describes self-injury developing later in the course of treatment in a patient diagnosed with catatonia, given the waxing and waning nature of catatonic symptoms over time.

CASE VIGNETTE

S is an 18-year-old youth with malignant catatonia previously described in the literature. His presenting catatonic symptoms were of profound psychomotor retardation, negativism, cardiovascular and thermoregulatory instability. Three years into his maintenance ECT course, he missed treatments due to travel. He developed extreme psychomotor agitation, requiring physical restraint during the flight home, and engaging in repetitive self-injury that resulted in bruises on all four extremities. En bloc ECT upon return to the United States resulted in rapid resolution of all catatonic symptoms (96).

Affective disturbance is the most common comorbidity of catatonia, and should be assessed given the unparalleled response of such to ECT, including when complicated by acute suicidality (55, 89, 97, 98).

CASE VIGNETTE

E is an 18-year-old autistic man, described in a previous publication, who presented with a 3-year history of intractable self-injury leading to significant face, head, torso, and arm injury. He also clearly endorsed 8/9 DSM-IV-TR symptoms for major depression, repeatedly stating that he wanted to die and go to heaven, and had attempted suicide on several occasions, which could have realistically caused death. He demonstrated multiple additional catatonic symptoms, including posturing, grimacing, grunting, and stupor (1).

As the second most common comorbidity of catatonia, psychotic pathology should similarly not be overlooked.

CASE VIGNETTE

Z. is a 12-year-old autistic female with intractable hand-head self-injury resulting in significant tissue injury and necessitating ongoing inpatient hospitalization. Z is additionally observed to engage in disorganized behavior and detailed, agitated conversations with invisible third parties, as well as posturing, grimacing, physical agitation, and echopraxia as if rowing a boat.

After evaluating for psychopathology, it is advisable to review and pursue psychopharmacological interventions that are known to be effective in catatonia. Lorazepam in increasing dosages is considered the first-line intervention for catatonia in the general psychiatric population as well as in patients with autism. It is suggested that the dose should be maximized, even up to 24 mg daily (55, 89, 99–101). Preliminary reports suggest, however, that lorazepam may be insufficient in some cases when the symptom severity is extreme, or the benefit conferred may be temporary before it becomes necessary to consider ECT (1, 4, 96, 102).

A decision may be made to first exhaust other possible psychotropic interventions for self-injury, catatonia, or additional concomitant psychopathology. The range of psychopharmacological options for self-injury is reviewed in a previous section of this chapter. It is generally reasonable to try some of these agents to ascertain for benefit. There are certain caveats that are important in clinical practice. For example, while atypical antipsychotics such as risperidone do indeed have research support and US Federal Drug Administration approval for self-injury in autism (36), antipsychotics can also significantly worsen baseline catatonia, or precipitate malignant catatonia, which can be a life-threatening situation necessitating intensive care and immediate implementation of frequent ECT (55, 89). In relation to other forms of psychopathology, such as affective and psychotic illness in intellectual disability, best practice recommendations from the American Association of Intellectual and Developmental Disability urge implementation of the same psychotropic paradigms as those used in the neurotypical population (17). Caution is given, however, regarding the propensity of individuals with intellectual disability to experience unusual and idiosyncratic reactions to psychotropic agents, which may limit treatment (103–105).

Behavioral Workup

As previously discussed, social factors may play into self-injury. Any patient being considered for ECT for self-injurious behavior should be comprehensively evaluated by an experienced clinician with expertise in applied behavioral analysis to explore any social contingencies to the patient's self-injurious behaviors and to develop appropriate behavioral treatment protocols. It is important for clinicians to be cognizant that SIB maintained by operant function may co-exist with high-frequency SIB conceptualized as an alternative sign of catatonia. It is also possible that operant SIB may become more amenable to interventions using behavioral paradigms after successful treatment of SIB of the catatonic variety.

CASE VIGNETTE

J is an 11-year-old boy with bipolar affective disorder, extreme, repetitive self-injury and aggression whose clinical course was effectively treated with ECT (3). J also demonstrated self-injury to access food, and was noted to begin biting his hands when seeing candy, then immediately stopping once the candy was provided. Once ECT resolved his affective disturbance and associated catatonic features, J was amenable to a behavioral protocol incorporating functional communication to access preferred food on a fixed schedule.

Medical Workup

All patients under consideration for ECT should receive a standard pre-ECT medical evaluation as dictated by regulations of the ECT facility, Practice Parameters for use of Electroconvulsive Therapy with adolescents (106), and any additional baseline health concerns in the individual patient. It is important to note that approximately 25–30% of autistic patients have concomitant seizure disorders; this may have implications for ECT and is discussed in some detail in Chapter 6, "ECT in Youth with Comorbid Medical and Neurological Disorders." Furthermore, patients with autism spectrum disorder and with other types of intellectual disability may suffer from additional medical pathology, particularly when autism is associated with a genetic syndrome. Such syndromes may be associated with other specific medical needs and concerns.

CASE VIGNETTE

An 18-year-old woman with Cornelia de Lange syndrome, autism, and self-injury was referred for ECT. Due to gastrointestinal and cardiac involvement in some patients with this syndrome, including gastroesophageal reflux disease, regurgitation, swallowing difficulties, bowel malrotation, and congenital heart defects, usually atrial or ventricular septal defects, additional evaluation by pediatric specialists was requested prior to starting ECT. This patient was not found to have any acute somatic issues, and there were no medical complications during ECT.

Patients with developmental disabilities may present with unusual comorbid medical conditions and, therefore, a comprehensive evaluation by appropriate specialists is necessary. One published report describes a youth with congenital cerebellar dysgenesis and multiple brain stem abnormalities who was fully evaluated by pediatric neurology prior to successfully receiving ECT for various symptoms of catatonia (102).

The presence of acute retinal damage and/or postoperative ophthalmological states is a uniquely challenging clinical situation that may arise in some patients with SIB who are being considered for ECT. Patients requiring ECT may present with repetitive self-injury directed toward the head, which is known to be associated with retinal detachment and can lead to vision loss without prompt detection and surgical repair (12). The primary clinical challenge in such patients with retinal detachment, as a result of SIB, is the expectation of rise in the intraocular pressure (IOP), although transient, during ECT (107, 108). However, experience from patients with glaucoma suggests that the changes in intraocular pressure during ECT appear to be benign in nature (109), and similarly the changes in the patients' IOP during the post-surgical period following ECT can be mitigated by ensuring adequate oxygenation and hyperventilation (110). The authors have preliminary experience with the safe use of ECT for intractable SIB that was commenced 15 days after bilateral retinal detachment repair; in this patient, measurements of intraocular pressure immediately preceding and 1–2 hours following ECT demonstrated minimal IOP elevation over the course of several weeks (73). While this matter may appear obscure, it is a safety issue, and also emphasizes the monumental impact that ECT may have in these patients, when repetitive SIB can be halted and vision saved. Blindness and frank upper motor neuron signs are known, tragic consequences of repeated head trauma in neurodevelopmentally disabled children (5, 12).

SALIENT MATTERS PRIOR TO COMMENCING ECT

Preparation of the Family, Patient and Staff

Appropriate preparation of the patient and family prior to commencement of ECT is essential (see Chapter 5, "A Practical Guide to Using ECT in Minors"). As highlighted in Chapter 4, "Ethical and Consent Aspects," stigma and negative perceptions regarding ECT are rampant in modern culture, and may significantly impact parental attitude toward this treatment. Education regarding ECT can significantly alleviate anxiety and improve a family's acceptance of the treatment (111).

CASE VIGNETTES

ECT was repeatedly suggested to the parent of an autistic child with multiple classic catatonic symptoms and severe SIB. This child would injure himself to the point of smashing several bones in his foot, yet the parent was significantly resistant to the idea, even though ECT was suggested after the child had failed to respond to high-dose benzodiazepines. After several weeks, the parent finally asked the clinician if it was true that ECT worked by "burning and destroying" neurons. Appropriate education and reading rapidly removed this frightening misperception.

The parent of another patient presented in the psychiatrist's office in tears over the mere thought of ECT, although his son's eyes were frequently swollen shut from repetitive SIB. The clinician discussed the procedure, and showed a brief video of another autistic patient receiving ECT. The parent was puzzled and asked "that's it?" after he observed the motor activity in the great toe of the cuffed leg. He was greatly relieved subsequently.

It is advisable to suggest many excellent written resources regarding ECT that are accessible to the lay public, as well as an educational video developed by Fink in the 1980s (112). Parents may further appreciate the opportunity to speak with other parents who have pursued ECT for their children in order to hear a "non-professional," but highly personal, perspective. Clinicians involved in ECT for this special patient population may choose to keep a running list of parental contacts to share with prospective patients and families.

Preparation of the patient is equally important, but may be more circumscribed given likely cognitive impairments. The ECT procedure should certainly be explained as fully as possible in terms that the patient can understand, similar to the models used for sharing medical information with pediatric patients of different ages. Use of pictures and developmentally appropriate social stories regarding the procedure may be very helpful and reduce patient anxiety, even if it is only to explain a trip to the hospital, having an IV placed, "going to sleep," waking up and having a snack in recovery. In our experience, the medical setting where this procedure is administered, the equipment, numerous unfamiliar faces, and the discomfort experienced during the placement of the IV are often the most distressing components of ECT for patients with intellectual disability. Reasonable adaptations should be considered; treatment of the "special needs" patient first, allowing parents to remain with their child as much as permitted by institutional regulations, and use of an inhalant anesthetic agent and topical application of lidocaine or numbing creams at the site of the IV placement are some of several steps suggested to ease discomfort. Parents may be encouraged to bring a child's preferred toy or a DVD to further distract him from the procedure; while admittedly unorthodox, the authors have seen their patients effectively distracted watching *Elmo*, *Fantasia*, and *Harry Potter* in the ECT pre- and post-treatment areas.

In addition to the preparation of the caregiver and the patient, preparing the staff may be equally important, when planning ECT for a youth with special needs. The steps may include education regarding the nature of the patient's disability and his or her impairments, ability to communicate, extent of damage from self-injury, and usage of protective equipment, when necessary. Aggression directed toward the staff may be an additional challenge and may confuse the direct care staff member, who may regard these behaviors as oppositional, intentional, or just plain "bad." Some staff members may be reminded about how they might handle unacceptable behaviors in their own children, thus contributing to their negative perceptions of the patient and/or the parents. In such instances, staff education plays a critical role, so that the behaviors can be conceptualized in alternative terms; instead of regarding the behavior as "bad" or "unacceptable," the role of operant conditioning, recognizing symptoms that are catatonic in nature, and the role of additional psychopathology (affective or psychotic) should be adequately recognized. It is also important to provide safety measures to minimize the risk of injury to staff. Health professionals who are not accustomed to working with individuals with disability and challenging behaviors may be appalled and overwhelmed by the patient's presentation, or even may be disturbed to observe frank physical injury. It can be unsettling for staff to see patients who arrive at the ECT suite wearing protective helmets or arm restraints. Nevertheless, our experience indicates that often these patients become widely accepted and the ECT staff may, in fact, over time enjoy interacting with them.

CASE VIGNETTE

An 18-year-old autistic male with major depression with catatonic features and acute suicidality, accompanied by intense hand-head SIB, began the ECT course while in a highly agitated state. At the first session, he threw his shoes at the ECT physician and slapped the anesthesiologist prior to anesthetic administration. Staff gradually learned to discuss preferred topics with the patient at each subsequent ECT and also to use support staff for safety. By the end of the acute course, the patient had developed pet names for both the anesthesia and ECT staff, and even taught them about car racing and his favorite children's authors. Discussing car colors was a preferred activity during preparation for ECT.

CASE VIGNETTE

A non-verbal 15-year-old patient with malignant catatonia accompanied by severe aggression and self-injury was instructed about the ECT process through the use of augmentative communication devices. After several ECTs, the patient added touch screen icons to his communication device for both the ECT and child psychiatry attending physicians, and used these regularly to discuss his experience.

Access to Appropriate Services

The lack of universal availability of quality ECT services has been described as violating the ethical principle of justice (113). This situation may be further compounded for youth, especially those with autism and other neurodevelopmental disabilities (74), particularly due to overwhelming stigma, misconception, and legal restrictions. In the United States, many individual states restrict ECT access to minors, while other states prevent legally appointed guardians of adult children from giving consent for procedures such as ECT. The following description of a young woman, although not a pediatric case, underscores some of the difficulties encountered across the age spectrum.

CASE VIGNETTE

A 25-year-old autistic woman was referred from a remote area for ECT because of frequent opisthotonus, stupor, negativism and intractable SIB toward the head that had already resulted in bilateral loss of vision. At the time of writing this chapter (2012), there was no ECT facility in her state. Patients in this state who need ECT are referred to an adjacent state, yet this state prevented the legal guardian from consenting to ECT. The family ultimately found appropriate services in a more distant state, yet treatment was delayed and the family suffered significant personal cost incurred due to travel.

Issues of ECT availability and affordability are crucial and should be fully explored prior to initiating treatment. Practical issues such as travel, cost, and any restrictions about reimbursement for treatment-costs incurred at an out-of-state facility should be clarified. Long-term cost of treatment is likely to be a critical and an ongoing issue, especially because many youth with SIB associated with catatonia, autism, and/or ID are likely to require continuation and maintenance ECT.

CONCOMITANT ADMINISTRATION OF MEDICATIONS

Many patients with intractable SIB who are being considered for a course of ECT are likely to be receiving one or more psychotropic medication. Therefore, a careful review of the medication regimen is imperative prior to commencing ECT. Children with concomitant seizure disorders may continue to receive the necessary antiepileptic medications, although the timing of administration prior to each ECT treatment should be reviewed and discussed with the patient's neurologist. The goal of adjusting the time when the antiseizure medication is administered is to ensure that the serum level of the antiepileptic agent is at its lowest and thereby less likely to interfere with an adequate seizure during ECT. Furthermore, in this patient group, it is more than likely that any pharmacological agent initiated to target SIB has not resulted in a robust response. Therefore, it is generally recommended that those pharmacological agents should be tapered off and discontinued. If a given psychotropic has conferred *some* therapeutic benefit, either for self-injury or for other forms of psychopathology, the decision may include that a given medication should be continued. For example, selective serotonin reuptake inhibitors (SSRIs) may be prescribed in individuals with intellectual disability to target self-injury, irritability, anxiety, repetitive or compulsive behaviors, and these would not necessarily be discontinued during ECT. Antipsychotics are also frequently prescribed for challenging behaviors in autism; however, if no benefit can be attributed to such medication, discontinuation is advisable given the propensity for antipsychotics to lower the seizure threshold, and also to worsen symptoms of catatonia (55, 89). The concomitant use of benzodiazepines during ECT is an additional key issue, as patients may be prescribed this group of agents for certain behaviors, anxiety, or as a first-line treatment for catatonia. If benzodiazepines have conferred benefit, there is no reason to discontinue the medication provided there is ready access to injectable flumazenil, a benzodiazepine antagonist, prior to stimulus application. Indeed, blueprints for treatment of autistic catatonia support concomitant use of benzodiazepines and ECT, and indicate that at times very high dosages of the former may be necessary (100, 101). It has also recently been proposed that flumazenil may augment ECT response in the benzodiazepine-naïve patient by altering endogenous GABA tone to elicit a higher-quality therapeutic seizure (114). The utility of this method may be particularly intriguing in patients with autism who have baseline abnormal expression of GABA in the brain, from a fetal stage onward (88), and is worthy of further investigation. For additional details regarding concomitant use of medications during ECT, the reader is referred to Chapter 6, "ECT in Youth with Comorbid Medical and Neurological Disorders."

GOAL SETTING PRIOR TO ECT

Setting treatment goals and response markers is critical, as it provides an objective method to monitor progress and assists in making sound clinical decisions during ongoing treatment. Most individuals with intellectual disabilities, especially those with intractable challenging behaviors, will have a large complement of behavioral health professionals as part of their treatment team. Therefore, it is important to work with all disciplines involved for monitoring treatment response to ECT. In some instances, the psychiatrist providing the ECT may encounter resistance from allied health care providers, especially those who may strictly ascribe to rigid behavioral paradigms in conceptualizing the etiology of self-injury, even when those paradigms have proved insufficient. In these instances, therefore, objective measures of response are additionally imperative so that subjective assessments can be minimized and the treatment team is more readily able to reach consensus. An ideal situation would allow the ECT physician to work closely with the treating psychiatrist and the behavioral professional to identify patient-specific topographies of self-injury and associated catatonic, affective, or psychotic symptoms that can be monitored on both frequency and intensity using 24-hour daily data collection. Family and other caregivers can easily be trained to collect such data, which can be saved and readily visualized in a computer graphic program like Excel; such data may be used for completing a trend analysis over time and would assist with medication and ECT parameter manipulation. Such data should also include scores from a standardized catatonia rating scale (BFCRS, KANNER), which should be completed at regular intervals and provide a useful, objective assessment of patient progress. For additional information, the reader is referred to Chapter 5, "A Practical Guide to Using ECT in Minors."

SUGGESTED MEASURES TO BE USED DURING INDEX ECT

Details regarding the technical aspects of ECT are described in Chapter 5, "A Practical Guide to Using ECT in Minors," and anesthesia parameters in pediatric patients are reviewed in Chapter 7, "Anesthesia." Certain issues, however, deserve special emphasis in considering ECT for intractable SIB.

First, bilateral electrode placement appears to be superior for the treatment of catatonia in autism and this placement mode has been recommended in prior blueprints for autistic catatonia (101, 115). Although current literature comparing electrode placement during ECT for adults with major depression does not find superiority of bilateral over unilateral electrode placement (116), cases reported in the literature involving ECT for autistic catatonia, both with and without SIB, support the superiority of bilateral placement. In fact, there are two published reports where the patients demonstrated delayed response when unilateral electrode placement was initially used (4, 96). Therefore, bilateral electrode placement is preferred in intractable self-injury, as one would consider this mode for other critical situations, such as in malignant catatonia or in cases of profound depression with acute suicidality, which also require rapid treatment response (48).

In addition to electrode placement, measures that optimize seizures should also be incorporated in patients with intractable SIB. As described in Chapter 2, "The Mechanism of Action of ECT," not all ECT is equal. The authors have found this matter to be exceptionally relevant in the autistic and intellectually disabled population, where adjustments of the ECT protocol to enhance seizure efficacy have been essential. These typically include well-known ECT augmentation strategies, such as pre-treatment IV hydration, hyperventilation, flumazenil administration prior to applying the electrical stimulus, and minimizing the use of anesthetic agents that have prominent antiepileptic properties, while using alternative agents such as remifentanil or ketamine (117, 118). There are no systematic studies, however, evaluating these measures in this unique patient population, but our nascent experience suggests that the benefit of ECT may be optimized. Ideally, these measures used to optimize treatment with ECT warrant systematic study in the special needs patient population, so that the most helpful components may be determined.

Adequate frequency of ECT appears to be another critical component of effective treatment for intractable SIB. Three times per week is the suggested starting schedule for most patients with self-injury, who have been described in this chapter and elsewhere in published reports. It should be noted that this initiation schedule is no different from what is used for patients with affective and/or psychotic pathology. Patients with SIB are generally continued on this schedule until benefit to treatment reaches a plateau; at that point, a gradual weaning process is initiated, while monitoring target symptoms to allow necessary flexibility in the schedule. An individually tailored ECT schedule should be continued, similar to that recommended for adults with major depression, to maximize stability of the response (119, 120); this strategy appears to be most useful when ECT is employed in the treatment of self-injury.

In some instances, a flexible treatment schedule may not be available. Reasons may include national or state policy—in the United Kingdom, for instance, ECT cannot be administered more than twice weekly, while in certain parts of United States, state law permits only a pre-approved number of treatments, which are required to be administered over a certain fixed period. Therefore, lack of access to a flexible, individually tailored schedule, either due to policy or legal issues or due to insurance-mandated reasons, may undermine effective treatment of intractable SIB using ECT.

CASE VIGNETTE

D is an 8-year-old autistic male, previously reported in the literature, who received ECT for intractable self-injury directed toward his head over several years. 24-hour data collection revealed an increasing frequency of SIB, which was noted as the ECT frequency was reduced from thrice weekly to twice weekly, then to once weekly and finally to twice monthly. However, the patient was discharged on twice monthly ECT due to the family's limited means for arranging more frequent transportation for out-of-state ECT. Twice monthly ECT nonetheless allowed sufficient SIB reduction and permitted D to reintegrate into his home, school and community, and also remain with minimal tissue damage.

MAINTENANCE ECT

An optimum duration of the acute, index course, until the SIB is stabilized, may be directly followed by maintenance ECT (M-ECT) in patients with intractable SIB. Experience, although limited, suggests that M-ECT has an important role in preventing symptom relapse (121, 122). This relapse is not limited to patients with SIB; rather, high rates of relapse have been noted in adults with major depression, especially when an acute ECT course is followed by a fixed-schedule rather than clinically determined frequency (119, 123). M-ECT has been shown in adult major depression to significantly reduce symptom relapse, rates of re-hospitalization, and total inpatient hospital days (119, 124, 125). Therefore, the current literature urges individually tailored M-ECT schedules, which should be based on symptom severity of each patient (119, 120, 126). Importantly, numerous histopathological, imaging, and cognitive studies of M-ECT have demonstrated lack of any deleterious effect or evidence of "brain damage," even in patients who have received treatment in excess of several hundred lifetime M-ECT. The growing literature regarding maintenance ECT in SIB similarly demonstrates that (1) regular, ongoing ECT treatment is necessary for symptom relief, and (2) there is no evidence of cognitive damage from such treatment, even when comprehensive neuropsychological testing is completed (121, 122, 127). It should be noted that prolonged M-ECT may offer sustained remission in SIB, and the reduced SIB appears to be inversely associated with ECT frequency, as described in the case vignette of D and visualized in Figure 12.5.

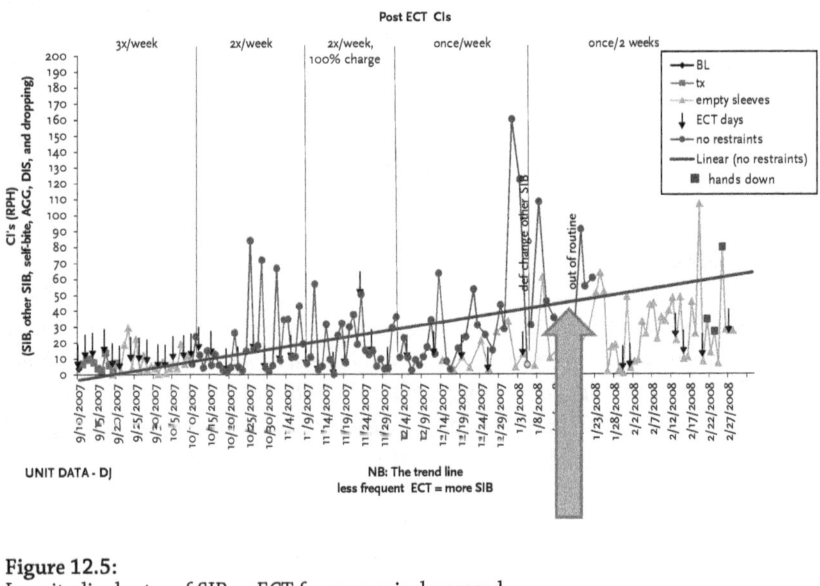

Figure 12.5:
Longitudinal rates of SIB as ECT frequency is decreased.

Some patients have required M-ECT at intervals as close as every 5 days and have demonstrated prompt symptom relapse at attempts at frequency reduction. The following cases are demonstrative of our experience.

CASE VIGNETTES

E is a 22-year-old autistic male whose acute and initial M-ECT courses for major depression with catatonic features, extreme self-injury and suicidality were previously reported. E continued to receive M-ECT every 5 days for 2 years, when a renewed attempt at frequency reduction was begun, alternating two every-fifth-day treatments with a third treatment at day 8. This schedule worked well for 4 weeks without any symptom relapse, yet at the beginning of the fifth week, E was noted to spend 20 consecutive hours posturing, and the next day attempted to both self-enucleate and scald himself. En bloc ECT consisting of five consecutive daily sessions and resumption of a fixed every fifth day schedule led to prompt symptom remission.

S is an 18-year-old autistic male whose acute and initial M-ECT courses for malignant catatonia have also been previously reported. After three years of weekly M-ECT, S traveled abroad and missed one M-ECT. Six days after the missed M-ECT, S developed insomnia, rapid speech, inappropriate laughing, giggling, and physical excitation associated with extreme aggression and self-injury, which rapidly deteriorated to frank delirious mania. He required physical restraint during his return journey and transfer to the ECT facility, with his body covered in bruises. All symptoms resolved with one week of en bloc ECT, followed by thrice weekly for one week, then twice weekly, then returning to the once weekly standing schedule.

The experiences with such patients are beginning to be replicated by other care providers (71) and pose critical questions given that such an exquisite sensitivity to withdrawal of M-ECT has not been reported in adult ECT patients with affective or other psychiatric disorders. Fink has proposed that optimal ECT practices for catatonia in autistic patients are likely different from accepted paradigms for typically developing adults with major depression, hypothesizing that the former are likely akin to ECT paradigms for malignant catatonia or delirious mania (128). In 1954, Bourne offered the term "convulsion dependence" to characterize patients who need "regular convulsions in order to maintain social adaptation." He identified patients who required ECT frequencies ranging from more than twice weekly to less than once monthly, and described three types of convulsion dependence: transient, protracted, and persistent. Thus far, our patients have fallen into the last category (129); we believe that this must be considered in the context of the unique underlying neuropsychiatric disturbance in these patients. Bourne also emphasized the painfully slow weaning of M-ECT frequency, which we have also observed in our patients. One patient, whose acute and initial M-ECT courses have

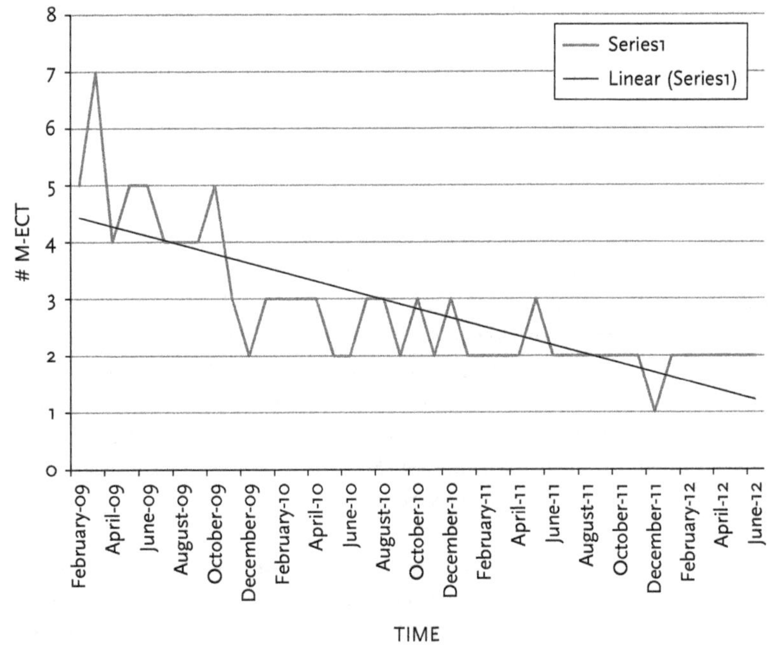

Figure 12.6:
Longitudinal decrease in necessary m-ECT over 3 years 5 months.

been previously published (102, 127), required an extremely gradual M-ECT frequency reduction to maintain symptom remission, as demonstrated in Figure 12.6.

The above findings have multiple, immediate, and delayed ramifications for the patient and family considering ECT for self-injurious behavior. It is imperative for all parties involved to understand that ECT is a treatment, not a cure, and that M-ECT will most likely be necessary. Unlike a fixed 10-day schedule of amoxicillin for an otitis media, M-ECT is better compared to ongoing use of insulin for diabetes or dialysis for renal failure. Such may pose practical questions, related to availability and convenience of ECT services, as well as long-term cost. M-ECT in this patient population is a longer-term commitment that needs to be recognized by providers, caregivers, and third party payers.

Maximization of concomitant medication therapies during M-ECT becomes critical in attempting to decrease the frequency of M-ECT, with particular emphasis on psychotropic targets of additional DSM affective, anxious, or psychotic pathology. Although we have found that many of these patients benefit from lithium therapy during M-ECT, our experience is nascent, and extensive future research is warranted. Long-term neuropsychological follow-up of these patients over years of receiving M-ECT is also necessary for determining optimum clinical practice.

JUSTIFICATION FOR M-ECT

Indeed, the need for ongoing ECT, the relative "unknowns" regarding ideal technical parameters of ECT in this group, and questions about long-term effects that have not been systematically studied may lead parents and providers to question the choice of treatment with ECT. The ethics of pediatric ECT in general are reviewed in Chapter 4, "Ethical and Consent Aspects,", including consideration for children who cannot provide informed consent. While the use of ECT for youth with affective, psychotic, and catatonic illness is endorsed by international organizations including the American Academy of Child and Adolescent Psychiatry (106), there are no clear guidelines for ECT specifically for self-injury, despite the strong connection to catatonic pathology and evidence for remarkable benefit.

It is likely that many readers of this chapter are seeking information because they are involved in treating a subgroup of patients who fail to respond to classic pharmacological, behavioral, and combined interventions. Many of these patients continue to suffer significant and frequent self-induced physical injury, may be confined to highly restrictive protective equipment, or have already incurred irreparable bodily damage. The global incapacitation of such a child, from physical, social, educational, family, and occupational perspectives, combined with the recent remarkable success of ECT in the termination of intractable self-injury, does tip the risk-benefit ratio in favor of an ECT trial for this group; anecdotal and published reports, albeit sparse, support that ECT may simply change their life for the better.

The father of a 16-year-old boy with a decade of SIB relieved by ECT described their experience:

> This process has been arduous at times and we are learning what a delicate balance it is to be consistently successful—but when we think of all the benefits and improvements that have been made, it is no sacrifice. (He) now has a chance. How great is that. He has a chance!

CONCLUSION

SIB can be a dangerous and distressing problem in many patients with autism or other intellectual disabilities. Following multidisciplinary assessment and generally when other approaches have failed, ECT has potential utility in those patients where the behavior appears internally driven and repetitive, and is occurring with extreme frequency and high intensity; in these cases, the SIB may be conceptualized as a movement disturbance and symptom of catatonia. The positive effects of ECT in this population can be dramatic. To optimize the outcome, there are certain aspects of the ECT procedure that warrant particular attention. Among other considerations, maintenance ECT will be required.

"Desperate illnesses wrought, by desperate appliance relieved, or sometimes not at all."
William Shakespeare, *Hamlet*

QUESTIONS AND ANSWERS

1. *Is ECT indicated for all autistic or intellectually disabled patients with self-injury?*
   No. Only a small subgroup of patients likely meets criteria for ECT.
2. *What causes SIB in patients with autism and other intellectual disability?*
   A complete understanding of the etiology of SIB in such patients is unknown. However, multiple potential etiological factors are suspected, which may include operant functions, concomitant psychiatric and medical pathology, and underlying neurochemical disturbance.
3. *Which patients are the best candidates for relief of intractable self-injury via ECT?*
   The best candidates are patients in whom self-injury occurs in a driven, repetitive fashion at extreme frequency and intensity, appearing as a motor disturbance and causing dangerous bodily injury. Furthermore, there is no evident operant function for this type of SIB in these patients, who have failed extensive prior behavioral and psychotropic interventions. However, operant-based SIB (associated with secondary gain) may coexist with SIB that resembles a stereotyped movement disturbance and is a likely symptom of catatonia.
4. *Should ECT be considered as a first-line intervention for SIB?*
   In most cases, no. Exceptions may include patients with concomitant catatonic deterioration, if the SIB poses an imminent risk of serious injury (trauma to eyes, among possible other types), or profound depression and/or suicidality where ECT would be acutely indicated.
5. *What type of assessment should occur prior to ECT consideration?*
   Comprehensive multidisciplinary assessment is recommended, which should include a psychiatrist, behavioral psychologist, and a pediatrician/internist, especially if there is suspicion for comorbid medical diagnoses.
6. *Is the ECT course time-limited?*
   No. Maintenance ECT is invariably necessary, and the frequency and the duration of treatment should be determined on a case-by-case basis.

7. *What modifications to the ECT protocol are recommended?*

   ECT implemented for self-injury is used in the same fashion as for other indications; however, specific recommendations include bilateral electrode placement, thrice weekly regimen during the acute treatment, and optimization of ECT parameters to maximize seizure efficacy. Additional modifications may be necessary in preparing the patient, family, and staff for ECT.

8. *Is ECT a replacement for pharmacotherapy for SIB?*

   No. Adjunctive psychotropics are generally necessary during the M-ECT phase, and must be optimized.

9. *Is self-injury a recognized indication for ECT?*

   Not yet. Future research is imperative in the service of these children.

DISCLOSURES

Dr. Lee E. Wachtel does not have any conflicts of interest or disclosures to report.

Dr. Dirk M. Dhossche does not have any conflicts of interest or disclosures to report.

REFERENCES

1. Wachtel L, Griffin M, Reti I. Electroconvulsive therapy in a man with autism experiencing severe depression, catatonia and self-injury. *J ECT.* 2010;26(1):70–3.
2. Wachtel L, Contrucci-Kuhn S, Griffin M, Thompson A, Dhossche D, Reti I. ECT for self-injury in an autistic boy. *Eur Child Adoles Psychiatry.* 2009;18(7):458–63.
3. Wachtel L, Jaffe R, Kellner C. Electroconvulsive therapy for psychotropic-refractory bipolar affective disorder and severe self-injury and aggression in an 11-year-old autistic boy. *Eur Child Adolesc Psychiatry.* Mar 2011;20(3):147–52.
4. Wachtel L, Kahng S, Dhossche D, Cascella N, Reti I. Electroconvulsive Therapy for catatonia in an autistic girl. *Am J Psychiatry.* 2008;165:329–33.
5. Bates W, Smeltzer D. Electroconvulsive treatment of psychotic self-injurious behavior in a patient with severe mental retardation. *Am J Psychiatry.* 1982;139:1355–6.
6. Fink M. Electroshock: Healing Mental Illness. London: Oxford University Press; 1999.
7. Baghdali A, Pascal C, Grisi S, Aussilloux C. Risk factors for self-injurious behaviors among 222 young children with autistic disorders. *J Intellect Disabil Res.* 2003;47:622–7.
8. Borthwick-Duffy SA. Epidemiology and prevalence of psychopathology in people with mental retardation. *J Consult Clin Psychol.* Feb 1994;62(1):17–27.

9. Eyman RK, Borthwick SA, Miller C. Trends in maladaptive behavior of mentally retarded persons placed in community and institutional settings. *Am J Ment Defic.* Mar 1981;85(5):473–7.
10. Yates T. The developmental psychopathology of self-injurious behavior: compensatory regulation in posttraumatic adaptation. *Clin Psychol Rev.* 2004;24:35–74.
11. Furniss F, Biswas A. Recent research on aetiology, development and phenomenology of self-injurious behavior in people with intellectual disabilities: a systematic review and implications for treatment. *J Intellect Disabil Res.* 2012;56(5):453–75.
12. Paclawskyj TR, Kurtz PF, O'Connor JT. Functional assessment of problem behaviors in adults with mental retardation. *Behav Modif.* Sep 2004;28(5):649–67.
13. Wachtel LE, Dhossche DM. Self-injury in autism as an alternate sign of catatonia: implications for electroconvulsive therapy. *Med Hypotheses.* 2010 Jul;75(1):111–4.
14. Eyman R, Call T. Maladaptive behavior and community placement of mentally retarded persons. *Am J Ment Defic.* Sep 1977;82(2):137–44.
15. Jacobson J. Problem behavior and psychiatric impairment within a developmentally disabled population I: behavior frequency. *Appl Res Ment Retard.* 1982;3(2):121–39.
16. Kahng S, Iwata B, Lewin A. Behavioral treatment of self-injury, 1964-2000. *Am J Ment Retard.* 2002 May, 2002;107(3):212–21.
17. AAMR. Treatment of psychiatric and behavioral problems in mental retardation. *Am J Ment Retard.* 2000;105:165–88.
18. Iwata B, Dorsey M, Slifer K, Bauman K, Richman G. Toward a functional analysis of self-injury. *JAppl Behav Anal.* 1982;27:197–209.
19. Rojahn J, Matson J, Naglieri J, Mayville E. Relationships between psychiatric conditions and behavior problems among adults with mental retardation. *Am J Ment Retard.* Jan 2004;109(1):21–33.
20. Emerson E, Moss S, Kiernan C. The relationship between challenging behaviour and psychiatric disorders in people with severe intellectual disabilities. In: Bouras N, ed. *Psychiatric and Behavioural Disorders in Mental Retardation.* Cambridge: Cambridge University Press; 1999, pp. 38–48.
21. Matson J, Sevin J. Theories of dual diagnosis in mental retardation. *J Consult Clin Psychol.* 1994;62(1):6–16.
22. Reiss, S. Assessment of psychopathology in persons with mental retardation. In: Matson J, ed. *Psychopathology of the Mentally Retarded.* Massachussetts: Allyn and Bacon.; 1993, pp. 17–39.
23. Moss S, Emerson E, Kiernan C, Turner S, Hatton C, Alborz A. Psychiatric symptoms in adults with learning disability and challenging behavior. *Br J Psychiatry.* 2000;177:452–6.
24. Saloviita T. The structure and correlates of self-injurious behavior in an institutional setting. *Res Dev Disabil.* 2000;21:501–11.
25. Hemmings C, Tsakanikos E, Underwood L, Holt G, Bouras N. Clinical predictors of severe behavioural problems in people with intellectual disabilities referred to a specialist mental health service. *Soc Psychiatry Psychiatr Epidemiol.* Oct 2008;43(10):824–30.
26. Hurley A. Depression in adults with intellectual disability: symptoms and challenging behaviour. *J Intellect Disabil Res.* Nov 2008;52(11):905–16.
27. Myrbakk E, von Tetzchner S. Psychiatric disorders and behavior problems in people with intellectual disability. *Res Dev Disabil.* 2008 Jul-Aug;29(4):316–32.

28. Harris J. *Developmental Neuropsychiatry*. Oxford UK: Oxford University Press; 1998, pp. 251–7.
29. Lesch M, Nyhan W. A familial disorder of uric acid metabolism and central nervous system function. *Am J Med.* 1964 Apr;36:561–70.
30. Breese G, Criswell H, Duncan G, Moy S, Johnson K, Wong D, et al. Model for reduced brain dopamine in Lesch-Nyhan syndrome: neurobiology of neonatal-6-hydroxydopamine lesioned rats. *Ment Retard Devl Disabil Res Rev.* 1995;1:111–9.
31. Schroeder S, Oster-Granite M, Berkson G, Bodfish J, Breese G, Cataldo M, et al. Self-injurious behavior: gene-brain-behavior relationships. *Ment Retard Dev Disabil Res Rev*. 2001;17:3–12.
32. Muehlmann A, Devine D. Glutamate-mediated neuroplasticity in an animal model of self-injurious behavior. *Behav Brain Res.* 2008;189:32–40.
33. Masi G. Pharmacotherapy of Pervasive Developmental Disorders in Children and Adolescents. *CNS Drugs*. 2004;18(14):1031–52.
34. Janowsky D, Barnhill L, Shetty M, Davis J. Minimally effective doses of conventional antipsychotic medications used to treat aggression, self-injurious and destructive behaviors in mentally retarded adults. *J Clin Psychopharmacol.* 2005;25(1):19–25.
35. Janowsky D, Barnhill L, Davis J. Olanzapine for self-injurious, aggressive and disruptive behaviors in intellectually disabled adults: a retrospective, open-label, naturalistic trial. *J Clin Psychiatry.* 2003;64(10):1258–65.
36. McDougle CJ SL, Aman MG, McCracken JT, Tierney E, Davies M, Arnold LE, Posey DJ, Martin A, Ghuman JK, Shah B, Chuang SZ, Swiezy NB, Gonzalez NM, Hollway J, Koenig K, McGough JJ, Ritz L, Vitiello B. Risperidone for the core symptoms of autism: results from the study by the autism network of the research units on pediatric psychopharmacology. *Am J Psychiatry.* 2005;162(6):1142–8.
37. McDougle C, Kem D, Posey D. Case series: use of ziprasidone for maladaptive symptoms in youth with autism. *J Am Acad Child Adolesc Psychiatry.* 2002;41(8):921–7.
38. Stigler K, Posey D, McDougle C. Aripiprazole for maladaptive behavior in pervasive developmental disorders. *J Child Adolesc Psychopharmacol.* 2004;14(3):455–63.
39. Hammock R, Levine W, Schroeder S. Brief report: effects of clozapine on self-injurious behavior of two risperidone nonresponders with mental retardation. *J Autism Dev Disord.* 2001;31(1):109–13.
40. Thalayasingam S, Alexander R, Singh I. The use of clozapine in adults with intellectual disability. *J Intellect Disabil Res.* 2004;48(6):572–9.
41. Gordon C, State R, Nelson J, Hamburger S, Rapoport J. A double-blind comparison of clomipramine, desipramine, and placebo in the treatment of autistic disorder. *Arch Gen Psychiatry.* 1993;50(441–447).
42. Janowsky D, Shetty M, Barnhill J, Elamir B, Davis J. Serotonergic antidepressant effects on aggressive, self-injurious and destructive/disruptive behaviors in intellectually disabled adults: a retrospective, open-label, naturalistic trial. *Intl J Neuropsychopharm.* 2005;8(37–48).
43. Mace F, Mauk J. Bio-behavioral Diagnosis and Treatment of Self-injury. *Ment Retard Dev Disabil.* 1995;1:104–10.
44. Symons F, Thompson A, Rodriguez MC. Self-injurious behavior and the efficacy of naltrexone treatment: a quantitative synthesis. *Ment Retard Dev Disabil.* 2004;10(3):193–200.

45. Kemp A, Fillmore P, Lenjavi M, Lyon M, Chicz-DeMet A, Touchette P, et al. Temporal patterns of self-injurious behavior correlate with stress hormone levels in the developmentally disabled. *Psychiat Res.* 2007;157:181–9.
46. Sandman C, Touchette P, Lenjavi M, Marion S, Chicz-DeMet A. B-endorphin and ACTH are dissociated after self-injury in adults with developmental disabilities. *Am J Men Retard.* 2003;108:414–24.
47. Tiefenbacher S, Novak M, Marinus L, Chase W, Miller J, Meyer J. Altered hypothalamic-pituitary-adrenocortical function in rhesus monkeys (Macaca mulatta) with self-injurious behavior. *Psychoneuroendocrinology.* 2004;29:501–15.
48. Fink M. *Electroconvulsive Therapy: A Guide for Professionals and Their Patients.* Oxford: Oxford University Press; 2009.
49. Shorter E, Fink M. *Endocrine Psychiatry: Solving the Riddle of Melancholia.* New York: Oxford University Press; 2010.
50. Casner J, Weinheimer B, Gualtieri C. Naltrexone and self-injurious behavior: a retrospective population study. *J Clin Psychopharmacol.* Oct 1996;16(5):389–94.
51. Symons F, Harper V, McGrath P, Breau L, Bodfish J. Evidence of increased non-verbal behavioral signs of pain in adults with neurodevelopmental disorders and chronic self-injury. *Res Dev Disabil.* May-Jun 2009;30(3):521–8.
52. Smith K, Matson J. Behavior problems: differences among intellectually disabled adults with co-morbid autism spectrum disorders and epilepsy. *Res Dev Disabil.* Sep-Oct 2010;31(5):1062–9.
53. Poppes P, van der Putten A, Vlaskamp C. Frequency and severity of challenging behaviour in people with profound intellectual and multiple disabilities. *Res Dev Disabil.* Nov-Dec 2010;31(6):1269–75.
54. Cooper SA, Smiley E, Allan LM, Jackson A, Finlayson J, Mantry D, et al. Adults with intellectual disabilities: prevalence, incidence and remission of self-injurious behaviour, and related factors. *J Intellect Disabil Res.* 2009 Mar;53(3):200–16.
55. Fink M, Taylor M. Catatonia. *A Clinician's Guide to Diagnosis and Treatment.* Cambridge: University Press; 2003.
56. Dhossche D, Wing L, Ohta M, Neumarker K-J, eds. *Catatonia in Autism Spectrum Disorders.* San Diego, CA, and London, UK: Elsevier Academic Press; 2006.
57. Hamilton M, ed. *Fish's Clinical Psychology Signs and Symptoms in Psychiatry.* Motor Disorders. Revised Reprint. Bristol: John Wright & Sons; 1974.
58. Bell L. *American Journal of Insanity.* 1849:97–127.
59. Kraepelin E. *Psychiatrie: Ein Lehrbuch fur Studirende und Aerzte.* 5th ed. Leipzig: Barth; 1896.
60. Stauder K. Die todliche Katatonie. *Arch Psychiatr Nervenkrank.* 1934;102:614–34.
61. Shulack N. Exhaustion syndrome in excited psychotic patients. *Am J Psychiatry.* 1946 1946;102:466–75.
62. Billig O, Freeman W. Fatal catatonia. *Am J Psychiatry.* 1944;100(March):633–8.
63. Aronson M, Thompson S. Complications of acute catatonic excitement. *Am J Psychiatry.* 1950 1950;107(3):216–20.
64. Ey H. *Catatonie. Etudes Psychiatriques.* Paris: Desclee de Brouwer & Cie; 1950.
65. Pivovarova G. Die Besonderheiten des Verlaufs der Hebephrenie im Jugendalter. *Psychiatrie, Neurologie, und medizinische Psychologie Leipzig.* 1965;189(17):185–91.
66. Leonhard K. The classification of endogenous psychoses. In: Robins E, ed. New York: Irvington Publications; 1979.

67. Carr V, Dorrington C, Schrader G, Wale J. The use of ECT for mania in childhood bipolar disorder. *Br J Psychiatry.* 1983;143:411–5.
68. Black D, Wilcox J, Stewart M. The use of ECT in children: case-report. *J Clin Psychiat.* 1985;46:98–9.
69. Chung A, Varghese J. Treatment of catatonia with electroconvulsive therapy in an 11 year-old girl. *Aust NZ J Psychiat.* 2008;42:251–3.
70. Cizadlo B, Wheaton A. Case study: ECT treatment of a young girl with catatonia. *J Am Acad Child Adoles Psychiatry.* 1995;34:332–5.
71. Siegel M, Milligan B, Robbins D, Prentice G. Electroconvulsive therapy in an adolescent with autism and bipolar I disorder. *J ECT.* 2012;28(4):252–5.
72. Consoli A, Cohen J, Bodeau N, Guinchat V, Wachtel L, Cohen D. Electroconvulsive therapy in adolescents with intellectual disability and severe self-injurious behavior and aggression: a retrospective study. *Eur Child Adolesc Psychiatry.* 2013;22(1):55–62.
73. Wachtel L, Griffin M, Reti I, Ying H. Stability of intraocular pressure after retinal re-attachment surgery during ECT for self-injury in a 12-year-old autistic boy. June, 27 epub ahead of print.
74. Wachtel L, Dhossche D. Challenges of electroconvulsive therapy for catatonia in youth with intellectual disabilities; another tomato effect? *J ECT.* 2012;28(3):151–3.
75. Wing L, Shah A. A systematic examination of catatonic-like clinical pictures in autism spectrum disorders. *Int Rev Neurobiol.* 2006;72:21–39.
76. Richman D, Lindauer S. Longitudinal assessment of stereotypic, proto-injurious, and self-injurious behavior exhibited by young children with developmental delays. *Am J Ment Retard.* Nov 2005;110(6):439–50.
77. Baron-Cohen S, Scahill VL, Izaguirre J, Hornsey H, Robertson MM. The prevalence of Gilles de la Tourette syndrome in children and adolescents with autism: a large scale study. *Psychol Med.* Sep1999;29(5):1151–9.
78. Canitano R, Vivanti G. Tics and Tourette syndrome in autism spectrum disorders. *Autism.* Jan 2007;11(1):19–28.
79. Gadow KD, Roohi J, DeVincent CJ, Hatchwell E. Association of ADHD, tics, and anxiety with dopamine transporter (DAT1) genotype in autism spectrum disorder. *J Child Psychol Psychiatry.* Dec 2008;49(12):1331–8.
80. Cavanna AE, Robertson MM, Critchley HD. Catatonic signs in Gilles de la Tourette syndrome. *Cogn Behav Neurol.* 2008 Mar;21(1):34–7.
81. Trivedi H, Mendelowitz A, Fink M. Gilles de la Tourette form of catatonia: response to ECT. *J ECT.* 2003;19:115–7.
82. Robertson MM, Cavanna AE. The many faces of Gilles de la Tourette syndrome. *J Psychosom Res.* Dec 2009;67(6):467–8.
83. Cavanna AE, Servo S, Monaco F, Robertson MM. The behavioral spectrum of Gilles de la Tourette syndrome. *J Neuropsychiatry Clin Neurosci.* 2009 Winter;21(1):13–23.
84. Cheung MY, Shahed J, Jankovic J. Malignant Tourette syndrome. *Mov Disord.* Sep 2007 15;22(12):1743–50.
85. Morais SL, Derenusson GN, Pinto JP, Hounie AG, Dursun SM, Wichert-Ana L, et al. Neurobiological substrates of electroconvulsive therapy for Tourette syndrome: a Serial SISCOM study. *J ECT.* Dec 2007;23(4):278–80.
86. Dhossche D, Reti I, Shettar S, Wachtel L. Tics as signs of catatonia: ECT response in two adolescents. *J ECT.* Oct 2010;26(4):266–9.

87. Gedye A. Serotonin-GABA treatment is hypothesized for self-injury in Lesch-Nyhan syndrome. *Med Hypotheses.* 1992 Aug;38(4):325–8.
88. Dhossche D, Song Y, Liu Y-M. Is there a connection between autism, Prader-Willi syndrome, catatonia, and GABA? *Int Rev Neurobiol.* 2005;71:189–216.
89. Caroff S, Mann S, Francis A, Fricchione G. Catatonia. *From Psychopathology to Neurobiology.* Washington, DC: American Psychiatric Publishing; 2004.
90. Wachtel L, Hagopian L. Psychopharmacology and applied behavioral analysis: tandem treatment of severe problem behaviors in intellectual disability and a case series. *Isr J Psychiatry Relat Sci.* 2006;43(4):265–74.
91. Bush G, Fink M, Petrides G, Dowling F, Francis A. Catatonia: I: Rating scale and standardized examination. *Acta Psychiatr Scand.* 1996;93:129–36.
92. Sienaert P, Rooseleer J, De Fruyt J. Measuring catatonia: a systematic review of rating scales. *J Affect Disord.* 2011;135(1–3):1–9.
93. Cohen D, Nicolas J, Flament M, Perisse D, Dubos P, Bonnot O, et al. Clinical relevance of chronic catatonic schizophrenia in children and adolescents: evidence from a prospective naturalistic study. *Schizophr Res.* 2005 Jul 15;76(2–3):301–8.
94. Cohen D, Flament M, Dubos P-F, Basquin M. Case series: catatanic syndrome in young people. *J Am Acad Child Adoles Psychiatry.* 1999;38:1040–6.
95. Carroll B, Kirkhart R, Ahuja N, Soovere I, Lauterbach E, Dhossche D, et al. Katatonia: a new conceptual understanding of catatonia and a new rating scale. *Psychiatry (Edgmont).* Dec 2008;5(12):42–50.
96. Wachtel L, Griffin M, Dhossche D, Reti I. Brief report: Electroconvulsive therapy for malignant catatonia in an autistic adolescent. *Autism.* 2010 Jul; 14(4):349–58.
97. Petrides G, Fink M, Husain M, Knapp R, Rush A, Mueller M, et al. ECT remission rates in psychotic versus nonpsychotic depressed patients: a report from CORE. *J ECT.* 2001;17:244–53.
98. Kellner CH, Fink M, Knapp R, Petrides G, Husain M, Rummans T, et al. Relief of expressed suicidal intent by ECT: a consortium for research in ECT study. *Am J Psychiatry.* May 2005;162(5):977–82.
99. Bush G, Fink M, Petrides G, Dowling F, Francis A. Catatonia. II. Treatment with lorazepam and electroconvulsive therapy. *Acta Psychiatr Scand.* 1996;93:137–43.
100. Fink M, Taylor M, Ghaziuddin N. Catatonia in autistic spectrum disorders: a medical treatment algorithm. *Int Rev Neurobiol.* 2006;72:233–44.
101. Dhossche D, Shah A, Wing L. Blueprints for the assessment, treatment, and future study of catatonia in autism spectrum disorders. *Int Rev Neurobiol.* 2006;72:267–84.
102. Wachtel L, Crawford T, Dhossche D, Reti I. Electroconvulsive therapy for pediatric malignant catatonia with cerebellar dysgenesis. *Pediatr Neurol.* Dec 2010;43(6):427–30.
103. Matson J, Bamburg J, Mayville E, Pinkston J, Bielecki J, Kuhn D, et al. Psychopharmacology and mental retardation: a 10 year review. *Res Dev Disabil.* 2000;21:263–96.
104. Mahan S, Holloway J, Bamburg J, Hess J, Fodstad J, JL M. An examination of psychotropic medicaiton side effects: does taking a greater number of psychotropic medications from different classes affect presentation of side effects in adults with ID? *Res Dev Disabil.* 2010;31(6):1561–9.
105. Matson J, Mahan S. Antipsychotic drug side effects for persons with intellectual disability. *Res Devel Disabil.* 2010;31:1570–6.

106. Ghaziuddin N, Kutcher S, Knapp P, Bernet W, Arnold V, Beitchman J, et al. Practice parameter for use of electroconvulsive therapy with adolescents. *J Am Acad Child Adoles Psychiatry.* 2004;43:1521–39.
107. Epstein H, Fagman W, Bruce D, Abram A. Intraocular pressure changes during anesthesia for electroshock therapy. *Anesth Analg.* 1975 Jul-Aug;54(4):479–81.
108. Edwards R, Stoudemire A, Vela M, Morris R. Intraocular pressure changes in nonglaucomatous patients undergoing electroconvulsive therapy. *Convuls Ther.* 1990;6(3):209–13.
109. Abrams R. *Electroconvulsive Therapy*. 4th edition. New York: Oxford University Press; 2002.
110. Saad D, Black J, Krahn L, Rummans T. ECT post eye surgery: two cases and a review of the literature. *J ECT.* Dec 2000;16(4):409–14.
111. Ghaziuddin N, Kaza M, Ghazi N, King C, Walter G, Rey J. Electroconvulsive therapy for minors: experiences and attitudes of child psychiatrists and psychologists. *J ECT.* 2001;17:109–17.
112. Fink M. *Informed ECT for Patients and Families*. Informational Videotape. Lake Bluff, IL: Somatics; 1986.
113. Ottosson J-O, Fink M. *Ethics of Electroconvulsive Therapy*. New York, Hove: Brunner-Routledge; 2004.
114. Yi J, Torres J, Azner Y, Vaidya P, Schiavi A, Reti I. Flumazenil pretreatment in benzodiazepine-free patients: a novel method for managing declining ECT seizure quality. *J ECT*. 2012;28(3):185–9.
115. Fink M, Taylor MA, Ghaziuddin N. Catatonia in autistic spectrum disorders: a medical treatment algorithm. *Int Rev Neurobiol.* 2006;72:233–44.
116. Kellner C, Knapp R, Husain M, Rasmussen K, Sampson S, Cullum M, et al. Bifrontal, bitemporal and right unilateral electrode placement in ECT: randomised trial. *Br J Psychiatry.* 2010 Mar;196(3):226–34.
117. Kranaster L, Kammerer-Ciernioch J, Hoyer C, Sartorius A. Clinically favourable effects of ketamine as an anaesthetic for electroconvulsive therapy: a retrospective study. *Eur Arch Psychiatry Clin Neurosci.* 2011;261(8):575–82.
118. Chen S. Remifentanil: a review of its use in electroconvulsive therapy. *J ECT.* 2011;27(4):323–7.
119. Kellner C, Knapp R, Petrides G, Rummans T, Husain M, Rasmussen K, et al. Continuation electroconvulsive therapy vs pharmacotherapy for relapse prevention in major depression: a multisite study from the Consortium for Research in Electroconvulsive Therapy (CORE). *Arch Gen Psychiat.* 2006;63:1337–44.
120. Odeberg H, Rodriguez-Silva B, Salander P, Martensson B. Individualized continuation electroconvulsive therapy and medication as a bridge to relapse prevention after an index course of electroconvulsive therapy in severe mood disorders: a naturalistic 3-year cohort study. *J ECT.* Sep 2008;24(3):183–90.
121. Wachtel L, Hermida A, Dhossche D. Maintenance electroconvulsive therapy in autistic catatonia: a case series review. *Prog Neuro-Psychoph.* May 2010 30;34(4):581–7.
122. Wachtel L, Reti I, Dhossche D, Slomine B, Sanz J. Stability of neuropsychological testing during two years of maintenance electroconvulsive therapy in an autistic man. *Prog Neuro-Psychoph.* Jan 15, 2010;35(1):301–2.
123. Wijkstra J, Nolen W, Algra A, Van Vliet I, Kahn R. Relapse prevention in major depressive disorder after successful ECT: a literature review and a naturalistic case series. *Acta Psychiatr Scand.* 2000;102:454–60.

124. O'Connor DW, Gardner B, Presnell I, Singh D, Tsanglis M, White E. The effectiveness of continuation-maintenance ECT in reducing depressed older patients' hospital re-admissions. *J Affect Disord.*2010;120(1–3):62–6.
125. Swoboda E, Conca A, Konig P, Waanders R, Hansen M. Maintenance electroconvulsive therapy in affective and schizoaffective disorder. *Neuropsychobiology.* Jan 2001;43(1):23–8.
126. Suzuki K, Awata S, Takano T, Ebina Y, Iwasaki H, Matsuoka H. Continuation electroconvulsive therapy for relapse prevention in middle-aged and elderly patients with intractable schizophrenia. *Psychiat Clin Neuros.* 2005;59:481–9.
127. Wachtel L, Dhossche D, Reti I, Hughes-Wheatland R. Stability of intellectual functioning during maintenance electroconvulsive therapy. *Pediatr Neurol.* Sep;47(3):219–21.
128. Fink M. Personal communication, 2012.
129. Bourne H. Convulsion Dependence. *Lancet.* 1954;267:1193–6.

INDEX